ICD-9-CM

Coding Handbook, with Answers

2007 REVISED EDITION

Faye Brown

In collaboration with the
Central Office on ICD-9-CM of the
American Hospital Association

HEALTH FORUM, INC.
An American Hospital Association Company
Chicago

The publisher gratefully acknowledges Nelly Leon-Chisen, RHIA, Anita Rapier, RHIT, CCS, and Gretchen Young-Charles, RHIA, Central Office on ICD-9-CM, for their assistance in preparing the final manuscript.

This publication is designed to provide accurate and authoritative information in regard to the subject matter covered. It is sold with the understanding that neither the author nor the publisher is engaged in rendering legal, accounting, or other professional service. If legal advice or other expert assistance is required, the services of a competent professional should be sought.

The views expressed in this publication are strictly those of the authors and do not necessarily represent official positions of the American Hospital Association.

At press time, additional guideline changes were anticipated for October 1, 2006, implementation. Please visit www.ahacentraloffice.org for guideline revisions.

AHA is a service mark of the American Hospital Association used under license by AHA Press.

Printed in the United States of America—08/06

Cover design by Tim Kaage

ISBN: 1-55648-337-6

Item Number: 148028

Contents

About the Author and Contributor   v

How to Use This Handbook   vii

**FORMAT AND CONVENTIONS AND
CURRENT CODING PRACTICES FOR *ICD-9-CM***

1 Introduction to the *ICD-9-CM* Classification   3

2 *ICD-9-CM* Conventions   11

3 Uniform Hospital Discharge Data Set   19

4 The Medical Record as a Source Document   27

5 Basic Coding Steps   31

6 Basic Coding Guidelines   35

7 Coding Guidelines for Operations and Procedures   47

USE OF SUPPLEMENTARY CLASSIFICATIONS

8 V and E Codes   63

CODING OF SIGNS AND SYMPTOMS

9 Symptoms, Signs, and Ill-Defined Conditions   75

**CODING OF INFECTIOUS AND PARASITIC DISEASES,
ENDOCRINE DISEASES AND IMMUNITY DISORDERS,
AND MENTAL DISORDERS**

10 Infectious and Parasitic Diseases   83

11 Endocrine, Metabolic and Nutritional Diseases and Immune-System Disorders   95

12 Mental Disorders   105

**CODING OF DISEASES OF THE BLOOD AND BLOOD-FORMING
ORGANS AND DISEASES OF THE NERVOUS SYSTEM**

13 Diseases of the Blood and Blood-Forming Organs   119

14 Diseases of the Nervous System and Sense Organs   127

**CODING DISEASES OF THE RESPIRATORY, DIGESTIVE,
AND GENITOURINARY SYSTEMS**

15 Diseases of the Respiratory System   141

16 Diseases of the Digestive System   157

17 Diseases of the Genitourinary System   171

CODING OF DISEASES OF THE SKIN AND DISEASES OF THE MUSCULOSKELETAL SYSTEM

18 Diseases of the Skin and Subcutaneous Tissue   187

19 Diseases of the Musculoskeletal System and Connective Tissue   195

CODING OF PREGNANCY AND CHILDBIRTH COMPLICATIONS, ABORTION, CONGENITAL ANOMALIES, AND PERINATAL CONDITIONS

20 Complications of Pregnancy, Childbirth, and the Puerperium   207

21 Abortion and Ectopic Pregnancy   225

22 Congenital Anomalies   235

23 Perinatal Conditions   241

CODING OF CIRCULATORY SYSTEM DISEASES AND NEOPLASTIC DISEASES

24 Diseases of the Circulatory System   253

25 Neoplasms   287

CODING OF INJURIES, BURNS, POISONING, AND COMPLICATIONS OF CARE

26 Injuries   309

27 Burns   331

28 Poisoning and Adverse Effects of Drugs   337

29 Complications of Surgery and Medical Care   345

PREVIEW OF *ICD-10-CM* AND *ICD-10-PCS*

30 Introduction to the *ICD-10-CM* and *ICD-10-PCS* Classifications   357

31 *ICD-10-CM*   361

32 *ICD-10-PCS*   369

33 Preparing for *ICD-10-CM* and *ICD-10-PCS*   377

34 Implementation Issues for *ICD-10-CM* and *ICD-10-PCS*   379

FINAL REVIEW EXERCISE   385

APPENDIX: Official Guidelines for Coding and Reporting   407

INDEX   497

About the Author and Contributor

In memoriam: Faye Brown, who was responsible for educating many generations of ICD-9-CM coders, died January 2, 2006. She was 86.

The first *ICD-9-CM Coding Handbook* was developed by the staff of the American Hospital Association's Central Office on ICD-9-CM and published in 1979 by American Hospital Publishing, Inc., now AHA Press. Mrs. Brown authored and revised subsequent editions of the handbook from 1989 through the 2006 edition, published in summer 2005. She also served as technical reviewer for several editions of the *ICD-9-CM Workbook for Beginning Coders,* also published by AHA Press.

Mrs. Brown was a nationally known consultant in medical record management and data quality evaluation. She worked extensively for national and international health care organizations, including the American Hospital Association (AHA), the Institute of Medicine, the Pan American Health Organization, and the World Health Organization.

Mrs. Brown was a member of the editorial advisory board for the *Coding Clinic for ICD-9-CM,* which is published by the AHA's Central Office. She served as acting director of the Central Office in 1990. She also participated in several coding teleconferences presented by the AHA.

In addition to having broad hospital experience in medical record administration, Mrs. Brown served as chairman of the Medical Record Administration Department in the School of Allied Health Sciences at Loma Linda University, Loma Linda, California. She was president of the American Medical Record Association during 1970–1971 and was named the association's distinguished member for 1978.

Revisions of more recent editions of the *ICD-9-CM Coding Handbook* and the *ICD-9-CM Workbook for Beginning Coders* have been produced in collaboration with the AHA's Central Office, following the Faye Brown tradition. In tribute to Mrs. Brown, the staff of the Central Office and AHA Press honor her legacy by carrying on her commitment to coding education through this and subsequent editions of the coding handbooks and workbooks.

Nelly Leon-Chisen, RHIA, is the director of coding and classification at the American Hospital Association (AHA), where she heads the Central Office on ICD-9-CM and the Central Office on HCPCS. She represents the AHA as one of the *ICD-9-CM* cooperating parties and is responsible for the development of *AHA Coding Clinic for ICD-9-CM* and *ICD-9-CM Official Guidelines for Coding and Reporting.*

Ms. Leon-Chisen's *ICD-10* activities include membership in the ICD-10-PCS Technical Advisory Panel, past co-chair of the Workgroup for Electronic Data Interchange (WEDI) ICD-10 Implementation Workgroup, and numerous testimonies on *ICD-10-CM* and *ICD-10-PCS* before the ICD-9-CM Coordination and Maintenance Committee and the National Committee on Vital and Health Statistics. She was also the AHA lead project manager on the joint AHA-AHIMA ICD-10-CM Field Study.

Ms. Leon-Chisen has lectured on coding, data quality, and *ICD-10* throughout the United States, Europe, and Latin America. She has broad health information management (HIM) experience in hospital inpatient and outpatient management, consulting, and teaching. She has been an instructor in the HIM and Health Information Technology Programs for the University of Illinois and Truman Community College, both in Chicago, Illinois. She is a past president of the Chicago Area Health Information Management Association and the recipient of its Distinguished Member Award. She is also the recipient of the Professional Achievement Award from the Illinois Health Information Management Association.

How to Use This Handbook

Like earlier editions of this handbook, this revision is designed to be used in several ways:

- As a textbook for academic programs in health information technology and administration
- As a text for in-service training programs
- As a self-instructional guide for individuals interested in learning coding outside a formal program or in refreshing their skills
- As a reference tool for general use in the workplace

This last usage prompted the inclusion of material that may be considered too advanced for the entry-level coder. More advanced material in chapters 9 through 29 can be omitted as needed to meet the requirements of various basic courses in the use of *ICD-9-CM*. General and basic information covered through chapter 8 should be understood before moving on to the study of individual chapters of *ICD-9-CM*, however, to provide a foundation for further study.

The handbook is designed to be used in conjunction with the three volumes of *ICD-9-CM*. The three volumes must be consulted throughout the learning process, and the material cannot be mastered without using them. The official versions published by the Government Printing Office are available only in CD-ROM format. Unofficial print versions are available from a number of publishers, often combined in one book with three divisions corresponding to the three volumes of the official version. If you are using a print version, there may be minor variations between the way material is displayed in this handbook and the way it is displayed in your version of the print classification.

The chapters in this handbook are not arranged in the same sequence as the chapters in *ICD-9-CM*. The first two sections of this handbook (chapters 1–8) provide discussions of the format and conventions followed in *ICD-9-CM* as well as basic coding guidelines and introductory material on the supplementary classifications (V codes and E codes). The next eight sections (chapters 9–29) work from the less complicated chapters to those that are more difficult. Faculty in either academic or in-service programs can rearrange this sequence to suit their particular course outlines.

Chapters 30–34 contain information on *ICD-10-CM* and *ICD-10-PCS*, the future replacements for *ICD-9-CM*. These chapters may be used as a reference tool for the workplace to prepare for future implementation. In addition, educational programs may feel a need to start informing their students about a potential replacement to the coding system they are currently studying.

The appendix, which provides official guidelines for coding and reporting, is a handy reference source.

To use this handbook effectively, readers should work through each example until they fully understand the coding principles under discussion. With the exception of a few examples cited in the first part of the handbook to illustrate basic coding conventions and practice, readers should be able to arrive at correct code assignments by following the instructions provided. An incorrect answer indicates that the reader needs to review the pertinent handbook material until it is fully understood. Exercises in the body of each chapter should be completed as they come up in the discussion rather than at the end of the chapter or part. Most chapters also provide a review exercise. There is also a final review exercise toward the end of the book that offers additional practice in coding.

The handbook follows three conventions:

- In some examples, a lowercase letter x is used to indicate a fourth or fifth digit that is required but cannot be assigned in the example given because certain information needed for assignment of these digits is not given. This is done to emphasize the concept and specific guideline without going too deeply into specific coding situations.
- The underlining of codes in text examples indicates correct sequencing; that is, the underlined code must be sequenced first in that particular combination of codes. When no code is underlined, there is no implicit reason why any of the codes in the series should be sequenced first. In actual coding, of course, other information in the health record may dictate a different sequence. This underlining convention is used in the handbook solely as a teaching device. It is not an element of the *ICD-9-CM* coding system.
- In the edition with answers, the underlining of words in exercise questions indicates the appropriate term to be referenced in using the alphabetic indexes. The underlining of codes in the answer column of the exercises indicates correct code sequencing, as it does in the examples in the main text.

Changes in Code Usage

Official coding guidelines and official coding advice, approved by the four cooperating parties responsible for administering the *ICD-9-CM* system in the United States (American Hospital Association, American Health Information Management Association, Centers for Medicare & Medicaid Services, and National Center for Health Statistics), are published quarterly in the *Coding Clinic for ICD-9-CM* by the Central Office on ICD-9-CM of the American Hospital Association. Such advice becomes effective as of the date of printing, although in some cases the information is merely a clarification of coding practice that is already in existence, in which case the date does not necessarily apply. In other cases, this official information may provide new advice on coding specific conditions or procedures and therefore require updating of some of the advice in this handbook or in previous issues of *Coding Clinic*.

Format and Conventions and Current Coding Practices for *ICD-9-CM*

1 Introduction to the *ICD-9-CM* Classification

The *International Classification of Diseases, Ninth Revision, Clinical Modification (ICD-9-CM),* is the medical classification system used in the United States for the collection of information regarding disease and injury. Volumes 1 and 2 consist of a clinical modification of the World Health Organization's *Manual of the International Statistical Classification of Diseases, Injuries, and Causes of Death, Ninth Revision (ICD-9).* *ICD-9-CM* is entirely compatible with *ICD-9* and maintains its statistical orientation. The clinical modification expands *ICD-9* codes to facilitate more precise coding of clinical diagnoses. Volume 3 of *ICD-9-CM* is a classification of operations and procedures developed for use in the United States; it is not a part of the World Health classification. For statistical purposes, the procedure classification system follows the same organization and principles on which volumes 1 and 2 are based.

A classification system is an arrangement of elements into groups according to established criteria. In *ICD-9* and *ICD-9-CM* these elements are diseases, injuries, surgeries, and procedures, which are grouped into appropriate chapters and sections. Three-digit categories are used in volumes 1 and 2, and two-digit categories are used in volume 3. These groups are the common basis of classification for general medical statistical use. They help to answer questions about groups of related causes and provide the capacity for the systematic tabulation, storage, and retrieval of disease-related data. Each numerical code represents a counting unit, with the three-digit categories forming the basis for data tabulation. In *ICD-9-CM* many disease and injury categories have been expanded by fourth- and fifth-digits that provide for additional specificity but remain collapsible to the three-digit category.

ICD-9-CM is a closed classification system—it provides one and only one place to classify each condition and procedure. Despite the large number of different conditions to be classified, the system must limit its size in order to be usable. Certain conditions that occur infrequently or are of low importance are frequently grouped together in residual codes labeled "other" or "not elsewhere classified." A final residual category is provided for diagnoses not stated specifically enough to permit more precise classification. Occasionally these two residual groups are combined in one code.

Medical coders must understand the basic principles behind the classification system in order to use *ICD-9-CM* appropriately and effectively. This knowledge is also the basis for understanding and applying the official coding advice provided through the *Coding Clinic for ICD-9-CM,* published by the Central Office on *ICD-9-CM* of the American Hospital Association. It is important for coders in all health care settings to keep current with the official coding guidelines as well as *Coding Clinic for ICD-9-CM.* This official advice is developed through the editorial board for the *Coding Clinic* and is approved by the four cooperating parties for *ICD-9-CM,* which include the American Hospital Association, the American Health Information Management Association, the Centers for Medicare & Medicaid Services (CMS, formerly the Health Care Financing Administration), and the National Center for Health Statistics. Revised codes and new codes are developed annually by the last two agencies and are implemented on October 1 of each year. Starting with Fiscal Year 2005, new *ICD-9-CM* codes may be implemented twice a year—April 1 and October 1 of each year. Only code proposals specifically requesting expedited approval and making a strong and convincing case for purposes of meeting the new technology process will be approved for April 1 implementation. There were no new codes implemented in April 2006.

ICD-9-CM is presented as three volumes:

- Tabular List of Diseases and Injuries (volume 1)
- Alphabetic Index of Diseases and Injuries (volume 2)
- Tabular List and Alphabetic Index of Procedures (volume 3) [Note: Volume 3 of the ICD-9-CM is intended for use only by hospitals for reporting of inpatient procedures.]

The official version of ICD-9-CM is available in CD-ROM format from the Superintendent of Documents, U.S. Government Printing Office (P.O. Box 371954, Pittsburgh, PA 15250-7954—telephone number 866/512-1800, or online at http://book store.gpo.gov). Printed versions are available from a number of commercial publishers.

TABULAR LIST OF DISEASES AND INJURIES (VOLUME 1)

The main classification of diseases and injuries in the Tabular List of Diseases and Injuries (volume 1) consists of 17 chapters. (See the table of contents reproduced in figure 1.1.) Approximately half of the chapters are devoted to conditions that affect a specific body system; the rest classify conditions according to etiology. Chapter 2, for example, classifies neoplasms of all body systems, while chapter 8 addresses diseases of the respiratory system only.

In addition, two supplementary classifications are included in volume 1. The first provides V codes that are used to code conditions that are not included in the main classification but may be recorded as diagnoses. The second provides E codes that are used as additional codes to indicate the external circumstances responsible for injuries and certain other conditions. V and E codes will be discussed briefly in chapter 8 of this handbook and in more detail in the chapters discussing the conditions to which they apply.

The variation in chapter titles in ICD-9-CM's table of contents represents the compromises made during the development of a statistical classification system based partially on etiology, partially on anatomical site, and partially on the circumstances of onset. The result is a classification system based on multiple axes. By contrast, a single-axis classification would be based entirely on the etiology of the disease, the anatomical site of the disease, or the nature of the disease process. Each chapter in the main classification is structured to provide the following subdivisions:

- Sections (groups of three-digit categories)
- Categories (three-digit code numbers)
- Subcategories (four-digit code numbers)
- Fifth-digit subclassifications (five-digit code numbers)

The basic code used to classify a particular disease or injury consists of three digits and is called a category. Most categories are expanded into subcategories by the addition of fourth digits; many subcategories include fifth-digit subclassifications that provide more specificity in coding. A decimal point is used to separate the basic three-digit category code from its subcategory and subclassifications (for example, 842.13).

Listings of fifth-digit subclassifications appear at the beginning of the chapter, section, or three-digit category code to which they apply. Fifth-digit subclassifications must be assigned for all of the codes within the chapter, section, or category that follows the listing. In other cases, fourth-digit subcategory codes are expanded to display applicable fifth digits.

Codes in the Tabular List appear in numerical order. References from the Alphabetical Index to the Tabular List are by code number, not by page number. Code numbers and titles appear in bold type in the Tabular List. Instructional notes that apply to the section, category, or subcategory are also included in the Tabular List.

In addition, volume 1 includes four appendices that provide further information:

- Appendix A, Morphology of Neoplasms, provides optional codes indicating the histological type and behavior of neoplasms.
- The classification no longer contains an Appendix B. Appendix B was a glossary of mental disorders. It was deleted in 2004. Instead, users are referred to the Diagnostic and Statistical Manual of Mental Disorders, fourth edition, text

FIGURE 1.1   Table of Contents from *ICD-9-CM*

TABLE OF CONTENTS

Preface .... *iii*
Acknowledgments .... *v*
Introduction .... *xiii*
Conventions Used in the Tabular List .... *xxi*
Guidance in the Use of ICD-9-CM .... *xxiii*

Classification of Diseases and Injuries
    1.   Infectious and Parasitic Diseases 1
    2.   Neoplasms 81
    3.   Endocrine, Nutritional, and Metabolic Diseases and
        Immunity Disorders 154
    4.   Diseases of the Blood and Blood-Forming Organs 188
    5.   Mental Disorders 204
    6.   Diseases of the Nervous System and Sense Organs 251
    7.   Diseases of the Circulatory System 358
    8.   Diseases of the Respiratory System 404
    9.   Diseases of the Digestive System 432
  10.   Diseases of the Genitourinary System 481
  11.   Complications of Pregnancy, Childbirth, and the
        Puerperium 527
  12.   Diseases of the Skin and Subcutaneous Tissue 569
  13.   Diseases of the Musculoskeletal System and
        Connective Tissue 593
  14.   Congenital Anomalies 639
  15.   Certain Conditions Originating in the Perinatal Period ... 683
  16.   Symptoms, Signs, and Ill-Defined Conditions 707
  17.   Injury and Poisoning 735

Supplementary Classification
    Classification of Factors Influencing Health Status and
    Contact with Health Service 880
    Classification of External Causes of Injury and Poisoning 930

Appendices
    A.   Morphology of Neoplasms 1055
    C.   Classification of Drugs by American Hospital
        Formulary Service List Number and Their *ICD-9-CM*
        Equivalents 1127
    D.   Classification of Industrial Accidents According to
        Agency 1137
    E.   List of Three-Digit Categories 1143

revision (*DSM-IV-TR*), for definitions of terms used in classifying mental disorders. *DSM-IV-TR* is published by the American Psychiatric Association.

- Appendix C, Classification of Drugs by the American Hospital Formulary Service List Number and Their ICD-9-CM Equivalents, provides help in determining appropriate E codes for use with certain types of drugs.
- Appendix D, Classification of Industrial Accidents According to Agency, is provided for use by external agencies but is rarely used in acute-care coding.

The coder should become familiar with the location and format of all three appendices because they often provide help in arriving at correct code assignment.

ALPHABETIC INDEX OF DISEASES AND INJURIES (VOLUME 2)

The Alphabetic Index of Diseases and Injuries (volume 2) includes entries for main terms, subterms, and more specific subterms. Main terms identify disease conditions or injuries. Subterms indicate site, type, or etiology for conditions or injuries. For example, acute appendicitis is listed under **Appendicitis,** acute, and stress fracture is listed under **Fracture,** stress. Occasionally, it is necessary for the coder to think of a synonym or other alternative term in order to locate the correct entry. There are, however, exceptions to this general rule, including the following:

- Congenital conditions are often indexed under the main term **Anomaly** rather than under the name of the condition.
- Conditions that complicate pregnancy, childbirth, or the puerperium are usually found under such terms as **Delivery, Labor, Pregnancy,** and **Puerperal.** They may also appear under the main term for the condition causing the complication by referencing the subterm "complicating pregnancy, childbirth, or puerperium." (An example of this type of entry appears under the main term **Diabetes, diabetic** in the Alphabetic Index.)
- Many of the complications of medical or surgical care are indexed under the term **Complications** rather than under the name of the condition.
- Late effects of an earlier condition can be found under **Late,** effect(s) (of).

A clear understanding of the format of the Alphabetic Index (volume 2) is a prerequisite for accurate coding. Understanding the indention pattern of the entries is a very important part of learning how to use the index. Now that a variety of vendors provide printed versions and others have computer programs for coding, the format is not as consistent as it was previously. In general, however, the following pattern is carried through:

- Main terms are set flush with the left-hand margin. They are printed in bold type and begin with a capital letter.
- Subterms are indented one standard indention (equivalent to about two typewriter spaces) to the right under the main term. They are printed in regular type and begin with a lowercase letter.
- More specific subterms are indented farther and farther to the right as needed, always indented by one standard indention from the preceding subterm and listed in alphabetical order.
- Carryover lines are indented two standard indentions from the level of the preceding line. Carryover lines are used only when the complete entry cannot fit on a single line. They are indented farther to avoid confusion with subterm entries.

In most printed versions, entries still continue to use two columns to a page, dictionary style. Most printed versions also use the basic three volumes, although they are now printed in one book rather than in three separate volumes. Printed versions for nonhospital settings (e.g., physician office, home health) usually consist of one book with only volumes 1 and 2 since volume 3 (procedure codes) does not apply to these settings.

The subterms listed under the main term **Rabies** in the following entry provide an example:

Rabies   071 [main term]
    contact   V01.5 [subterm]
    exposure to   V01.5 [subterm]
    inoculation   V04.5 [subterm]
        reaction—*see* Complications, [more specific subterm]
            vaccination [carryover line]
    vaccination, prophylactic (against)   V04.5 [subterm]

Each of the subterms (contact, exposure to, inoculation, and vaccination) is indented one standard indention from the level of the main term and is listed in alphabetical order. The fifth line is a more specific entry ("reaction") under the subterm "inoculation," and the sixth line is a carryover line indented two standard indentions from the preceding line.

Exercise 1.1

A reproduction of a page from volume 2 is shown below. Label the indicated lines as either main terms, subterms, or carryover lines.

1.	Main term	**Racket nail** 757.5
2.	Carryover line	**Radial nerve**—*see* condition **Radiation effects and sickness**—*see also* Effect, adverse, radiation
3.	Subterm	cataract 366.46 dermatitis 692.89
4.	Main term	sunburn 692.71 **Radiculitis** (pressure) (vertebrogenic) 729.2
5.	Subterm	accessory nerve 723.4 anterior crural 724.4 arm 723.4 brachial 723.4 cervical NEC 723.4 due to displacement of intervertebral disc
6.	Carryover line	—*see* Neuritis, due to, displacement intervertebral disc
7.	Subterm	leg 724.4 lumbar NEC 724.4 lumbosacral 724.4 rheumatic 729. syphilitic 094.89 thoracic (with visceral pain) 724.4 **Radiculomyelitis** 357.0 toxic, due to Clostridium tetani 037
8.	Carryover line	Corynebacterium diphtheriae 032.89 **Ramsay Hunt syndrome** (herpetic geniculate ganglionitis) 053.11
9.	Subterm	meaning dyssynergia cerebellaris

10.	Subterm	myoclonica 334.2
		Ranke's primary infiltration (*see also*
		  Tuberculosis) 010.0
		Ranula 527.6
		congenital 750.26
		Rape (*see also* nature and site of injury)
		  alleged, observation or examination V71.5

Alphabetization Rules

In order to locate main terms and subterms quickly and efficiently, it is important to understand the alphabetization rules followed in the Alphabetic Index. Letter-by-letter alphabetization is used both in volume 2 and in the alphabetical portion of volume 3. The system of alphabetization ignores the following:

- Single spaces between words
- Single hyphens within words
- The final "s" in the possessive forms of words

The following list shows an example of letter-by-letter alphabetization with these modifications:

- Beer-drinkers' heart (disease)   425.5 [ignores hyphen]
- Bee sting (with . . .)   989.5 [ignores space between words]
- Brailsford's disease   732.3 [ignores possessive form]
- Brailsford-Morquio disease or syndrome   277.5 [ignores hyphen]

Numerical Entries

Subterm entries for numerical characters and words indicating numbers appear first under the appropriate main term or subterm. These are listed in numerical order rather than being alphabetized in their spelled-out form. Such characters and words include Roman numerals, such as "II"; Arabic numerals, such as "2"; and adjectival terms, such as "second." For example, in volume 2, **Paralysis**, nerve, third, comes before, rather than after, **Paralysis**, nerve, fourth. Here are more examples:

Anomaly, anomalous . . .
    chromosomes, chromosomal   758.9
        13 . . .
        18 . . .
        21 . . .
Disorder . . .
    coagulation . . .   286.9
        factor VIII . . .
        factor IX . . .
        neonatal . . .
Disorder . . .
    nerve   349.9 . . .
        cranial   352.9
            first
            second
            third

Connecting Words

Words such as "with," "in," "due to," and "associated with" are used to express the relationship between the main term or a subterm indicating an associated condition or etiology. Subterms preceded by "with" or "without" are not listed in alphabetical order but appear immediately below the main term or appropriate subterm entries; subterms beginning with other connecting words appear in alphabetical order. Coders who fail to remember this feature of the alphabetization rules often make coding errors by overlooking the appropriate subterm. Review the following subterm entries under the main term **Bronchitis** using the instructions at the end of this example:

Bronchitis (diffuse) (hypostatic) (infectious)
(inflammatory) (simple) 490

1	with
2	emphysema—*see* Emphysema
3	influenza, flu, or grippe 487.1
4	obstruction airway, chronic 491.20

> with
>> acute bronchitis 491.22
>> exacerbation (acute) 491.21
> tracheitis 490
>> acute or subacute 466.0
>>> with bronchospasm or obstruction
>>> 466.0
>> chronic 491.8

5	acute or subacute 466.0
6	with

> bronchospasm 466.0
> obstruction 466.0
> tracheitis 466.0

7	chemical (due to fumes or vapors)

> 506.0

8	due to

> fumes or vapors 506.0
> radiation 508.8

9	allergic (acute) (*see also* Asthma) 493.9
10	arachidic 934.1

1. Refer to lines 1, 5, 9, and 10 as indicated in the example. Note that the subterms preceded by the connecting word "with" immediately follow the main term **Bronchitis** and precede the subterms beginning with the letter "a" (lines 5, 9, and 10).
2. Refer to lines 6, 7, and 8 as indicated in the example. Note that the more specific subterms preceded by the connecting word "with" immediately follow the subterm acute or subacute. In this case, the subterms beginning with the word "with" precede the subterms beginning with the letters "c" and "d" (lines 7 and 8).
3. Also note that, in both cases, the subterms indented under the connecting word "with" are listed in alphabetical order. For example, lines 2, 3, and 4 indicated in the example are in alphabetical order.

Index Tables

The main body of the volume 2 Alphabetic Index uses tables for the systematic arrangement of subterms under the main entries of **Hypertension** and **Neoplasm.** These tables simplify access to complex combinations of subterms.

Section 2 of volume 2 contains a Table of Drugs and Chemicals that begins with the code for poisoning and followed by E codes. The use of this table will be discussed later in this handbook in the chapter on poisoning and adverse effects of drugs (chapter 28).

The format and alphabetization rules used within the tables are the same as those followed in the rest of the Alphabetic Index. The use of these tables will be discussed in detail later in this handbook, but it would be useful for the reader to become familiar with the location and format of the tables at this point of the discussion.

TABULAR LIST AND ALPHABETIC INDEX OF PROCEDURES (VOLUME 3)

Volume 3 contains both the Alphabetic Index and the Tabular List for surgery and procedures. The format for the Tabular List section of volume 3 is the same as that for volume 1, except that procedure codes consist of two digits, followed by a decimal point and one or two additional digits (for example, 54.11). The format and alphabetization rules for the Alphabetic Index section of volume 3 are the same as those followed for volume 2, with the exception that subterms beginning with the words "as," "by," and "for" sometimes immediately follow the main term or subterm rather than appearing in the usual alphabetical sequence; otherwise the words "with" and "without" remain in the first position. For example:

Arthrotomy   80.10
    as operative approach—*omit code*
    with
        arthrography—*see* Arthrogram
        arthroscopy—*see* Arthroscopy
        injection of drug   81.92
        removal of prosthesis (*see also* Removal, prosthesis, joint structures)   80.00
    ankle   80.17
    elbow   80.12

As the preceding example shows, subterms beginning with "as" and "with" precede the subterms ankle and elbow. Main term entries are the names of procedures and operations, with many listed under more general terms such as "repair," "removal," "insertion," and so on.

Exercise 1.2

Without referring to the handbook material or any volume of *ICD-9-CM,* answer the following questions either true or false.

   F   1. The main classification consists of 17 chapters, which refer to types of conditions, anatomical systems, E codes, and V codes.

   T   2. In the Classification of Diseases and Injuries, three-digit code numbers are referred to as categories.

   T   3. For code numbers in disease classification, the decimal point appears between the third and the fourth digits, whereas in procedure classification, the decimal point appears between the second and the third digits.

   F   4. The Table of Drugs and Chemicals is found in volume 1 of *ICD-9-CM.*

   T   5. When the subterms "with" and "without" appear under a main term entry in the Index of Diseases and Injuries, they immediately follow the main term and precede all other subterms except numerical entries at the same indention level.

Incorrect answers to any of the questions in the preceding exercise indicate a need to go back and review the first section of this chapter of the handbook before proceeding further.

---

2 *ICD-9-CM* Conventions

ICD-9-CM follows certain conventions in order to provide large amounts of information in a succinct and consistent manner. Most conventions are used in all three volumes. Slight variations used in volume 3 are discussed in chapter 7 of this handbook. A thorough understanding of these conventions is fundamental to accurate coding. *ICD-9-CM* conventions include the following:

- Instructional notes
- Abbreviations
- Cross-reference notes
- Punctuation marks
- Relational terms ("and," "with," "due to")

INSTRUCTIONAL NOTES

A variety of notes appear in all three volumes as instructions to the coder. These include general notes, inclusion and exclusion notes, code first notes, and use additional code notes.

General Notes

Most general notes in the Tabular List of diseases provide information regarding fifth digits that must be used; a few provide general information on usage in a specific section such as code 250 that explains the fourth and fifth digits. General informational notes are used in a similar way in the alphabetic indexes for diseases and procedures. Index notes are usually enclosed in boxes and printed in italic type. For example, the main term **Fracture** in volume 2 includes an informational note that explains the diagnostic terms used to designate open and closed fractures. A similar note occurs in volume 3 under the main term **Examination.**

Inclusion and Exclusion Notes

Codes in a classification system must be mutually exclusive, with no overlapping of content. In *ICD-9-CM*, therefore, it is sometimes necessary to indicate when certain conditions are or are not included in a given subdivision. This is accomplished by means of inclusion and exclusion notes.

The location of inclusion and exclusion notes is extremely important. When this type of note is located at the beginning of a chapter or a section in *ICD-9-CM*, that advice applies to all codes within the chapter or section and is not repeated with individual categories or specific codes. The coder must keep in mind that instructional notes affecting the code under consideration may be located on a previous page.

Inclusion Notes

Inclusion notes are introduced by the word "includes" when placed at the beginning of a chapter or section; the word "includes" is not used when the inclusion note applies only to a category or subcategory code. Conditions listed in an inclusion note may be synonyms or conditions similar enough to be classified to the same code. Inclusion notes are not exhaustive; rather, they list certain conditions to reassure the coder, particularly when the title in the Tabular List may not seem to apply.

An example of an inclusion note can be found in volume 1, category **216, Benign neoplasm of skin.** The inclusion notes listed under category 216 apply to all codes listed from 216.0 through 216.9. Another list appears under code 216.5; here the additional terms apply to this code only.

Exclusion Notes

Exclusion notes are introduced by the word "excludes," and in most printed versions are usually enclosed in a box or shaded. Excluded conditions are listed in alphabetical order, with the code number or code range shown in parentheses.

Exclusion notes are the opposite of inclusion notes; they indicate that a particular condition is not assigned to the code to which the note applies. The basic message of an excludes note is "code this condition elsewhere."

The most common type of exclusion note, and the most clear-cut, is an indication that another code must be used if there is a specific associated condition. An example can be found in volume 1, with the exclusion note under code **575.0, Acute cholecystitis.** This note indicates that code 575.0 is not assigned for acute cholecystitis when cholelithiasis is also present; code 574.0x should be used instead.

575.0 Acute Cholecystitis

> Excludes   *that with:*
>> *choledocholithiasis* (574.3)
>> *acute and chronic choleystitis* (575.12)
>> *choledocholithiasis* (574.3)
>> *choledocholithiasis and cholelithiasis* (574.6)
>> *cholelithiasis* (574.0)

A second type of exclusion note indicates that two conditions that appear to be similar actually have entirely different codes. For example, the same condition may have separate codes depending on whether it is acquired or congenital, or whether it occurs in an adult or a newborn. The correct interpretation in such cases is that one code or the other should be used, but not both.

For example, observe the exclusion note under code **622.3, Old laceration of cervix,** in volume 1. The exclusion note indicates that code 665.3x should be assigned when the laceration is the result of current obstetrical trauma. Also, code **734, Flat foot,** excludes flat feet described as congenital, rigid, or spastic, and refers the coder to 754.61 for such conditions.

"Code First Underlying Condition"

The instructional note "Code first underlying condition" is used in the Tabular List to identify a code for a condition that is a manifestation of an underlying disease. It indicates that the code for the underlying condition must be sequenced before the code for the manifestation. In the Alphabetic Index this convention is indicated by listing the underlying code first, followed by the manifestation code in brackets. The code for the underlying disease will also have an instructional note in the Tabular List to "use additional code" for the manifestation. When the instruction notes and Alphabetic Index provide these instructions, the manifestation code must always follow the code for the underlying condition and can never be designated as a principal diagnosis. The use of two codes in this prescribed way is referred to as "dual classification" or "dual coding." The goal of this usage in ICD-9-CM is to maintain conformity with ICD-9.

Some instructions of this type indicate that a specific code must be assigned first. In volume 1, an example of this instructional note can be found under code **484.5,** *Pneumonia in anthrax,* which specifies that code **022.1, Pulmonary anthrax,** must be assigned before code 484.5. Other notes of this type provide a list introduced by the word "as"—meaning that any of the listed codes or any other appropriate code can be assigned first. Code **595.4,** *Cystitis in diseases classified elsewhere,* provides a list of conditions that may be the underlying condition.

"Use Additional Code"

The instruction to "use additional code" indicates that another code may be needed to include a complete statement of the condition. If the condition mentioned in the note is documented as present, the additional code should always be assigned.

For example, volume 1 includes an instructional note under category **595, Cystitis.** The note indicates that an additional code should be assigned to identify the organism responsible for the cystitis when it has been identified. Very occasionally, this instruction indicates that the manifestation should be listed first with an additional code for the underlying condition. The logic for this instruction is that a life-threatening condition should be listed before the chronic underlying condition. See code **337.3, Autonomic dysreflexia,** for an example of this instruction.

"Code, If Applicable, Any Causal Condition First"

The instruction to "Code, if applicable, any causal condition first" indicates that if a causal condition were present, it would be sequenced before the code to which this note is attached. In volume 1, an example of this instructional note can be found under subcategory **707.1, Ulcer of lower limbs, except decubitus.** This instruction indicates that if a causal condition is documented, then the causal condition should be sequenced first (in this example, chronic venous hypertension with ulcer, postphlebetic syndrome with ulcer, etc.). However, unlike the instructional note "code first underlying condition," code 707.1x may be sequenced as a first-listed code or principal diagnosis, if no causal condition is applicable or known.

ABBREVIATIONS

ICD-9-CM uses two main abbreviations:

- NEC for not elsewhere classified
- NOS for not otherwise specified

Although their meanings appear simple, these abbreviations are often misunderstood and misapplied by coders. It is very important to understand not only their meanings, but also their differences, because they provide guidelines for correct code selection.

NEC

The abbreviation NEC (not elsewhere classified) is used in the Alphabetic Index to indicate that there is no separate code for the condition even though the diagnostic statement may be very specific. In the Tabular List, such conditions are ordinarily classified to the final digit 8 with a title that includes the words "other specified" or "not elsewhere classified." This permits the grouping of related conditions to conserve space and limit the size of the classification system. For example, a cardiac dysrhythmia specified as atrioventricular (AV) or interference is included in code **426.89, Other specified cardiac dysrhythmia.**

NOS

The abbreviation NOS (not otherwise specified) is the equivalent of "unspecified" and is used only in the tabular lists. Codes so identified are to be used only when neither the diagnostic statement nor the medical record provides information that permits classification to a more specific code. The codes in these cases are ordinarily classified to the final digit 9; conditions listed as both "not elsewhere classified" and "unspecified" are sometimes combined in one code. Note that a main term followed by a list of subterms in the alphabetic indexes usually displays the unspecified code; the subterms must always be reviewed to determine whether a more specific code can be assigned.

For example, the main term **Conduction disorder, unspecified,** displays code 426.9; subterms such as "heartblock, not otherwise specified" are provided for more specific conduction disorders. Code 426.9 should be assigned only when there is no information in the medical record to identify one of these subterms.

CROSS-REFERENCE NOTES

Cross-references are used in the alphabetic indices to advise the coder to look elsewhere before assigning a code. The cross-reference instructions include "*see,*" "*see also,*" "*see* category," and "*see* condition."

"See"

The "see" cross-reference indicates that the coder must refer to an alternative term. This instruction is mandatory; coding cannot be completed without following this advice. For example, the entry for **Hemarthrosis, traumatic,** uses this cross-reference to advise the coder to reference the entry for "sprain" by site.

"See Also"

The "see also" cross-reference advises the coder that there is another place in the Alphabetic Index to which the coder must refer when the entries under consideration do not provide a code for the specific condition or procedure. It is not necessary to follow this cross-reference when the original entries provide all the information necessary.

For example, the cross-reference for the term **Psychosis, schizophrenia, schizophrenic,** advises the coder to "*see also* Schizophrenia" when none of the specific subterms provides a code. If a coder is attempting to locate the code for catatonic schizophrenia, it would not be necessary to follow this cross-reference because there is a subterm catatonic under the subterm schizophrenic. If the diagnosis were undifferentiated schizophrenia, however, the code could be located only by following the "*see also*" reference.

"See Category"

The "see category" variation of the "see" cross-reference provides the coder with a category number. The coder must refer to that number in the Tabular List and select a code from the options provided there. For example, a cross-reference under the index entry for late effect of intracranial abscess refers the coder to category 326.

"See Condition"

Occasionally, the index advises the coder to refer to the main term of a condition. For example, if a coder references the main term **Arterial** for arterial thrombosis, the index advice is to "see condition" and the coder should then go to the main term **Thrombosis.** This cross-reference ordinarily appears when the coder has referenced the adjective rather than the term (in noun form) for the condition itself.

PUNCTUATION MARKS

Several punctuation marks are used in *ICD-9-CM*, most of which have a specialized meaning in addition to the usual English language usage.

Parentheses

Parentheses are used in *ICD-9-CM* to enclose supplementary words or explanatory information that may be either present or absent in the statement of diagnosis or procedure without affecting the code to which it is assigned. Such terms are considered to be "nonessential modifiers" and are used to suggest that the terms in parentheses are included in the code but need not be stated in the diagnosis or procedure. This is a significant factor in correct code assignment. Terms enclosed in parentheses in either the Tabular List (volume 1) or the Alphabetic Index (volume 2) do not affect the code assignment in any way; they serve only as reassurance that the correct code has been located.

For example, refer to the main term **Pneumonia,** which has numerous nonessential modifiers enclosed in parentheses. Unless a more specific subterm is located, this code will be assigned for pneumonia described by any of the terms in parentheses. Diagnoses of acute pneumonia and Alpenstich pneumonia, for instance, are both coded 486 because both terms appear in parentheses as nonessential modifiers. Pneumonia not otherwise specified is also assigned to code 486 because none of the terms in parentheses is required for this code assignment.

It is important to distinguish between the use of nonessential and essential modifiers. Essential modifiers are listed as subterms in the alphabetic indices, not in parentheses, and they do affect code assignment. However, words in parentheses are nonessential and do not affect the code assignment. For example, scoliosis described as acquired or postural is classified as 737.30 as these words are nonessential modifiers and do not affect the code; on the other hand, the term congenital is an essential modifier and the code for this term is 754.2.

Exercise 2.1.

Referring only to the title and inclusion notes for code 490, mark an "X" in front of each of the diagnostic statements listed below that is included in code 490.

__X__	Catarrhal bronchitis NOS
_____	Chronic bronchitis
_____	Allergic bronchitis
__X__	Tracheobronchitis NOS
_____	Asthmatic bronchitis

Square Brackets

Square brackets are often used in the tabular lists to enclose synonyms, alternative wordings, abbreviations, and explanatory phrases that provide additional information—for example, paroxysmal atrial tachycardia [PAT]. They are similar in that they are not required of the statement of diagnosis or operation. Square brackets are also used to indicate that the number in the bracket can only be a manifestation and the other number must be assigned first for the underlying code. The code in the brackets in this situation indicates that both conditions must be used, and the code in the brackets can never be assigned as the principal diagnosis. In most printed versions of the manuals, both the brackets and the second code are printed in italics. In the following example from volume 2, the first code represents an underlying disease, and the second code enclosed in brackets manifestation:

Cystitis . . .
    actinomycotic   039.8 [*595.4*]

Colons

Colons are used in both inclusion and exclusion notes to indicate that one of the modifiers from the list indented below the entry must be present in order for the statement to apply. The exclusion statement under code 518.5 in volume 1 is an example of this usage; here the colon following the subterm pneumonia indicates that it is described as aspiration pneumonia or hypostatic pneumonia is excluded.

518.5 Pulmonary insufficiency following trauma or surgery
        Adult respiratory distress syndrome
        Pulmonary insufficiency following:
            shock
            surgery
            trauma
        Shock lung
        Excludes   *adult respiratory distress syndrome associated with other conditions*
                (518.82)
                pneumonia:
                    aspiration *(507.0)*
                    hypostatic *(514)*
                respiratory failure *(518.81)* *(518.83–518.84)*

Exercise 2.2

Referring only to the title and inclusion notes provided for the four-digit code 39.29, mark an "X" in front of each procedure listed below that is included in code 39.29.

__X__	Brachial bypass
__X__	Bypass graft of femoropopliteal arteries
__X__	Vascular bypass, not otherwise specified
_____	Bypass graft
__X__	Popliteal bypass graft

RELATIONAL TERMS

Words such as "and," "due to," "with," "associated with," "without," and "in" are used to indicate various types of relationships expressed in *ICD-9-CM*, and are used as subterms in the alphabetic indexes. These words have special meanings in *ICD-9-CM* and in the discussion of coding principles.

"And"

The word "and" should be interpreted to mean either "and" or "or" when it appears in a title. For example, code 415.1x in volume 1 includes pulmonary embolism and/or pulmonary infarction. In volume 3, code 38.5x includes ligation and/or stripping of varicose veins.

"Due To"

The words "due to" in either the alphabetic indexes or the tabular lists indicate that a causal relationship between two conditions is present. *ICD-9-CM* occasionally makes such an assumption when both conditions are present. In other combinations, however, the diagnostic statement must indicate this relationship. For example, certain conditions affecting the mitral valve are assumed to be rheumatic in origin, whether or not the diagnostic statement makes this distinction. In other cases, the Alphabetic Index provides a subterm "due to," which must be followed when the physician's statement indicates a causal relationship. The coder should be guided by the index entry.

"With"

Words such as "with," "with mention of," "associated with," and "in" indicate that both elements in the title must be present in the diagnostic or procedural statement. Although these terms do not necessarily indicate a cause-effect relationship, they occur together much of the time and the classification system indicates this relationship. The main term **Pneumonia** provides a good example of this use of the subterm "in" psittacosis 073.0.

3 Uniform Hospital Discharge Data Set

The Uniform Hospital Discharge Data Set (UHDDS) is used for reporting inpatient data in acute-care, short-term, and long-term care hospitals. It uses a minimum set of items based on standard definitions that could provide consistent data for multiple users. Only those items that met the following criteria were included:

- Easily identified
- Readily defined
- Uniformly recorded
- Easily abstracted from the medical record

Its use is required for reporting Medicare and Medicaid patients. In addition, many other health care payers also use most of the UHDDS for the uniform billing system.

DATA ITEMS

The UHDDS requires the following items:

- Principal diagnosis
- Other diagnoses that have significance for the specific hospital episode
- All significant procedures

The four cooperating parties responsible for maintaining *ICD-9-CM* have developed official guidelines for designating the principal diagnosis and for identifying other diagnoses that should be reported in certain situations. The UHDDS also contains a core of general information that pertains to the patient and to the specific episode of care, such as the age, sex, and race of the patient; the expected payer; and the hospital's identification.

The UHDDS definitions were originally developed in 1985 for hospital reporting of inpatient data elements. Since that time, the application of UHDDS definitions has been expanded to include all non-outpatient settings. In addition to acute care short-term and long-term care hospitals, the definitions for principal diagnosis and other (secondary) diagnoses also apply to psychiatric hospitals, home health agencies, rehabilitation facilities, nursing homes, and other settings. Guidelines for selection of principal diagnosis and other diagnoses discussed below apply to all these settings.

Principal Diagnosis

The principal diagnosis is defined as the condition established after study to be chiefly responsible for admission of the patient to the hospital. It is important that the principal diagnosis be designated correctly because it is significant in cost comparisons, in care analysis, and in utilization review. It is crucial for reimbursement because many third-party payers (including Medicare) base reimbursement primarily on principal diagnosis. It is ordinarily listed first in the physician's diagnostic statement, but this is not always the case; the coder must always review the entire medical record to determine the condition that should be designated as the principal diagnosis.

The words "after study" in the definition of principal diagnosis are important, but they are sometimes confusing. It is not the admitting diagnosis but rather the diagnosis found after workup or even after surgery that proves to be the reason for admission. For example:

- A patient admitted with urinary retention may prove to have hypertrophy of the prostate, which is causing the urinary retention. In this case, the prostatic hypertrophy is the principal diagnosis unless treatment was directed only to the urinary retention.
- A patient may be admitted because of unstable angina, and a percutaneous transluminal angioplasty may be carried out to clear arteriosclerotic blockage of the coronary artery in order to abort what appears to be an impending myocardial infarction. In this case, the coronary arteriosclerosis is the principal diagnosis because, after study, it was determined to be the underlying cause of the angina and the reason for admission.
- A patient was admitted with severe abdominal pain. The white blood cell count was elevated to 16,000, with shift to the left. The patient was taken to surgery, where an acute ruptured appendix was removed. After study, the principal diagnosis is acute ruptured appendicitis.
- A patient was admitted with severe abdominal pain in the right lower quadrant and an admitting diagnosis of probable acute appendicitis. The white blood cell count was slightly elevated. The patient was taken to surgery, where a normal appendix was found but an inflamed Meckel's diverticulum was removed. After study, the principal diagnosis is Meckel's diverticulum.

The circumstances of inpatient admission always govern the selection of the principal diagnosis, and the coding directives in the *ICD-9-CM* manuals, volumes 1, 2, and 3, take precedence over all other guidelines. The importance of consistent, complete documentation in the medical record cannot be overemphasized. Without such documentation, the application of all coding guidelines is a difficult, if not impossible, task.

There are special instructions related to the selection of principal diagnosis when a patient is admitted as an inpatient from the hospital's observation unit or from outpatient surgery. For example:

Admission following medical observation: A patient may be treated in a hospital's observation unit to determine if the condition improves sufficiently for the patient to be discharged. If the condition either worsens or doesn't improve, the physician may decide to admit the patient as an inpatient. The principal diagnosis reported would be the medical condition that led to the hospital admission.

Admission following postoperative observation: A patient undergoing outpatient surgery may require postoperative admission to an observation unit to monitor a condition (or complication) that develops postoperatively. If the patient subsequently requires inpatient admission to the same hospital, the UHDDS definition of principal diagnosis applies: "that condition established after study to be chiefly responsible for occasioning the admission of the patient to the hospital for care."

Admission from outpatient surgery: A patient undergoing outpatient surgery may be subsequently admitted for continuing inpatient care at the same hospital. The following guidelines should be followed in selecting the principal diagnosis for the inpatient admission:

- If the reason for the inpatient admission is a complication, assign the complication as the principal diagnosis.
- If no complication or other condition is documented as the reason for the inpatient admission, assign the reason for the outpatient surgery as the principal diagnosis.
- If the reason for the inpatient admission is another condition unrelated to the surgery, assign the unrelated condition as the principal diagnosis.

The following official guidelines for designating the principal diagnosis apply to all systems and etiologies. (Guidelines that apply only to specific body systems or etiologies are discussed in the relevant chapters of this handbook. The complete *Official Guidelines for Coding and Reporting* may be found in this book's appendix.)

1. *Two or more diagnoses that equally meet the definition for principal diagnosis:* In the unusual situation in which two or more diagnoses equally meet the criteria for prin-

cipal diagnosis as determined by the circumstances of the admission and the diagnostic workup and/or therapy provided, either may be sequenced first when neither the Alphabetic Index nor the Tabular List directs otherwise. However, it is not simply the fact that both conditions exist that makes this choice possible. When treatment is totally or primarily directed toward one condition, or when only one condition would have required inpatient care, that condition should be designated as the principal diagnosis. Also, if another coding guideline (general or disease-specific) provides sequencing direction, that guideline must be followed.

Example 1: A patient was admitted with unstable angina and acute congestive heart failure. The unstable angina was treated with nitrates, and intravenous Lasix was given to manage the heart failure. Both diagnoses meet the definition of principal diagnosis equally, and either may be sequenced first.

Example 2: A patient was admitted with acute atrial fibrillation with rapid ventricular response and was also in heart failure with pulmonary edema. The patient was digitalized to reduce the ventricular rate and given intravenous Lasix to reduce the cardiogenic pulmonary edema. Both conditions meet the definition of principal diagnosis equally, and either may be sequenced first.

Example 3: A patient was admitted with severe abdominal pain, nausea, and vomiting due to acute pyelonephritis, 590.10, and diverticulitis, 562.11. Both underlying conditions were treated, and the physician believed both equally met the criteria for principal diagnosis. In this instance, either condition may be listed as principal diagnosis.

2. *Two or more comparable or contrasting conditions:* In the rare instance where two or more comparable or contrasting conditions are documented as either/or (or similar terminology), both diagnoses are coded as though confirmed and the principal diagnosis is designated according to the circumstances of the admission and the diagnostic workup and/or therapy provided. When no further determination can be made as to which diagnosis more closely meets the criteria for principal diagnosis, either may be sequenced first. Note that this does not apply for outpatient encounters.

Example 1: A patient with the same complaints as those outlined in example 3 above was admitted with a final diagnosis of acute pyelonephritis versus diverticulum of the colon. The patient was treated symptomatically and discharged for further studies. In this case, both conditions meet the criteria for principal diagnosis equally and either can be designated as the principal diagnosis.

Example 2: The treatment of another patient with the same symptoms and the same final diagnoses was directed almost entirely toward the acute pyelonephritis, indicating that the physician considered this the more likely problem and that, after study, it was the condition that occasioned the admission. In this case, both conditions would be coded, but the acute pyelonephritis would be sequenced first because of the circumstances of the admission.

3. *A symptom followed by contrasting/comparative diagnoses:* When a symptom is followed by contrasting/comparative diagnoses, the symptom code is sequenced first. However, if the symptom code is integral to each of the conditions listed, no additional code for the symptom is reported. Codes are assigned for all listed contrasting/comparative diagnoses.

Example 1: A patient was admitted for workup because of severe fatigue. The discharge diagnosis was recorded as fatigue, due to either depressive reaction or hypothyroidism. In this case, the symptom code for fatigue is designated the principal diagnosis, with additional codes assigned for both the depressive reaction and the hypothyroidism.

Example 2: The discharge diagnosis is stated as gastrointestinal bleeding, due to either acute gastritis or angiodysplasia. In this case, the diagnoses are coded as contrasting/comparative diagnoses and no separate code is assigned for the bleeding because the codes for both conditions include any associated bleeding.

4. *Original treatment plan not carried out:* In a situation in which the original treatment plan cannot be carried out due to unforeseen circumstances, the criteria for designation of the principal diagnosis do not change. The condition that occasioned the admission is designated as principal diagnosis even though the planned treatment was not carried out.

Example 1: A patient with benign hypertrophy of the prostate was admitted for the purpose of a transurethral resection of the prostate (TURP). Shortly after admission, but before the patient was taken to the operating suite, the patient fell and sustained a fracture of the left femur. The TURP was canceled; hip pinning was carried out on the following day. The principal diagnosis remains hypertrophy of the prostate even though that condition was not treated.

Example 2: A patient with a diagnosis of carcinoma of the breast confirmed from an outpatient biopsy was admitted for the purpose of modified radical mastectomy. Before the preoperative medications were administered the next morning, the patient indicated that she had decided against having the procedure until she was able to consider possible alternative treatment more thoroughly. No treatment was given, and she was discharged. The carcinoma of the breast remains the principal diagnosis because it was the condition that occasioned the admission even though no treatment was rendered.

Other Diagnoses

Other reportable diagnoses are defined as those conditions that coexist at the time of admission or develop subsequently or affect patient care for the current hospital episode. Diagnoses that have no impact on patient care during the hospital stay are not reported even when they are present. Diagnoses that relate to an earlier episode and have no bearing on the current hospital stay are not reported.

For UHDDS reporting purposes, the definition of "other diagnosis" includes only those conditions that affect the episode of hospital care in terms of any of the following:

- Clinical evaluation
- Therapeutic treatment
- Further evaluation by diagnostic studies, procedures, or consultation
- Extended length of hospital stay
- Increased nursing care and/or other monitoring

All these factors are self-explanatory except the first. Clinical evaluation means that the physician is aware of the problem and is evaluating it in terms of testing, consultations, and close clinical observation of the patient's condition. In most cases, a patient who is being evaluated clinically will also fit into one of the other criteria. Note that a physical examination alone does not qualify as further evaluation or clinical evaluation; the physical examination is a routine part of every hospital admission. No particular order is mandated for sequencing other diagnoses. The more significant ones should be sequenced early in the list when the number of diagnoses that may be reported is limited.

Reporting Guidelines for Other Diagnoses

The following guidelines and examples should be studied carefully in order to understand the rationale for determining other diagnoses that should be reported:

1. *Previous conditions stated as diagnoses:* Physicians sometimes include in the diagnostic statement historical information or status post procedures performed on a previous admission that have no bearing on the current stay. Such conditions are not reported. However, history codes (V10–V19) may be used as secondary codes if the historical condition or family history has an impact on current care or influences treatment.

Example: A patient was admitted with acute myocardial infarction; the physician noted in the history that the patient was status post cholecystectomy and had been hospitalized one year earlier for pneumonia. At discharge, the physician documented the final diagnoses as acute myocardial infarction, status post cholecystectomy, and history of pneumonia. Only the acute myocardial infarction is coded and reported; the other conditions included in the diagnostic statement had no bearing on the current episode of care.

2. *Other diagnosis with no documentation supporting reportability:* If the physician has included a diagnosis in the final diagnostic statement, it should ordinarily be coded. If there is no supporting documentation in the medical record, however, the physician should be consulted as to whether the diagnosis meets reporting criteria; if so, the physician should be asked to add the necessary documentation. Reporting of conditions for which there is no supporting documentation is in conflict with UHDDS criteria.

Example 1: A 10-year-old boy was admitted with open fracture of the tibia and fibula following a bicycle accident. On physical examination, the physician noted that there was a nevus on the leg and that the patient had a small asymptomatic inguinal hernia. All these diagnoses were documented on the face sheet. The fracture was reduced with internal fixation, but neither the nevus nor the hernia was treated or further evaluated on this admission. The nevus and hernia are not reported because there is nothing to indicate that they had any effect on the episode of care.

Example 2: A patient was admitted with an acute myocardial infarction. The physician also included in the diagnostic statement a strabismus and a bunion noted on the physical examination. Review of the medical record revealed that no further reference to these conditions was made in terms of further evaluation or treatment; therefore, no codes for either the strabismus or the bunion would be assigned.

3. *Chronic conditions that are not the thrust of treatment:* A patient was admitted for treatment of his uncontrolled Type II diabetes. He also has a current chronic obstructive pulmonary disease as well as Parkinson's disease. Although these chronic conditions were not treated specifically, these chronic conditions are reported because they also required evaluation and monitoring of them.

Example 1: A patient was admitted following a hip fracture, and a diagnosis of Parkinson's disease was noted in the history and physical examination. Nursing notes indicate that the patient required additional care because of the Parkinsonism. Both diagnoses are reported.

Example 2: A patient was admitted with pneumonia, and the presence of diabetes mellitus was documented in the record. Blood sugars were monitored by laboratory studies, and nursing personnel also checked blood sugars before each meal. The patient was continued on his diabetic diet. Although no active treatment was provided, ongoing monitoring was required and the condition is reported.

Example 3: A patient was admitted with acute diverticulitis, and the physician documented in the admitting note a history of hypertension. Review of the medical record indicates that blood pressure medications were given throughout the stay. The hypertension is reportable, and the physician should be asked to add it to the diagnostic statement.

Example 4: A patient was admitted in congestive heart failure. She had known hiatal hernia and degenerative arthritis. Neither condition was further evaluated or treated; by their nature, the conditions do not require continuing clinical evaluation. Only the code for the congestive heart failure is assigned; the other conditions are not reportable.

Example 5: A 60-year-old diabetic patient was transferred from an extended care facility for treatment of a decubitus ulcer. The physician noted in the history and physical exam that the patient was status post left below-the-knee amputation due to peripheral vascular disease. This condition required additional nursing assistance and is reported.

4. *Conditions that are an integral part of a disease process should not be reported as additional diagnoses.*

Example 1: A patient was admitted with nausea and vomiting due to infectious gastroenteritis. Nausea and vomiting are common symptoms of infectious gastroenteritis and are not reported.

Example 2: A patient was admitted with severe joint pain and rheumatoid arthritis. Severe joint pain is a characteristic part of rheumatoid arthritis and is not reportable.

5. *Conditions that are not an integral part of a disease process should be coded when present.*

Example 1: A patient was admitted by ambulance following a cerebrovascular accident suffered at work. The patient was in a coma but gradually recovered consciousness. Diagnosis at discharge was reported as cerebrovascular thrombosis with coma. In this case, coma is coded as an additional diagnosis because it is not implicit in a cerebrovascular accident and is not always present.

Example 2: A 5-year-old boy was admitted with a 104-degree fever associated with acute pneumonia. During the first 24 hours, the patient also experienced convulsions due to the high fever. Both the pneumonia and the convulsions are reported because convulsions are not routinely associated with pneumonia. Fever is commonly associated with pneumonia, however, and no code is assigned.

6. *Abnormal findings:* Codes from sections 790–796 for nonspecific abnormal findings (laboratory, radiology, pathology, and other diagnostic results), should be assigned only when the physician has not been able to arrive at a related diagnosis but indicates that the abnormal finding is considered to be clinically significant by listing it in the diagnostic statement. This differs from the coding practices in the outpatient setting when coding encounters for diagnostic tests that have been interpreted by a physician.

The coder should never assign a code on the basis of an abnormal finding alone. To make a diagnosis on the basis of a single lab value or abnormal diagnostic finding is risky and carries the possibility of error. A value reported as either lower or higher than the normal range does not necessarily indicate a disorder. Many factors influence the values in a lab sample; these include the collection device, the method used to transport the sample to the lab, the calibration of the machine that reads the values, and the condition of the patient. For example, a patient who is dehydrated may show an elevated hemoglobin due to increased viscosity of the blood. When findings are clearly outside the normal range and the physician has ordered other tests to evaluate the condition or has prescribed treatment without documenting an associated diagnosis, it is appropriate to ask the physician whether a diagnosis should be added or whether the abnormal finding should be listed in the diagnostic statement. Incidental findings on X-ray such as asymptomatic hiatal hernia or a diverticulum should not be reported unless further evaluation or treatment is carried out.

Example 1: A low potassium level treated with intravenous or oral potassium is clinically significant and should be brought to the attention of the physician if no related diagnosis has been recorded.

Example 2: A hematocrit of 28 percent, even though asymptomatic and not treated, was evaluated with serial hematocrits. Because the finding is outside the range of normal laboratory values and has been further evaluated, the physician should be asked whether an associated diagnosis should be documented.

Example 3: A routine preoperative chest X-ray on an elderly patient reveals collapse of a vertebral body. The patient was asymptomatic, and no further evaluation or treatment was carried out. This is a common finding in elderly patients and is insignificant for this episode.

Example 4: In the absence of a cardiac problem, an isolated electrocardiographic finding of bundle branch block is ordinarily not significant, whereas a finding of a Mobitz II block may have important implications for the patient's care and would warrant asking the physician whether it should be reported for this admission.

Example 5: The physician lists an abnormal sedimentation rate as part of the diagnostic statement. The physician has been unable to make a definitive diagnosis during the hospitalization in spite of further evaluation and considers the abnormal finding a significant clinical problem. **Code 790.1, Elevated sedimentation rate,** should be assigned.

Admitting Diagnosis

Although the admitting diagnosis is not an element of the UHDDS, it must be reported for some payers and may also be useful in quality-of-care studies. Ordinarily, only one admitting diagnosis can be reported. The inpatient admitting diagnosis may be reported as one of the following:

- A significant finding (symptom or sign) representing patient distress or an abnormal finding on outpatient examination
- A possible diagnosis based on significant findings (working diagnosis)
- A diagnosis established on an ambulatory care basis or during a previous hospital admission
- An injury or poisoning
- A reason or condition not actually an illness or injury, such as a follow-up examination or pregnancy in labor

If the admitting diagnosis is reported, the code should indicate the diagnosis provided by the physician at the time of admission. Although the admitting diagnosis may not agree with the principal diagnosis on discharge, the admitting diagnosis should not be changed to conform with the principal diagnosis. Examples of admitting diagnoses and subsequent principal diagnoses follow:

- Admitting: Gastrointestinal bleeding   578.9
  Principal: Acute duodenal ulcer with hemorrhage   532.00
- Admitting: Lump in breast   611.72
  Principal: Carcinoma of breast   174.9
- Admitting: Acute cholecystitis   575.0
  Principal: Acute cholecystitis with cholelithiasis   574.00
- Admitting: Congestive heart failure   428.0
  Principal: Acute myocardial infarction, anterior wall
              (initial episode of care)   410.11
- Admitting: Suspected myocardial infarction   410.90
  Principal: Dissecting thoracic aneurysm of aorta   441.01

PROCEDURES

The UHDDS requires that all significant procedures be reported. The UHDDS definitions of significant procedures and other reporting guidelines are discussed in chapter 7 of this handbook, along with other information on coding operations and procedures.

RELATIONSHIP OF UHDDS TO OUTPATIENT REPORTING

The UHDDS definition of principal diagnosis does not apply to the coding of outpatient encounters. In contrast to inpatient coding, no "after study" element is involved because ambulatory care visits do not permit the continued evaluation ordinarily needed to meet UHDDS criteria. If the physician does not identify a definite condition or problem at the conclusion of a visit or encounter the coder should report the documented chief complaint as the reason for the encounter/visit.

For Medicare reporting, a special rule applies for reporting hospital admissions that occur within 72 hours of outpatient care at the same facility. In this situation the UHDDS definition of principal diagnosis does apply and the principal diagnosis is the condition responsible for the admission, not the condition responsible for the outpatient encounter. Additional codes are assigned for other reportable diagnoses or procedures performed during the 72-hour period. Note that this rule applies for all outpatient care provided during the 72-hour period prior to admission, not only outpatient surgery.

ETHICAL CODING AND REPORTING

While coded medical data is used for a variety of purposes, it has become increasingly important in determining payment for health care. Medicare reimbursement depends on the correct designation of the principal diagnosis, the presence or absence of additional codes that represent complications or comorbidities as defined by the DRG system, and procedures performed. Other third-party payers may follow slightly different reimbursement methods, but the accuracy of *ICD-9-CM* coding is always vital.

Accurate and ethical *ICD-9-CM* coding depends on correctly following all instructions in the coding manuals as well as all official guidelines developed by the cooperating parties and published in the American Hospital Association's quarterly *Coding Clinic for ICD-9-CM*. Accurate and ethical reporting requires the correct selection of those conditions that meet the criteria set by the UHDDS and the official guidelines mentioned above. Over-coding and over-reporting may result in higher payment, but it is unethical and may be considered fraudulent. On the other hand, it is important to be sure that all appropriate codes are reported, as failure to include all diagnoses or procedures that meet reporting criteria may result in financial loss for the health care provider.

Occasionally certain codes are identified by Medicare as being unacceptable as the principal diagnosis. This does not mean that the code should not be assigned when it is correct; it means that the third-party payer may question or deny payment. It is important to code correctly, and then make whatever adjustment is required for reporting. Otherwise, the coder runs the risk of developing incorrect coding practices that will distort data used for other purposes.

Hospitals sometimes feel a need to code nonreportable diagnoses or procedures for internal use; this is acceptable if the facility has a system for maintaining this information outside the reporting system.

4 The Medical Record as a Source Document

The source document for coding and reporting diagnoses and procedures is the medical record. Although discharge diagnoses are usually recorded on the face sheet or the discharge summary, further review of the medical record is needed to ensure complete and accurate coding. Operations and procedures are frequently not listed on the face sheet or are not described in sufficient detail, making a review of operative reports, pathology reports, and other special reports imperative. The entire record should be reviewed to determine the specific reason for the encounter and the conditions treated.

Physicians sometimes fail to list reportable conditions that developed during the stay but were resolved prior to discharge. Conditions such as urinary tract infection or dehydration, for instance, are often not included in the diagnostic statement even though progress notes, physicians' orders, and laboratory reports make it clear that such conditions were treated. It is inappropriate for coders to assign a diagnosis based solely on physician orders for prescribed medications without the physician documenting the diagnosis being treated. If there is enough information to make it likely that an additional diagnosis should be reported, the physician should be consulted; no diagnosis should be added without the approval of the physician. Because diagnostic statements sometimes include diagnoses that represent past history, or existing diagnoses that do not meet the Uniform Hospital Discharge Data Set (UHDDS) guidelines for reportable diagnoses, a review of the medical record is required to determine whether these diagnoses should be coded for this encounter.

It is customary to list the principal diagnosis first in the diagnostic statement. Many physicians, however, are not aware of coding and reporting guidelines and consequently, this custom is not consistently followed. Because the correct designation of the principal diagnosis is of critical importance in reporting diagnostic information, the coder must be sure that medical record documentation supports the designation of principal diagnosis. If it appears that another diagnosis should be designated as principal diagnosis, or if conditions not listed should be reported, the coder should follow the health care facility's procedures for obtaining a corrected diagnostic statement.

Medical records contain a variety of reports that document the reason the patient came to the hospital, the tests performed and their findings, the therapies provided, descriptions of any surgical procedures, and daily records of the patient's progress. Each report contains important information needed for accurate coding and reporting of the principal diagnosis, other diagnoses, and the procedures performed.

A number of standard reports can be found in almost any medical record, but other reports will appear depending on the condition for which the patient is being treated, the extent of workup and therapy provided, and the attending physician's style of documentation. For example, a physician may list final diagnoses on the admission record (face sheet), progress notes or on the discharge summary. Consultants occasionally record their consultation notes in the progress notes rather than on separate reports.

Review of the inpatient medical record should begin with the discharge summary because it provides a synopsis of the patient's hospital stay, including the reason for admission, significant diagnostic findings, treatment given, the patient's course in the hospital, follow-up plan, and final diagnostic statement. The history section usually indicates the reason for admission (principal diagnosis), which may require confirmation by review of the history and physical examination and admitting and emergency department records.

The section of the discharge summary that describes the course in the hospital usually indicates treatment given and any further workup that has been done. It is particularly useful in determining whether all listed diagnoses meet the criteria for reporting and identifying other conditions that may merit reporting.

Conditions mentioned elsewhere in the body of the discharge summary do not necessarily warrant reporting but may provide clues for more specific review to make a final determination. The medical record should be reviewed further to determine whether such conditions meet the criteria for reportable diagnoses as defined in the UHDDS. The medication record is often helpful in indicating that therapeutic treatment may have been administered, but the coder must not assume a diagnosis solely on the basis of medication administration or abnormal findings in diagnostic reports. In addition, recorded diagnoses do not always contain sufficient information for providing the required specificity in coding. For example, a diagnosis of pneumonia may not indicate the organism responsible for the infection; a review of diagnostic studies of the sputum may provide this information. The physician should be asked to confirm that the organism discovered on the positive culture is the causative agent. The physician should indicate confirmation by documenting in the medical record before a code identifying the specific type of pneumonia can be assigned. A diagnosis of fracture may indicate which bone was fractured, but not the particular part of the bone, information that is necessary for accurate code assignment. The X-ray or the operative report should supply these data.

Some facilities may develop their own additional coding guidelines to provide assistance in determining when a physician query is appropriate. If the test findings are outside the normal range and the physician has ordered other tests to evaluate the condition or prescribed treatment, it is appropriate to ask the physician whether the diagnosis should be added. However, a facility's internal guidelines may not interpret abnormal findings to replace physician documentation or physician query.

The following examples illustrate diagnoses that are often recorded with less-than-complete information but can be coded more specifically by referring to diagnostic reports within the medical record. Note the variation in code assignment when more information is available after physician confirmation:

- Diagnosis: Cancer of cervix   180.9
  Pathology report: Carcinoma, in situ, of cervix   233.1
- Diagnosis: Urinary tract infection   599.0
  Laboratory report: E. coli in urine   599.0 + 041.4
- Diagnosis: Fracture of femur   821.00
  X-ray report: Open fracture of subtrochanteric neck of the femur   820.32

Code assignment is generally based on the attending physician's documentation. It is also appropriate to base code assignment on the documentation of other physicians involved in the care and treatment of the patient, as long as there is no conflicting information from the attending physician. A physician query is not necessary if a physician involved in the care and treatment of the patient, including consulting physicians, has documented a diagnosis and there is no conflicting documentation from another physician. If documentation from different physicians conflicts, the attending physician should be queried for clarification since he or she is ultimately responsible for the final diagnosis.

In some institutions, there are mid-level providers, such as nurse practitioners and physician assistants, who are involved in the care of the patient and document diagnoses in the health record. It is appropriate to base code assignments on the documentation of mid-level providers if they are considered legally accountable for establishing a diagnosis within the regulations governing the provider and the facility. The *Official Guidelines for Coding and Reporting* use the term *provider* to mean physician or any qualified health care practitioner who is legally accountable for establishing the patient's diagnosis.

Not all reportable services or procedures during an encounter or admission are performed or documented by physicians. It is appropriate to assign a procedure code based on documentation by the nonphysician professional who provided the service. This applies only to procedure coding where there is documentation to substantiate the code. It does not apply to diagnosis coding. The documentation from the nonphysician professional who provided the service may be the only evidence that the service was provided. This is true of services such as infusions carried out by nurses and therapies provided by physical, respiratory, or occupational therapists.

Outpatient records generally contain less information than inpatient records. Nevertheless, all available reports for the encounter should be reviewed prior to code assignment. Code assignment is dependent on the information available at the time of code assignment. For ambulatory records, an additional data element called "patient's reason for visit" is usually reported. This data element, also called "Form Locator 76" (FL76), has a dual use on claims. For inpatient claims, FL76 represents the "Admitting Diagnosis," while for outpatient claims it represents the "Patient's Reason for Visit."

FL76 is reported on unscheduled outpatient visits (e.g., emergency department or urgent care visits) to identify the main reason the patient sought treatment. The reason may differ from the physician's final diagnosis at the end of the encounter. Only one diagnosis code can be reported in this field. If there are multiple conditions present, the code most likely to justify the patient encounter should be reported.

In 2006, a new data element called "present on admission (POA) indicator" was approved by the National Uniform Billing Committee (NUBC) for inpatient reporting. The POA indicator applies to the diagnosis codes for claims involving inpatient admissions to general acute-care hospitals or other facilities. This element applies in states where it may be required by law or regulation for public health reporting. The POA indicator is intended to identify principal and secondary diagnoses that were present at the time the order for inpatient admission occurs. Conditions that develop during an outpatient encounter, including the emergency encounter immediately preceding the inpatient admission, are considered as present on admission.

There are five options for reporting all diagnoses:

Code	Definition
Y	Yes
N	No
U	No information available in the record
W	Clinically undetermined
Unreported/not used	Exempt from POA reporting

At press time, the list of *ICD-9-CM* codes for which the POA indicator does not apply (left blank on paper claims, "not used" on electronic claims) was not available. The list, along with guidelines for reporting the POA indicator, are under development by the *ICD-9-CM* cooperating parties and are expected in the October 2006 revision of the *Official Guidelines for Coding and Reporting*.

5 Basic Coding Steps

Once the medical record has been reviewed to determine the principal diagnosis and other reportable diagnoses and procedures, the following steps in locating the codes to be assigned should be undertaken, using the three volumes of *ICD-9-CM:*

1. Locate the main term in the Alphabetic Index.

   ■ Review subterms and nonessential modifiers related to the main term.
   ■ Follow any cross-reference instructions.
   ■ Refer to any notes in the Alphabetic Index.

2. Verify the code number in the Tabular List.

   ■ Read the code title.
   ■ Read and be guided by any instructional notes. Refer to other codes as instructed.
   ■ Determine whether a fifth digit must be added.

3. Assign the verified code or codes.

It is imperative that these steps be followed without exception; the condition or procedure to be coded must first be located in the Alphabetic Index and then verified in the Tabular List. Relying on memory or using only the index or Tabular List may lead to incorrect code assignment.

LOCATE THE CODE ENTRY IN THE ALPHABETIC INDEX

The first step in coding is to locate the main term in the Alphabetic Index. In volume 2, the condition is listed as the main term, usually expressed as a noun. General terms such as "admission," "encounter," and "examination" are used to locate code entries for the supplementary V code section. In volume 3, the main term may be the specific title of a procedure, or a general term such as "excision," "incision," or "removal." Some conditions and procedures are indexed under more than one main term. For example, anxiety reaction can be located in either of the following index entries:

Anxiety (neurosis) (reaction) (state)   300.00
Reaction . . .
  anxiety   300.00

In volume 3, adenoidectomy can be located by referring to the main term **Adenoidectomy** or by referring to the main term **Excision,** as follows:

Adenoidectomy (without tonsillectomy)   28.6
Excision . . .
  adenoids (tag)   28.6
    with tonsillectomy   28.3

If a main term cannot be located, the coder should consider a synonym, eponym, or other alternative term. Once the main term is located, a search should be made of subterms, notes, or cross-references. Subterms provide more specific information of many types and must be checked carefully, following all the rules of alphabetization. The main term code entry should not be assigned until all subterm possibilities have been exhausted. During this process, it may be necessary to refer again to the medical record to determine whether any additional information is available to permit assignment of a more specific code. If a subterm cannot be located, the nonessential modifiers following the main term should be reviewed to see whether the subterm may be included there. If not, alternative terms should be considered.

Exercise 5.1

Without referring to the Alphabetic Index of Diseases, underline the word in items 1–7 that indicates the main term for each diagnosis. In items 8–15, underline the main term for the procedure in the Alphabetic Index of Procedures. In some cases, more than one word in a statement of a diagnosis or procedure is to be underlined.

1. Acute myocardial <u>infarction</u>
2. Chronic <u>hypertrophy</u> of tonsils and adenoids
3. Acute suppurative <u>cholecystitis</u>
4. Syphilitic aortic <u>aneurysm</u>
5. Normal, spontaneous <u>delivery</u>, full-term infant
6. Drug <u>overdose</u> due to barbiturates
7. Urinary tract <u>infection</u> due to E. coli
8. Type II <u>tympanoplasty</u>, left ear
9. <u>Incision</u> and <u>drainage</u> of abscess, neck
10. Open fracture <u>reduction</u>, left femur, with nail
11. Scleral <u>buckling</u>, left eye
12. Magnet <u>extraction</u> of metallic sliver from right eye
13. Bowel <u>resection</u> with transverse <u>colostomy</u>
14. Right inguinal <u>herniorrhaphy</u> and right <u>hydrocelectomy</u>
15. Intracapsular cataract <u>extraction</u>, right eye

VERIFY THE CODE NUMBER IN THE TABULAR LIST

Once a code number entry has been located in the Alphabetic Index, the coder must refer to that number in the Tabular List; a code should not be assigned without such verification. In addition to the title for the code entry, it may be necessary for coders to review the title for the chapter, section, and category in order to be sure the correct code has been identified. Although the title in the Tabular List does not always match the Alphabetic Index entry exactly, it is usually clear whether it applies. For example:

- Appendicitis (541) has an additional modifier of "unqualified" in the Tabular List. This alerts the coder to look elsewhere when the type of appendicitis is stated in the medical record.
- Menorrhalgia (625.3) has the title **Dysmenorrhea** in the Tabular List. Although the title in Volume 1 is not identical to the term in the Alphabetic Index, it is clear that it is the right code for this condition.

Any significant discrepancy between the index entry and the tabular listing should alert the coder to the need to review the Alphabetic Index for a more appropriate term.

All instructional terms and notes should be read and followed when they apply, with particular attention to exclusion notes. Ordinarily the code number listed with the main term entry in the index is for an unspecified condition. It is important to review other codes in the related area to determine whether a more specific code can be assigned.

CODING DEMONSTRATIONS

Follow the steps outlined above to determine the correct code for each of the diagnostic statements listed below:

- **Bunion, right great toe**
  Refer to main term **Bunion,** which provides a code of 727.1. Note that there are no subterms. Verify this by referring to code 727.1 in the Tabular List. In this case, the index entry and Tabular List title are identical and code 727.1 should be assigned.

- **Sciatica due to herniated lumbar disc**

  Refer to the main term **Sciatica** in the Alphabetic Index, and the subterms for displacement or herniation of nucleus pulposus. An inclusion note in the Tabular List indicates "lumbago or sciatica due to displacement of intervertebral disc," 722.10. If you are uncertain whether herniation and displacement are the same for purposes of coding, check the index for the main term **herniation.**

- **Acute bronchitis due to Staphylococcus**

  Look up the main term **Bronchitis** and then the subterm acute. The code entry is 466.0. Read the "use additional code" note that advises you to also assign a code to identify the responsible organism. Look up **Infection,** staphylococcal, and find code 041.10, which is assigned in the Tabular List. The code title is Staphylococcal infection, unspecified. Review the medical record to see whether there is any mention of the specific type of Staphylococcus. If there is, consider 041.11 or 041.19; if not, assign code 041.10 as an additional code.

- **Aberrant pulmonary artery**

  Refer to the main term **Aberrant.** Check the subterms, and note that there is no entry for pulmonary artery but that there is a cross-reference note to "*see also* Malposition, congenital." Follow the cross-reference advice and refer to **Malposition.** You immediately see a more specific subterm for "Artery, pulmonary," with code entry 747.3. The title for this code in the Tabular List is Anomalies of the pulmonary artery, and it is clearly the correct code for this condition.

- **Acute bronchopneumonia due to aspiration of oil**

  Locate the main term **Bronchopneumonia** in volume 2. Note the cross-reference instruction to "*see* Pneumonia, broncho." Follow the cross-reference by turning to the main term **Pneumonia** (acute) (Alpenstich) (benign) . . . . Note that the term acute is a nonessential modifier enclosed in parentheses under the main term **Pneumonia.** This applies also to the subterm, and so this term has now been accounted for but does not directly affect code assignment. Refer to the following subterms listed under the main term:

  Pneumonia (acute) (Alpenstich) (benign) . . .
     broncho-, bronchial (confluent) (croupous)
       (diffuse) (disseminated) (hemorrhagic) . . .
     aspiration (*see also* Pneumonia, aspiration)
       507.0

  Search through the main term and subterms cited above and underline the component parts of the diagnostic statement that have been located so far. Note that all component parts of the diagnostic statement except "of oil" have been located. Refer back to the subterm aspiration and note the cross-reference to "*see also* Pneumonia, aspiration." When you refer to **Pneumonia,** aspiration, you see that there are additional subterms here under the connecting words "due to" with a subterm for oils and essences, that takes you to code 507.1. Refer to code 507.1 in the Tabular List, and note that the title for this code is Pneumonitis due to inhalation of oils and essences. Although the title is not worded exactly the same as the diagnosis, there is such a close correlation that it is clear that this is the code that should be assigned. Assign code 507.1 because it covers all elements of the diagnosis and no instructional notes contradict its use.

Review Exercise 5.2

Using the Alphabetic Indexes and the Tabular Lists, code the following diagnoses and procedures.

	Code(s)
1. Chronic hypertrophy of tonsils and adenoids	474.10
Tonsillectomy and adenoidectomy	28.3
2. Fibrocystic disease of breasts	610.1
3. Acute suppurative mastoiditis with subperiosteal abscess	383.01
4. Recurrent direct left inguinal hernia with gangrene	550.01
Herniorrhaphy	53.01
5. Acute upper respiratory infection with influenza	487.1
6. Benign cyst of breast	610.0
Aspiration of cyst, left breast	85.91

6 Basic Coding Guidelines

The basic coding guidelines discussed in this chapter apply throughout the *ICD-9-CM* classification system. Following these principles is vital to accurate code selection and correct sequencing. Guidelines that apply to specific chapters of *ICD-9-CM* will be discussed in the relevant chapters of this handbook. The most current version of the complete *ICD-9-CM Official Guidelines for Coding and Reporting* available at press time is included in the appendix. For a revised version of the guidelines available after publication of this handbook, please visit www.ahacentraloffice.org. Adherence to these guidelines when assigning *ICD-9-CM* diagnosis and procedure codes is required under the Health Insurance Portability and Accountability Act of 1996 (HIPAA).

USE BOTH THE ALPHABETIC INDEXES AND THE TABULAR LISTS

The first coding principle is that both the Alphabetic Indexes and the Tabular Lists must be used to locate and assign appropriate codes. The condition or procedure to be coded must first be located in the index, and the code provided there must then be verified in the Tabular List. The coder must follow all instructional notes to determine that more specific subterms or important instructional notes are not overlooked. Experienced coders sometimes rely on their memory for commonly used codes, but consistent reference to the Alphabetic Index and the Tabular Lists is imperative, no matter how experienced the coder is.

ASSIGN CODES TO THE HIGHEST LEVEL OF DETAIL

A second basic principle is that codes must be used to the highest number of digits available. This can be accomplished by following these steps:

- Assign a three-digit disease code only when there are no four-digit codes within that category.
- Assign a four-digit code only when there is no fifth-digit subclassification for that category.
- Assign a fifth digit for any category for which a fifth-digit subclassification is provided.

The same principles apply to the selection of a procedure code. No two-digit procedure codes are provided, and three digits can be used only when no four-digit code is provided.

All digits must be used. None can be omitted and none can be added. The one exception to this rule is that a zero (0) should be added as a fourth digit to the rare code that requires a fifth digit when no fourth digit is provided. The following examples demonstrate these basic coding principles:

1. Refer to volume 1, category **490, Bronchitis, not specified as acute or chronic.** Code 490 has no fourth-digit subdivisions; therefore, the three-digit code is assigned.
2. Refer to volume 1, category **540, Acute appendicitis.** This category includes fourth digits that indicate the presence of peritonitis or peritoneal abscess. Because fourth-digit subdivisions are provided, code 540 cannot be assigned.

3. Refer to volume 1, category **493, Asthma.** Category 493 has five fourth-digit subdivisions (493.0, 493.1, 493.2, 493.8, and 493.9). It also uses a fifth-digit subclassification to specify whether there is any mention of status asthmaticus or acute exacerbation. Any code assignment from category 493 must have five digits to ensure coding accuracy.
4. Turn to the Tabular List in volume 3, code **50.4, Total hepatectomy.** This code is complete with only three digits because there are no subdivisions.
5. Turn to the Tabular List in volume 3, category **80, Incision and excision of joint structures.** Fourth-digit subdivisions to specify the anatomical site appear at the beginning of category 80, indicating that a four-digit code for the site will be required.

ASSIGN RESIDUAL CODES (NEC AND NOS) AS APPROPRIATE

The main term entry in the Alphabetic Index is usually followed by the code number for the unspecified condition. This code should never be assigned without a careful review of subterms to determine whether a more specific code can be located. When the coder's review does not identify a more specific code entry in the index, titles and inclusion notes in the subdivisions under either the three-digit or the four-digit code in the Tabular List should be reviewed. The residual NOS code should never be assigned when a more specific code is available. The following examples demonstrate this basic coding principle:

1. Refer to the Alphabetic Index in volume 2 for nontraumatic hematoma of breast, which is classified as 611.8. This is listed as "other" specified conditions of the breast. Even though the diagnosis is very specific, no separate code is provided.
2. Refer to the Alphabetic Index for phlebitis. Note that phlebitis, not otherwise specified, is assigned to code 451.9, Phlebitis, of unspecified site. Further review of the medical record reveals that this is a phlebitis of the lower extremity and therefore is more appropriately assigned to code 451.2, Phlebitis of lower extremities.

ASSIGN COMBINATION CODES WHEN AVAILABLE

A single code used to classify either two diagnoses, or a diagnosis with an associated secondary condition, or a diagnosis with an associated complication is called a combination code. Combination codes can be located in the index by referring to subterm entries, with particular reference to subterms that follow connecting words such as "with," "due to," "in," and "associated with." Other combination codes can be identified by reading inclusion and exclusion notes in the Tabular Lists.

Only the combination code is assigned when that code fully identifies the diagnostic conditions involved or when the Alphabetic Index so directs. For example:

- Acute cholecystitis with cholelithiasis   574.00
- Acute pharyngitis due to streptococcal infection   034.0
- Bilateral recurrent femoral hernia with gangrene   551.03
- Glaucoma with increased episcleral venous pressure   365.82

Exercise 6.1

Code the following diagnoses.

	Code(s)
1. Influenza with pneumonia	487.0
2. Acute cholecystitis with cholelithiasis and choledocholithiasis	574.60
3. Meningitis due to salmonella infection	003.21

Occasionally, a combination code lacks the necessary specificity in describing the manifestation or complication; in such cases, an additional code may be assigned. The coder should be guided by directions in the Tabular List for the use of an additional code or codes that may provide more specificity. For example, code 648.2x classifies anemia complicating pregnancy, delivery, or the puerperium. Because it does not indicate the type of anemia, an additional code can be assigned for this purpose.

ASSIGN MULTIPLE CODES AS NEEDED

Multiple coding is the use of more than one code to fully identify the component elements of a complex diagnostic or procedural statement. A complex statement is one that involves connecting words or phrases such as "with," "due to," "incidental to," "secondary to," or similar terminology. The coder should be guided by directions in the Tabular List for the use of an additional code or codes that may provide more specificity. When no combination code is provided, multiple codes should be assigned as needed to fully describe the condition regardless of whether there is advice to that effect.

Mandatory Multiple Coding

The term "dual classification" is used to describe the required assignment of two codes to provide information about both a manifestation and the associated underlying disease. Mandatory multiple coding is identified in the Alphabetic Index by the use of a second code in brackets. The first code identifies the underlying condition and the second identifies the manifestation. Both codes must be assigned and sequenced in the order listed.

In the Tabular List the need for dual coding is indicated by the presence of a "use additional code" note with the code for the underlying condition, and a "code first underlying condition" note with the manifestation code. In printed versions of the manuals, the manifestation code is in italics. Manifestation codes cannot be designated as the principal diagnosis and a code for the underlying condition must always be listed first except for an occasional situation where other directions are provided. A code in brackets in the Alphabetic Index can be used only as a secondary code for the specific condition or procedure indexed in this way. For example:

- Diabetic type 1, on insulin, polyneuropathy   250.61 + 357.2 + V58.67
  [Note: V58.67 is not required for type 1 diabetics. However, *Coding Clinic,* Fourth Quarter 2004, p. 55, indicated that V58.67 may be assigned for type 1 diabetics, if desired. The Editorial Advisory Board felt that although V58.67 was not required, it was useful information to capture. This textbook has followed that advice.]
- Arthritis due to mumps   072.79 + 711.50

Exercise 6.2

Code the following diagnoses according to the coding principles for correct sequencing of codes.

	Code(s)
1. Diabetic retinitis	250.50
	362.01
2. Chondrocalcinosis of shoulder region due to calcium pyrophosphate	275.49
	712.21
3. Arbovirus meningitis	066.9
	321.2
4. Rheumatoid arthritis with polyneuropathy	714.0
	357.1
5. Cataract due to chalcosis	360.24
	366.34

Discretionary Multiple Coding

The "code, if applicable, any causal condition first" note indicates that multiple codes should be assigned only if the causal condition is documented as being present. An example is ulcer of lower limbs, except decubitus (707.1x) requires the code to identify postphlebetic syndrome with ulcer (459.11) be assigned as the first-listed code or principal diagnosis, but only if it is documented as being the cause of the ulcer.

The instruction to "use additional code" indicates that multiple codes should be assigned only if the condition mentioned is documented as being present. Examples include the following:

- Raynaud's syndrome (443.0) requires an additional code to identify gangrene (785.4), but only when gangrene is mentioned in the diagnosis or documented in the medical record.
- Urinary tract infection (599.0) requires an additional code to identify the organism, if it is documented, such as positive culture of E. coli (041.4).

Exercise 6.3

Code the following diagnoses.

	Code(s)
1. Acute cystitis due to E. coli infection	595.0
	041.4
2. Alcoholic gastritis due to chronic alcoholism	535.30
	303.90
3. Diverticulitis of colon with intestinal hemorrhage	562.13
4. Diabetic neuritis due to type 1 diabetes mellitus, patient on insulin	250.61
	357.2
	V58.67

Exercise 6.3 *(continued)*

---

5. Reiter's syndrome with arthritis   099.3

                                                      711.10

---

6. Fulminant hepatitis, type A, with hepatic coma   070.0

Avoid Indiscriminate Multiple Coding

Indiscriminate coding of irrelevant information should be avoided. For example, codes for symptoms or signs characteristic of the diagnosis and integral to it should not be assigned. Codes are never assigned solely on the basis of findings of diagnostic tests, such as laboratory, X-ray, or electrocardiographic tests, unless the diagnosis is confirmed by the physician. This differs from the coding practices in the outpatient setting when coding encounters for diagnostic tests that have been interpreted by a physician. Codes should not be assigned for conditions that do not meet Uniform Hospital Discharge Data Set (UHDDS) criteria for reporting. For example, diagnostic reports often mention such conditions as hiatal hernia, atelectasis, and right bundle branch block with no further mention to indicate any relevance to the care given. Assigning a code is inappropriate for reporting purposes unless the physician provides documentation to support the condition's significance for the episode of care.

Codes designated as unspecified are never assigned when a more specific code for the same general condition is assigned. For example, diabetes mellitus with unspecified complication would never be assigned when a code for diabetes with renal complication (250.4x) is assigned for the same episode of care.

CODE UNCONFIRMED DIAGNOSES AS IF ESTABLISHED

When a diagnosis for an inpatient at the time of discharge is qualified as "possible," "probable," "suspected," "likely," "questionable," "?," or "rule out," the condition should be coded and reported as though the diagnosis were were established. Other terms that fit the definition of a probable or suspected condition are: "consistent with," "compatible with," "indicative of," "suggestive of," and "comparable with." Note that the exception to this guideline is the coding of HIV infection/illness. Code only cases confirmed by physician documentation. The guideline regarding unconfirmed diagnoses does not apply to coding or reporting for an outpatient as if the diagnosis is established. For these patients the principal diagnosis is the highest degree of certainty such as symptoms, signs, or abnormalities.

- Outpatient is admitted with severe generalized abdominal pain. The physician's diagnostic statement is: abdominal pain, probably due to acute gastritis (535.00). Only the code for gastritis is assigned as the pain is implicit in the diagnosis.
- Patient admitted with a diagnosis of probable peptic ulcer   533.90
- Patient diagnosed with possible posttraumatic brain syndrome, nonpsychotic   310.2

Caution should be used in coding unconfirmed diagnoses of conditions such as epilepsy, AIDS, and multiple sclerosis as if they were established. Incorrect reporting of such conditions can have serious personal consequences for the patient, such as the inability to obtain a driver's license and possible social and job discrimination. Physicians are often unaware that official coding guidelines require a diagnosis qualified as unconfirmed to be coded as if established; therefore, the coder should consult the physician before assigning codes for such unconfirmed conditions.

Rule Out vs. Ruled Out

It is important to distinguish between the terms "rule out," which indicates that a diagnosis is still considered to be possible, and "ruled out," which indicates that a diagnosis originally considered as likely is no longer a possibility.

Diagnoses qualified by the term "rule out" are coded as if established for inpatient episodes of care in the same way that diagnoses described as possible or probable are coded. A diagnosis described as "ruled out" is never coded. If an alternative condition has been identified, that diagnosis should be coded; otherwise, a code for the presenting symptom or other precursor condition should be assigned. Here are some examples of codes assigned according to this coding principle:

- Rule out gastric ulcer . . .   531.90 [condition is coded]
- Acute appendicitis, ruled out; Meckel's diverticulum found at surgery . . .   751.0 [code only the diverticulum]
- Rule out angiodysplasia of the colon . . .   569.84 [condition is coded]

ACUTE AND CHRONIC CONDITIONS

When the same condition is described as both acute (or subacute) and chronic, it should be coded according to the Alphabetic Index subentries for that condition. If separate subterms for acute (or subacute) and chronic are listed at the same indention level in the Alphabetic Index, both codes are assigned, with the code for the acute condition sequenced first. (Note that a condition described as subacute is coded as acute if there is no separate subterm entry for subacute.) For example, refer to the Alphabetic Index entry for acute and chronic bronchitis:

Bronchitis . . .
    acute or subacute . . .   466.0 . . .
    chronic . . .   491.9

Because both subterms appear at the same indention level, both codes are assigned, with code 466.0 sequenced first.

When only one term is listed as a subterm, with the other in parentheses as a nonessential modifier, only the code listed for the subterm is assigned. For example, for a diagnosis of acute and chronic poliomyelitis, the Alphabetic Index entry is as follows:

Poliomyelitis (acute) (anterior) (epidemic)   045.9 . . .
    chronic   335.21

The only code assigned in this situation is **335.21, Progressive muscular atrophy.**

In some cases, a combination code has been provided for use when the condition is described as both acute and chronic. For example, code 518.84 includes both acute and chronic respiratory failure. When there are no subentries for acute (or subacute) or chronic, these modifiers are disregarded in coding the condition. For example, refer to **Fibrocystic** disease, breast. Neither acute nor chronic is listed as a subterm, and so code 610.1 is assigned.

Exercise 6.4

Code the following diagnoses.

	Code(s)
1. Acute and chronic <u>appendicitis</u>	540.9
	542
2. Subacute and chronic <u>pyelonephritis</u>	590.10
	590.00
3. Acute and chronic <u>cervicitis</u>	616.0

IMPENDING OR THREATENED CONDITION

Selection of a code for a condition described at the time of discharge or at the conclusion of an outpatient encounter as impending or threatened depends first on whether the condition actually occurred. If so, the threatened/impending condition is coded as a confirmed diagnosis.

For example, the medical record shows a diagnosis of threatened premature labor at 28 weeks gestation. Review of the medical record indicates that a stillborn was delivered during the hospital stay. This is coded as **644.21, Early onset of labor, delivered,** because the threatened condition did occur.

If neither the threatened/impending condition nor a related condition occurred, however, the coder must refer to the Alphabetic Index to answer the following two questions: Is the condition indexed under the main term threatened or impending? Is there a subterm for impending or threatened under the main term for the condition? If such terms appear, the coder should assign the code provided. There are several subterms under each of the main terms **Impending** and **Threatened,** as well as several main terms with such subentries. For example, if a patient is admitted with threatened abortion but the abortion is averted, the code **640.0x, Threatened abortion,** is assigned, because there is an index entry for "threatened" under the main term **Abortion.**

When neither term is indexed, the precursor condition that actually existed is coded; a code is not assigned for the condition described as impending or threatened. For example: A patient is admitted with a diagnosis of impending gangrene of the lower extremities, but the gangrene was averted by prompt treatment. Because the gangrene did not occur and there is no index entry for impending gangrene, a code must be assigned for the presenting situation that suggested the possibility of gangrene, such as redness or swelling of the extremity.

LATE EFFECTS

A late effect is a residual condition that remains after the termination of the acute phase of an illness or injury. Such conditions may occur at any time after an acute injury or illness. There is no set period of time that must elapse before a condition is considered to be a late effect. Some late effects are apparent early; others may make an appearance long after the original injury or illness has been resolved. Certain conditions due to trauma, such as malunion, nonunion, and scarring, are inherent late effects no matter how early they occur.

Late effects include conditions reported as such or as sequela of a previous illness or injury. The fact that a condition is a late effect may be inferred when the diagnostic statement includes terms such as the following:

- Late
- Old
- Due to previous injury or illness
- Following previous injury or illness
- Traumatic, unless there is evidence of current injury

Exercise 6.5

Write an "X" in front of each diagnostic statement given below that identifies a late effect of an injury or illness. For each such statement underline the residual condition once and the cause of the late effect twice.

   X   1. Hemiplegia due to previous cerebrovascular accident

   X   2. Malunion of fracture, right femur

   X   3. Scoliosis due to old infantile paralysis

           4. Laceration of tendon of finger two weeks ago; admitted now for tendon repair

   X   5. Keloid secondary to injury nine months ago

   X   6. Mental retardation due to previous viral encephalitis

Locating Late Effect Codes

Codes that indicate the cause of a late effect can be located by referring to the main term **Late** and the subterm effects in the Alphabetic Index of Diseases and Injuries (volume 2). Note that *ICD-9-CM* provides only a limited number of codes to indicate the cause of a late effect:

- Late effects of tuberculosis   137.0–137.4
- Late effects of acute poliomyelitis   138
- Late effects of other infectious and parasitic diseases   139.0–139.8
- Late effect of rickets   268.1
- Late effects of intracranial abscess or pyogenic infection   326
- Late effects of cerebrovascular disease   438.0–438.9
- Late effects of complications of pregnancy, childbirth, and the puerperium   677
- Late effects of musculoskeletal and connective tissue injuries   905.0–905.9
- Late effects of injuries to the skin and subcutaneous tissues   906.0–906.9

- Late effects of injuries to the nervous system   907.0–907.9
- Late effects of other and unspecified injuries   908.0–908.9
- Late effects of other and unspecified external causes   909.0–909.9

Two Codes Required

Complete coding of late effects requires two codes:

- Residual condition or nature of late effect
- Cause of the late effect

The residual condition is sequenced first, followed by the code for the cause of the late effect, except in a few instances where the Alphabetic Index or the Tabular List directs otherwise. If the late effect is due to injury, a late effect E code should also be assigned. For example:

- Traumatic arthritis of right shoulder due to old fracture of right humerus
  716.11 + 905.2 + E929.9
- Paralysis of left leg due to old poliomyelitis   344.30 + 138
- Scoliosis due to poliomyelitis at age 12   138 + 737.43

There are three exceptions to the coding principle that requires two codes for late effect:

- When the residual effect is not stated, the cause of late effect code is used alone.
- When no late effect code is provided in *ICD-9-CM* but the condition is described as being a late effect, only the residual condition is coded. Note that conditions described as due to previous surgery are not coded as late effects but are classified as history of or complications of previous surgery, depending on the specific situation.
- When the late effect code has been expanded at the fourth- or fifth-digit level to include the residual condition, only the cause of the late effect code is assigned. At present only category 438, Late effect of cerebrovascular disease, has been expanded in this way.

LATE EFFECT VS. CURRENT ILLNESS OR INJURY

A late effect code is not used with a code for a current injury or illness of the same type, with one exception. A code from category **438, Late effects of cerebrovascular disease,** is assigned as an additional code when a patient with residual effects from an earlier cerebrovascular disease is seen because of current cerebrovascular disease. For example, a patient with residual aphasia due to subdural hemorrhage two years ago who is admitted because of acute cerebral thrombosis would have the following codes assigned:

434.0   Cerebral thrombosis
438.11   Late effect of cerebrovascular disease, with speech and language deficits, aphasia

Exercise 6.6

Code the following diagnoses.

	Code(s)
1. Residuals of <u>poliomyelitis</u> 　　　　　　　　or <u>Late</u>	138
2. Sequela of old <u>crush</u> injury to left foot 　　　　　　　　or <u>Late</u>	906.4
3. Cerebrovascular <u>accident</u> two years ago with 　residual hemiplegia of the dominant side	438.21
4. <u>Contracture</u> of hip following partial hip 　replacement one year ago	718.45

Review Exercise 6.7

Code the following diagnoses.

	Code(s)
1. Traumatic <u>arthritis</u>, right ankle, following 　<u>fracture</u>, right ankle	716.17 905.4
2. Cicatricial <u>contracture</u> of left hand due to <u>burn</u>	709.2 906.6
3. Brain <u>damage</u> following cerebral abscess 　seven months ago 　　　　　　　　<u>Late</u>	348.9 326

Review Exercise 6.7 *(continued)*

4. Flaccid <u>hemiplegia</u> due to old cerebrovascular
   <u>accident</u>   438.20

5. Bilateral neural <u>deafness</u> resulting from childhood   389.12
   measles 10 years ago   139.8

6. <u>Mononeuritis</u>, median nerve, resulting   354.1
   from previous <u>crush</u> injury to right arm   906.4
                                          or <u>Late</u>

7. Posttraumatic, painful <u>arthritis</u>, left hand   716.14
                                          <u>Late</u>   908.9

8. Residuals of previous severe <u>burn</u>, left wrist   906.6
                                          or <u>Late</u>

9. Locked-in state (paralytic syndrome) due to old   438.50
   cerebrovascular accident   344.81

7 Coding Guidelines for Operations and Procedures

General information on volume 3 of *ICD-9-CM* is provided in this chapter, and guidelines for coding operations and procedures are discussed. Procedures specific to certain body systems will be covered in the relevant chapters of this handbook.

UNIFORM HOSPITAL DISCHARGE DATA SET FOR REPORTING PROCEDURES

The Uniform Hospital Discharge Data Set (UHDDS) requires all significant procedures to be reported. In addition, Medicare requires the reporting of any procedure that affects payment, whether or not it meets the definition of significant procedure. Other procedures may be reported at the hospital's discretion.

A significant procedure is defined as one that meets any of the following conditions:

- Is surgical in nature
- Carries an anesthetic risk
- Carries a procedural risk
- Requires specialized training

Surgery includes incision, excision, destruction, amputation, introduction, insertion, endoscopy, repair, suturing, and manipulation. Any procedure performed under anesthesia other than topical carries an anesthetic risk. Procedural risk is more difficult to define, but any procedure that has a recognized risk of inducing functional impairment, physiologic disturbance, or possible trauma during an invasive procedure is included in this group. Procedures requiring specialized training are those that are performed by specialized professionals, qualified technicians, or clinical teams specifically trained to perform certain procedures or whose services are directed primarily to carrying them out. This implies training over and above that ordinarily provided in the education of physicians, nurses, or technicians. For Medicare reporting, the surgeon who performs the procedure must be identified by a number that is unique within the hospital, and the date of the procedure must also be reported. Electronic claim formats may accept up to 25 procedure codes. However, at the present time, Medicare reporting provides space to report six procedures; if more than six have been performed, all therapeutic procedures, particularly those related to the principal diagnosis, should be reported to the extent possible. Under the Health Insurance Portability and Accountability Act of 1996 (HIPAA), for administrative simplification purposes, standard code sets have been designated for electronic claim transactions. This regulation went into effect in 2003.

ICD-9-CM is the standard for hospitals when reporting surgery and procedures for inpatients. The American Medical Association's *Current Procedural Terminology (CPT)* and the *Health Care Procedure Coding System (HCPCS)* level II codes rather than the *ICD-9-CM* volume 3 codes are the standards for hospital reporting of outpatient procedures and physician reporting. Many hospitals also code outpatient procedures using the *ICD-9-CM* system for their own internal use.

Principal Procedure

The principal procedure as described by the UHDDS is one performed for definitive treatment (rather than for diagnostic or exploratory purposes) or one that is necessary to care for a complication. If two or more procedures appear to meet this definition, the one most related to the principal diagnosis is designated as the principal procedure. If both are equally related to the principal diagnosis, the most resource-intensive or complex procedure is usually designated as principal. When more than one procedure is reported, the principal procedure should be identified by the one that relates to the principal diagnosis. Coders are advised to follow UHDDS definitions for reporting unless a particular payer has substantially different reporting requirements.

FORMAT AND ORGANIZATION

Volume 3 of *ICD-9-CM* contains both a Tabular List and Alphabetic Index for classifying procedures. The format and organization discussed earlier in this handbook in relation to volumes 1 and 2 of *ICD-9-CM* also apply to volume 3.

Most chapters in the Tabular List of Procedures in volume 3 deal with a specific body system. The four exceptions are chapters 00, 13, 16 and 17. Chapter 13 classifies obstetrical procedures, and chapter 16 classifies diagnostic and therapeutic procedures not generally considered to be surgical in nature.

Chapters 00 and 17 capture a diverse group of procedures and interventions affecting all body systems. This deviation from the normal structure of *ICD-9-CM* is an attempt to accommodate new technology when there are no available slots in the appropriate body system chapters. Chapters 00 and 17 were identified as unused chapters that could be utilized to create new codes when the corresponding specific body system chapter was full. The plan is to exhaust all codes in chapter 00 first and then start populating chapter 17 when chapter 00 is no longer available. There are currently no chapter 17 codes.

Procedure codes consist of three or four digits, with two digits preceding a decimal and one or two digits following the decimal. With the exception of the four chapters mentioned above, the two-digit axis is the body system or site, with the digits following the decimal indicating a more specific site, the type or purpose of the procedure, or the operative technique used.

CONVENTIONS

The conventions followed in Volume 3 are essentially the same as those used in the disease classification, with minor differences in certain instructional notes.

"Code Also"

This instructional note is used to indicate that an additional code should be assigned if the referenced procedure was performed. It also applies to two specific situations:

- To advise the coder that individual components of a procedure, or two procedures that might be considered as a unit, must be coded; this is expressed as "Code also any synchronous . . . ." For example:
  - —13.1   Intracapsular extraction of lens
    Code also any synchronous insertion of pseudophakos (13.71)
  - —42.6x   Antesternal anastomosis of esophagus
    Code also any synchronous:
      esophagectomy (42.40–42.42)
      gastrostomy (43.1–43.2)

- To advise the coder that an additional code is to be assigned when certain adjunct procedures are performed, or certain equipment is used. This type of instruction is often found at the beginning of a category or subcategory and applies to all subdivisions. For example:
    —35.3   Operations on structures adjacent to heart valves
      Code also cardiopulmonary bypass [extra corporeal circulation] [heart-lung machine] (39.61)

The need to assign codes for two closely related procedures is sometimes indicated in the index by the use of slanted brackets enclosing the second code in the entry. This convention indicates that both codes must be assigned and sequenced as indicated.

LOCATING PROCEDURE TERMS IN THE ALPHABETIC INDEX

Main terms in the Alphabetic Index usually indicate the general type of procedure (for example, incision, excision, graft, implant, insertion, or removal), although a few are also indexed by the common name of the procedure, such as hysterectomy or appendectomy. Subterms introduced by the words "with" and "without" ordinarily immediately follow the main term, with a few exceptions. Other connecting words include "by," "for," and "to"; these terms are usually listed in alphabetical order.

Cross-reference terms are used in the procedure index just as they are in the Alphabetic Index of Diseases, but the volume 3 index is not as thoroughly cross-referenced as the volume 2 index. Therefore, it is often necessary to refer to a synonym or a general term to locate the appropriate code assignment.

Eponyms

Surgical procedures are sometimes identified by eponyms, usually the name of the surgeon (or surgeons) who developed the procedure. Eponyms may be indexed in any of three ways:

- Under the eponym itself:
    Davis operation (intubated ureterotomy)   56.2
- Under the main term **Operation:**
    Operation
       Davis (intubated ureterotomy)   56.2
- Under a main term or subterm(s) that describes the operation:
    Ureterotomy   56.2

When there is no entry for the eponym, the coder should refer to the main term that describes the procedure. For example, there is no index entry for the procedure "insertion of LeVeen shunt," but the code can be located by referring to **Shunt,** peritoneovascular, 54.94.

Excision of Organ or Lesion

Removal of an organ is usually listed by site under the main terms **Excision** or **Resection.** When only a lesion of the organ is removed, however, it is necessary to check the main term **Excision,** the subterm "lesion," and the more specific subterm that indicates the site of the lesion. For example, no entry for abdominal wall can be located under the main term Excision, but it can be located by referring to the subterm "lesion" under the main term Excision.

Bilateral Procedures

Some codes make a distinction to indicate if a procedure is performed unilaterally or bilaterally. This is not true for certain major procedures such as joint replacements. In these cases, the code is assigned twice when the procedure is performed on both sides. This guideline was developed primarily because joint replacement codes do not provide information that defines whether the procedure was unilateral or bilateral. The additional procedure has an impact on patient care and represents a significant use of resources. Codes for less significant procedures can also be assigned twice when the additional procedure meets similar criteria, but in most cases it is not useful to do so, particularly for minor procedures such as excision of skin lesions.

CODING OPERATIVE APPROACHES AND CLOSURES

The operative approach is ordinarily considered to be an integral part of the procedure. No code is assigned when a definitive procedure is carried out, except for the rare situation when the code for the surgery does not imply the approach. Both the Alphabetic Index and the Tabular List often instruct the coder to "omit code" when it represents an operative approach. However, this is not performed consistently enough for the coder to rely on it as the means of identifying which approach codes should not be assigned. Codes are not assigned for closure or anesthesia.

The operative approach is coded, however, when an opening into a body cavity is followed only by a diagnostic procedure such as a biopsy. For example, an exploratory laparotomy is performed for the purpose of removing an abdominal mass. When the cavity is opened, it is clear that a malignant lesion has spread through the abdominal cavity to the extent that a therapeutic resection is inappropriate. The surgeon removes samples of tissue to confirm the diagnosis and closes the abdominal incision. In this case, the laparotomy is coded and sequenced first, with an additional code for the biopsy. The reasoning behind this is that a procedure such as an exploratory laparotomy is a more significant procedure than a biopsy and therefore should be sequenced first.

Laparoscopic, Thoracoscopic, and Arthroscopic Approaches

Laparoscopic, thoracoscopic, and arthroscopic approaches are now being used for a number of procedures that were formerly carried out only by an open approach, and new codes have been developed to include these techniques. Such approaches permit the removal of tissue or organs under videoscopic guidance through a very small incision. These procedures are less invasive than open surgery and usually result in less trauma to the patient, earlier discharge from the hospital, and more rapid recovery. The laparoscopic, thoracoscopic, or arthroscopic approach is not always successful, however, and it is sometimes necessary to shift to an open approach in order to complete the surgery. When conversion to an open approach becomes necessary, only the open procedure is coded; no code is assigned for the laparoscopic, thoracoscopic, or arthroscopic approach. Code **V64.41, Laparoscopic surgical procedure converted to open procedure;** code **V64.42, Thoracoscopic surgical procedure converted to open procedure;** or code **V64.43, Arthroscopic surgical procedure converted to open procedure,** is assigned as an additional diagnosis in this situation. This advice applies even when no separate code indicating this approach is provided in *ICD-9-CM.*

Other Endoscopic Approaches

Other endoscopic approaches are coded, unless the Alphabetic Index directs otherwise or the code title indicates that the procedure was performed by endoscopy. When an endoscope is passed through more than one body cavity, the code for the endoscopy identifies the most distant site. For example, the procedure identified as esophagogastroduodenoscopy is classified as **45.13, Other endoscopy of small intestine.**

Exercise 7.1

Code the following procedures. Do not assign diagnosis codes.

	Code(s)
1. Arthrotomy of right knee with partial <u>patellectomy</u>	77.86
2. Craniotomy <u>Resection</u> of brain tumor, right frontoparietal area	01.59
3. Laminectomy with <u>excision</u> of herniated lumbar disc	80.51
4. Exploratory laparotomy with partial <u>resection</u> of small intestine with end-to-end anastomosis	45.62
5. Exploratory laparotomy with <u>appendectomy</u>	47.09
6. Transurethral <u>removal</u> of ureteral calculus	56.0
7. <u>Urethroscopy</u> to <u>control</u> postoperative hemorrhage, prostate	60.94
8. <u>Cystoscopy</u> with left retrograde ureteral <u>pyelogram</u>	87.74

Exercise 7.1 *(continued)*

9. Laparoscopic <u>cholecystectomy</u>	51.23

10. <u>Cholecystectomy</u>, open, following attempt by laparoscopy	<u>51.22</u> V64.41

CODING BIOPSIES

A biopsy is defined as the taking of tissue from a living person for the purpose of microscopic study. A biopsy code is not assigned when a lesion removed for therapeutic purposes is sent to the laboratory for examination, even though the term biopsy may be used in describing the procedure. Surgical specimens are routinely sent to the pathology laboratory for study; this is not considered a biopsy, and assigning a biopsy code is inappropriate. The two basic types of biopsies are open and closed.

Closed Biopsy

Closed biopsies are performed percutaneously by needle, by brush, by aspiration, or by endoscopy. Although most biopsy codes have been revised to identify an endoscopic biopsy, a few codes still do not make this distinction. For example, the code for biopsy of the urethra (58.23) does not indicate how it is performed; if it is done by endoscopy, codes for both the endoscopic approach and the biopsy are assigned. In this situation, the code for the endoscopy is sequenced first; it is considered the more significant procedure because it poses more risk for the patient.

In a brush biopsy, mucous or exfoliative tissue is removed by using a brush or bristle to collect cells for cytological examination. The procedure classification provides a separate code for a brush biopsy of a few anatomical locations; otherwise, the code for closed biopsy of the specified site is assigned. An aspiration biopsy collects cells for examination by aspiration; this procedure is also included in the code for closed biopsy.

Open Biopsy

When an open biopsy is performed by way of an incision, the incision is implicit in the biopsy code. When the approach is implied, as with biopsy of bone, no additional code for incision of the skin is required. When a biopsy is incidental to the removal of other tissue during a procedure, both the procedure and the biopsy are coded, with the more definitive procedure sequenced first. For example, a biopsy of the liver or pancreas may be performed when the main procedure is a colon resection or an appendectomy. When a diagnostic exploratory procedure, such as an exploratory transpleural thoracoscopy (34.21) is performed along with a biopsy (for example, biopsy of the pleura, 34.24), both the biopsy and thoracoscopy are coded.

A needle biopsy for the removal of a small sample of tissue performed during an open surgical procedure is coded as a closed biopsy even though the body cavity was opened. The type of biopsy is determined by the technique used to obtain tissue for study; the terms open and closed in this connection do not refer to the surgical approach used to obtain access to an internal organ. The code for the definitive procedure is sequenced first, with an additional code for the needle biopsy. For example, a total cholecystectomy was performed by means of abdominal incision. During the course of the procedure, the pancreas was noted to be slightly enlarged and a needle biopsy of the pancreas was performed to provide tissue for pathological examination. In this case, code **51.22 Cholecystectomy** and code **52.11, Closed (aspiration) (needle) (percutaneous) biopsy of pancreas,** are assigned as sequenced.

Occasionally, a biopsy is performed immediately before the definitive procedure is begun. This permits the pathologist to perform a rapid-frozen section examination to determine whether malignancy is present and allows the surgeon to modify the extent of surgery as necessary. The biopsy is then followed by more definitive surgery during the same operative episode. In this case, both a biopsy code and a code for the therapeutic procedure are assigned, with the therapeutic code sequenced first. For example:

- Biopsy (open) of transverse colon for frozen section, followed by transverse colectomy   45.74 + 45.26
- Open biopsy of breast tumor for rapid-frozen section; no malignancy found; lumpectomy carried out   85.21 + 85.12

Exercise 7.2

Code the following procedures. Do not assign diagnosis codes.

	Code(s)
1. Frozen-section examination of open biopsy of left breast mass followed by left radical mastectomy	85.45 85.12
2. Exploratory laparotomy with needle biopsy of pancreas	54.11 52.11
3. Open biopsy of nasal sinus	22.12
4. Needle biopsy of liver	50.11
5. Transurethral biopsy of bladder	57.33

Exercise 7.2 *(continued)*

6. Percutaneous biopsy of prostate   60.11

7. Endoscopic biopsy of bile duct   51.14

CODING DIAGNOSIS-RELATED PROCEDURES

Certain procedures are performed only for very specific conditions; in these cases, care should be taken that the associated diagnosis code is also assigned. For example, a solitary kidney cannot be removed unless the patient has only a solitary kidney; therefore, the presence of this procedure code without a related diagnosis code would clearly be in error. Other examples include the following:

- Procedure: Repair of retinal detachment
  Diagnosis: Retinal detachment
- Procedure: Reduction of nasal fracture
  Diagnosis: Nasal fracture

CODING CANCELED PROCEDURES

Sometimes a decision to cancel a planned procedure is made after the patient has been admitted. In this case, a code from category **V64, Persons encountering health services for specific procedures not carried out,** is assigned to account for the cancellation; no procedure code is assigned. Without the canceled procedure code, the admission might be questioned in utilization or quality-of-care studies. Note that a code from category V64 cannot be assigned as the principal diagnosis. Planned surgery may be canceled for one of several reasons, including any of the following:

- The patient may develop a condition that contraindicates the surgery (V64.1). For example, a patient was admitted for a mastectomy because of carcinoma in situ of breast discovered on previous examination. Surgery was canceled because the patient was found to have an E. coli urinary tract infection. This situation would be coded as follows:
  - Carcinoma in situ of breast   233.0
  - Urinary tract infection   599.0
    - due to E. coli   041.4
  - Surgery canceled/contraindication   V64.1
- The patient may decide not to have the planned surgery (V64.2). For example, a patient was admitted for a mastectomy because of carcinoma in situ discovered previously. Before the procedure was begun, the patient decided to postpone the surgery in order to investigate other forms of treatment before proceeding with surgery. This situation would be coded as follows:
  - Carcinoma in situ of breast   233.0
  - Surgery canceled/patient decision   V64.2

- Problems in scheduling, illness of key staff, or some other situation may necessitate the cancellation of scheduled surgery (V64.3). For example, a patient was admitted for a mastectomy because of carcinoma in situ previously discovered. Surgery was canceled because the anesthesiologist assigned to the case was involved in an auto accident and no other anesthesiologist was available. The patient was discharged, to be readmitted for the mastectomy three days later. This situation would be coded as follows:

    Carcinoma in situ of breast   233.0
    Surgery canceled/other reason   V64.3

CODING INCOMPLETE PROCEDURES

Except for a code for the obstetrical procedure of failed forceps (73.3), the procedure classification makes no provision for indicating that a procedure has not been completed. When a planned procedure is begun but cannot be completed, it is coded to the extent to which it was actually performed according to the following principles:

- If incision only, code to incision of site.
- If endoscopic approach is unable to reach site, code endoscopy only.
- If cavity or space was entered, code to exploration of site.
- Code V64.x indicates that procedure codes are not completed as follows:
    V64.00   Vaccination not carried out, unspecified reason
    V64.01   Vaccination not carried out because of acute illness
    V64.02   Vaccination not carried out because of chronic illness or condition
    V64.03   Vaccination not carried out because of immune compromised state
    V64.04   Vaccination not carried out because of allergy to vaccine or component
    V64.05   Vaccination not carried out because of caregiver refusal
    V64.06   Vaccination not carried out because of patient refusal
    V64.07   Vaccination not carried out for religious reasons
    V64.08   Vaccination not carried out because patient had disease being vaccinated against
    V64.09   Vaccination not carried out for other reason
    V64.1   Surgical or other procedure not carried out because of contraindication
    V64.2   Surgical or other procedure not carried out because of patient decision
    V64.3   Surgical or other procedure not carried out because of other reason

The following are examples of coding incomplete procedures:

- Patient was admitted for transurethral removal of ureteral stone. Scope was passed as far as the bladder, but the surgeon was unable to pass it into the ureter. Code the cystoscopy only.
- Patient was admitted for cholecystectomy with exploration of common duct. When the abdominal cavity was entered, extensive metastatic malignancy involving the stomach and duodenum with probable primary neoplasm in the pancreas was found. The procedure was discontinued, and the operative wound was closed. Assign only code **54.11, Exploratory laparotomy,** because that was the extent of the procedure actually performed.
- A patient was admitted for cholecystectomy. When the abdominal incision had been made, the patient suddenly developed an accelerating hypertension. Surgery was discontinued, the incision was closed, and the patient was returned to the nursing unit for care. Code only **54.0, Incision of the abdominal wall.**

When a procedure is considered to have "failed" in that it did not achieve the hoped-for result or because every objective of the procedure could not be accomplished, the procedure is coded as performed. For example, occasionally there is an almost immediate re-occlusion of the coronary artery after the completion of a percutaneous coronary angioplasty, which makes it necessary to return to the operating room to perform a coronary artery bypass to correct the problem. The angioplasty might be described as a failed procedure, but, in fact, the procedure was performed and should be coded. Note that failure to achieve the therapeutic objective is not classified as a complication of the procedure.

CODING SHUNT PROCEDURES

Although shunt procedures are often identified by the name of the device (for example, Denver or LeVeen shunt), these devices are usually used for a variety of purposes. Codes are assigned on the basis of the therapeutic intent and the procedure involved rather than on the name of the shunt. Codes can be found in the index under the main terms Creation, Formation, or Shunt.

Ventriculoperitoneal shunts are inserted to drain cerebrospinal fluid to the peritoneal cavity when the normal cerebrospinal pathway is obstructed. When a procedure is described as a revision of a ventriculoperitoneal shunt, the coder must review the operative report to determine which portion of the shunt is involved. If only the peritoneal site is revised, code **54.95, Incision of the peritoneum,** is assigned. If the ventricular site is revised, code **02.42, Replacement of ventricular shunt,** is assigned. If both sites are involved in the revision, both codes should be assigned.

Sometimes, a ventriculoperitoneal shunt may undergo externalization because of recurrent infections. This procedure may be performed at bedside and involves incising the skin at the anterior chest wall. The shunt is externalized and connected to an external drainage system. Assign code **86.09, Other incision of skin and subcutaneous tissue,** for this type of procedure.

CODING STENT INSERTIONS

Intravascular stents are tubular metal implants designed to restore blood flow by reopening or enlarging a blood vessel and maintaining patency. Stents are also valuable in treating threatened or abrupt vessel closure, thus reducing the need for emergency surgery. Drug-eluting stents are a new type of stent created to address the common problem of vessel restenosis post stent insertion. Drug-eluting stent refers to a stent with an active drug (such as sirolimus, taxol or paclitaxel) that is released in a controlled manner. Care must be taken to review the medical record documentation to determine the type of stent used. The insertion of conventional stents, drug covered or drug coated stents is assigned to **36.06, Insertion of coronary artery stent(s),** or **39.90, Insertion of non-drug-eluting peripheral vessel stent(s).** The insertion of drug-eluting stents is coded to **36.07, Insertion of drug-eluting coronary artery stent(s)** or **00.55, Insertion of drug-eluting peripheral vessel stent(s).** Coronary angioplasty performed by any technique is inherent in the placement of a coronary stent; the appropriate code for the angioplasty (00.66 or 36.03) is assigned with an additional code of 36.06 or 36.07 for the stent insertion. Code 39.90 or 00.55 is assigned for peripheral vessel stent insertion. Codes are provided for other stent insertions. For example, code 51.43 is assigned for insertion of a stent into a bile duct; if insertion is by endoscopy, code 51.87 is assigned. Code 51.98 is assigned for pancreatic transhepatic insertion.

Additional codes are used to provide information on the number of vessels treated (00.40–00.43) and the number of stents inserted (00.45–00.48) if multiple stents are inserted. These codes apply to both coronary and peripheral vessels. If the procedure involves a vessel bifurcation, code **00.44, Procedure on vessel bifurcation,** is used to identify the presence of a vessel bifurcation. Code 00.44 does not describe a specific bifurcation stent. This code may be used only once per operative episode regardless of the number of vessel bifurcations.

STEREOTACTIC RADIOSURGERY

Stereotactic radiosurgery is performed as a treatment for brain lesions and tumors such as acoustic neuroma, pituitary adenoma, and skull-based meningioma. It is also used for treating atriovenous malformations and has been used in the treatment of functional disorders such as Parkinson's disease, epilepsy, and intractable pain. Indications for treatment by this technique include lesions inaccessible to open surgery, medical contraindications for open surgery, elderly or very young patients, or recurrent lesions after open surgery or radiation therapy.

Treatment begins by taking the patient to the radiology department where a stereotactic head frame is placed to provide for target coordination determination. Code **93.59, Other immobilization, pressure, and attention to wound,** is assigned for placement of the head frame. Imaging studies such as CT or MRI scanning or angiography are then carried out. Computer imaging is used to develop an individual radiation dosage plan for the patient and identifying the precise location to be treated. When the imaging is complete, the patient is placed in the head frame and radiation is focused on the lesion. Subcategory **92.3, Stereotactic radiosurgery,** has been expanded by adding a fourth digit (92.30–92.39) that indicates the source of radiation.

COMPUTER ASSISTED SURGERY

Recent advances in technology have resulted in diagnostic and therapeutic procedures being performed with the assistance of computer technology. These may include computed tomography-free navigation and image-guided navigation, as well as imageless navigation. Computer assisted surgeries are reported with the code for the specific diagnostic or therapeutic procedure performed, along with a code from subcategory 00.3, Computer assisted surgery [CAS]. Computer assisted surgery is classified on the basis of the different imaging modalities used, such as computed tomography (00.31), magnetic resonance (00.32), fluoroscopy (00.33), imageless computer assisted surgery (00.34), multiple datasets (00.35), and other modalities (00.39).

Review Exercise 7.3

Code the following procedures. Do not assign diagnosis codes.

	Code(s)
1. Revision of peritoneal portion of ventriculoperitoneal shunt	54.95
2. Arthrotomy of right knee with excision of right medial meniscus and patellar shaving	80.6 77.66

Review Exercise 7.3 *(continued)*

3. Right frontal craniotomy with resection of osteoma of
   frontal bone   01.6

4. Dilation and curettage, uterus   69.09
   Cervical biopsies, punch   67.12
   Multiple vulvar biopsies   71.11

5. Atherectomy of iliac artery with injection of thrombolytic   39.50
   agent and stent insertion   99.10
                                                                   39.90
                                                                   00.40
                                                                   00.45

6. Esophagoscopy with biopsy of esophagus   42.24

7. Submucous septectomy, nasal, and nasal septoplasty   21.5

8. Exploratory laparotomy   51.22
   Cholecystectomy   51.51
   Incidental appendectomy   51.81
   Intraoperative cholangiogram   47.19
   Common bile duct exploration with dilation of
   sphincter of Oddi   87.53

9. Laparoscopic appendectomy   47.01

10. Reclosure of operative wound of abdominal wall   54.61

Review Exercise 7.3 *(continued)*

11. Partial laparoscopic cholecystectomy   51.24

12. Craniotomy with plastic repair of encephalocele   02.12
    cranioplasty

13. Single-vessel percutaneous coronary angioplasty with use   00.66
    of thrombolytic agent and insertion of stent   36.06
                                                                             00.40
                                                                             00.45
                                                                             99.10

14. Endoscopic insertion of stent in pancreatic duct   52.93

15. Removal of acoustic neuroma via Stereotactic Cobalt-60 radiosurgery   92.32
    Placement of head frame   93.59
    Computerized axial tomography of brain   87.03

Use of Supplementary Classifications

8 V and E Codes

In addition to the main classification (001–999), two supplementary classifications are provided in *ICD-9-CM*:

- Factors influencing health status and contact with health service (V codes: V01–V86)
- External causes of injury and poisoning (E codes: E800–E999)

USING THE SUPPLEMENTARY CLASSIFICATIONS

Certain V codes are designated as the principal (or first-listed) diagnosis in specific situations; others are assigned as additional codes when it is important to indicate a history, status, or problem that may affect health care. Some V codes can be used as either the principal (or first-listed) diagnosis or as an additional code. (See the list at the end of this chapter.) E codes are assigned as additional codes to indicate the responsible medication for any condition described as an adverse effect of the correct use of a drug or other medicinal or biological substance. E codes are also used to report the external cause of an injury. Because V codes and E codes must be used throughout the classification, this chapter provides a general introduction to understanding such use before going on to other chapters in the handbook.

LOCATING V CODES AND E CODES

The format and conventions used throughout the main classification are also used in the indexes and tabular lists for these supplementary classifications. Index entries for V codes are included in the main Alphabetic Index (volume 2). These are the key main terms:

- Admission
- Examination
- History
- Observation
- Aftercare
- Problem
- Status

The Tabular List for V codes follows immediately after the final chapter of the main classification in volume 1.

E codes for poisoning and adverse effects of therapeutic drugs are located in the Table of Drugs and Chemicals in section 2 of volume 2. Names of drugs and other substances are listed alphabetically in the left-hand column of the table, with the E codes listed in the right-hand column arranged by intent of use. E codes that indicate the correct use of a prescribed drug are selected from the right-hand column labeled therapeutic use. Other E codes are assigned to indicate the external cause of injuries and poisoning. The use of E codes in this situation will be discussed in chapters 26–28.

V CODES

V codes are used as the principal (or first-listed) diagnosis in the following situations:

- To indicate that a person with a resolving disease or injury or a chronic condition is being seen for specific aftercare, such as the removal of orthopedic pins
- To indicate that the patient is seen for the sole purpose of special therapy, such as radiotherapy, chemotherapy, or dialysis

- To indicate that a person not currently ill is encountering the health service for a specific reason, such as to act as an organ donor, to receive prophylactic care, or to receive counseling
- To indicate the birth status of newborns

V codes are assigned as additional diagnosis codes in the following situations:

- To indicate that a patient has a history, health status, or other problem that is not in itself an illness or injury but may influence patient care. Note that the following V codes can be listed first if the fact of the history itself is the reason for admission or encounter:
    - V10.x   Personal history of malignant neoplasm
    - V12.4   Personal history of disorders of nervous system and sense organs
    - V16–V19   Family history
- To indicate the outcome of delivery for obstetric patients

Admission or Encounter for Aftercare Management

Aftercare visit codes (V51–V58) are used when the initial treatment of a disease or injury has been completed but the patient requires continued care during the healing phase or for long-term consequences of the disease. The aftercare code is not assigned when treatment is directed at a current acute disease or injury. The exceptions to this rule are encounters for the sole purpose of dialysis (V56.x), chemotherapy (V58.11), immunotherapy (V58.12), or radiotherapy (V58.0). When the encounter is for the purpose of both radiotherapy and chemotherapy, both codes are assigned and either can be sequenced first. (Chapter 17 discusses the correct use of dialysis codes; chapter 25, chemotherapy codes.)

Admission for aftercare management ordinarily involves planned care, such as the fitting and adjustment of a prosthetic device (V52.x), attention to an artificial opening (V55.x), or removal of an internal fixation device (V54.01). A code from category **V57, Care involving use of rehabilitation procedures,** is assigned as the principal diagnosis when the patient is admitted for the purpose of rehabilitation following previous illness or injury, with the fourth digit indicating the focus of treatment. An additional code is assigned for the residual condition requiring rehabilitation. No code for the original injury or illness that led to the disability is assigned.

Coding guidelines require that fracture codes be used only for the initial treatment encounter and that subsequent encounters be reported with the use of an orthopedic aftercare code. Subcategories **V54.1, Aftercare for healing traumatic fracture,** and **V54.2, Aftercare for healing pathologic fracture,** are used to provide greater specificity in identifying the fracture site being treated. These codes are particularly useful in the post acute care setting such as home health services.

There are also codes to report aftercare following surgery for neoplasms (V58.42), injury and trauma (V58.43) and for specific body systems (V58.71–V58.78). These codes should be reported along with any other aftercare codes or other diagnosis codes to provide more detail regarding an aftercare visit.

Aftercare codes are generally listed first to explain the reason for the encounter. They can be used occasionally as additional codes when aftercare is provided during an encounter for treatment of an unrelated condition but no applicable diagnosis code is available (for example, the closure of a colostomy during an admission to treat an injury sustained in an automobile accident). The sequencing of multiple aftercare codes is discretionary. When the patient is admitted because of a complication of previous care, the appropriate code from the main classification is assigned rather than the aftercare V code. (See chapter 29 of this handbook.)

Admission for Follow-Up Examination

A code from category V67 is assigned as the principal diagnosis or reason for encounter when a patient is admitted for the purpose of surveillance after the initial treatment of a disease or injury has been completed. For example:

- Examination following treatment of healed fracture   V67.4
- Examination following surgical excision of tumor followed by radiotherapy   V67.1

If a recurrence, extension, or related condition is identified, the code for that condition is assigned as the principal diagnosis rather than a code from category V67. For example:

- An asymptomatic patient who had a resection of the descending colon a year earlier is admitted for colonoscopy to evaluate the anastomosis and determine whether there is any recurrence of malignancy. Colonoscopy proved the anastomosis to be normal, and there was no evidence of cancer recurrence. In this case, code **V67.0, Follow-up examination, Following surgery,** is coded as the principal diagnosis, with an additional code of **V10.05, History of malignant neoplasm of large intestine,** and a code for the colonoscopy.
- An asymptomatic patient who had a resection of the descending colon a year earlier is admitted for colonoscopy to evaluate the anastomosis and determine whether there is any recurrence of malignancy. Colonoscopy showed the anastomosis to be normal, and there was no evidence of cancer recurrence. A polyp was found distal to the anastomosis, however, and it was removed; pathology examination showed it to be benign. Code **211.3, Benign polyp of colon,** is assigned as the principal diagnosis, with code **V10.05, History of malignant neoplasm, large intestine,** assigned as an additional code. In this case, no code from category V67 is assigned because a related condition was identified.
- A patient who had a colon resection for removal of carcinoma of the descending colon one year ago is now seen for follow-up examination to evaluate the anastomosis and determine whether there is any recurrence of disease. Colonoscopy showed normal anastomosis but revealed a recurrence of cancer at the primary site. Code **153.2, Malignant neoplasm of descending colon,** is assigned as the principal diagnosis. No code from category V67 is assigned.
- A patient who had surgical excision of a malignant neoplasm of the ovary one year ago, followed by chemotherapy, is admitted for follow-up examination. There is no evidence of recurrence or metastasis, and no other pathologic condition was identified. Code **V67.2, Follow-up examination following chemotherapy,** is assigned along with a code of V10.43 to indicate the history of ovarian cancer as the reason for the examination.
- A patient who had benign polyps of the colon removed one year ago is now complaining of pain in the left lower abdomen. A colonoscopy performed to determine whether there is any recurrence of colon polyps proved to be entirely normal. In this case, code **789.04, Abdominal pain, left lower quadrant,** is assigned rather than a code from category V67 because the abdominal pain was the reason for the admission.

Code **V67.51, Follow-up examination following treatment with high-risk medication, not elsewhere classified,** is assigned as the reason for encounter only when the patient is no longer on the medication.

Codes from subcategory V58.6 are assigned when the patient is currently receiving long-term anticoagulant therapy (V58.61), antibiotic therapy (V58.62), antiplatelets/antithrombotics (V58.63), nonsteroidal anti-inflammatories (V58.64), steroids (V58.65), aspirin (V58.66), insulin (V58.67), or long-term therapy for other high-risk medications that require continued monitoring and evaluation. Codes from subcategory V58.6 are assigned if the patient is receiving a medication for an extended period. For example:

- as a prophylactic measure (e.g., to prevent deep venous thrombosis)
- as treatment of a chronic condition (e.g., arthritis)
- for a disease requiring a lengthy course of treatment (e.g., cancer)

An additional code is assigned for the conditions for which the medication is prescribed. Do not assign a code from subcategory V58.6 when the medication is to treat an acute illness or injury and is being given for a brief period of time (e.g., antibiotics to treat bronchitis).

Code V58.83 is used to report encounters for therapeutic drug monitoring. If the drug being monitored is one that the patient has been receiving on a long-term basis, a code from subcategory V58.6 should be added. Coding guidelines do not provide a definition or time frame for long-term drug therapy. If a patient receives a drug on a regular basis and has multiple refills available for a prescription then it is appropriate to document long-term drug use. Documentation of long-term drug use is at the discretion of the health care provider.

Admission for Observation and Evaluation

A code from category **V71, Observation and evaluation for suspected conditions not found,** is assigned when inconclusive symptoms, signs, or other evidence of disturbed physiology warrant clinical observation and evaluation but neither the suspected condition nor an alternative is identified, and no additional evaluation or treatment appears to be required at the current level of care. Outpatient referral for surveillance or for further diagnostic studies does not contradict the use of a code from this category. When a related diagnosis is established, the code for that condition is assigned instead of a code from category V71. Codes from category V29 are used for observation of a newborn. (See chapter 23 of this handbook.)

A code from category V71 can be assigned only as the principal diagnosis or reason for encounter, never as a secondary diagnosis. A code from category V71 is ordinarily assigned as a solo code, with two exceptions:

- When a chronic condition requires care or monitoring during the stay, a code for that condition can be assigned as an additional code. Codes for chronic conditions that do not affect the stay are not assigned.
- When admission is for the purpose of ruling out a serious injury, such as concussion, codes for minor injuries such as abrasions or contusions may be assigned as additional codes. This exception is based on the fact that such minor injuries in themselves would not require hospitalization.

The following examples may help the coder to better understand the use of category V71:

- A physician, family member, or law enforcement representative refers the patient for evaluation of a suspected mental disorder. None is found, and no other condition is identified. Code **V71.09, Observation for suspected mental condition,** is assigned.
- A patient is seen in the emergency department because of alleged rape. Observation and examination reveal no physical findings, such as hemorrhage or laceration. Code **V71.5, Observation following alleged rape or seduction,** is assigned as the principal diagnosis. Code V71.5 covers the collection of specimens, advice given for prophylaxis of pregnancy, and any other provision of counseling services. When physical findings suggest that a rape has occurred, code V71.5 is not assigned; the condition identified is coded and designated as the principal diagnosis. Rape is not a medical diagnosis, but a matter of jurisprudence.
- The patient presents with generalized complaints involving nonspecific abdominal pain, minimal weight loss, and change of bowel habits. Because of a strong family history of colon cancer, the patient is admitted for evaluation for suspected malignancy. The presence of a neoplasm is ruled out, and no alternative diagnosis is made; it seems obvious that the symptoms reported are largely subjective. Code **V71.1, Observation for suspected malignant neoplasm,** is assigned with an additional code of **V16.0, Family history of malignant neoplasm of gastrointestinal tract.**

Note that a code from category V71 is not assigned when a patient is admitted to the observation unit of the hospital immediately following same-day (outpatient) surgery, even though the medical record may suggest that the admission is for observation. In this case, code the reason for the surgery as the first reported diagnosis (reason for the encounter). If the patient develops complications during the outpatient encounter, including during the observation stay, code these complications as secondary diagnoses. Continue to report the reason for the surgery as the reason for the overall encounter. Additional codes are assigned for the procedures performed. For example:

- A patient is admitted following outpatient surgery for a unilateral direct inguinal hernia repair for "continued observation." Review of the medical record indicates that the patient was admitted to observation because he was experiencing severe nausea and vomiting. Code **550.90, Inguinal hernia, without mention of obstruction or gangrene, unilateral or unspecified (not specified as recurrent),** is assigned as the first-listed diagnosis, not a code from category V71. In addition, code **787.01, Nausea with vomiting,** is assigned as the secondary diagnosis, and code **53.01, Repair of direct inguinal hernia,** for the procedure.

If a patient is admitted after a period in the outpatient observation unit for further evaluation unrelated to surgery, the principal diagnosis is the condition that provided the original reason for the outpatient observation. If a patient is admitted to an observation unit for a medical condition, and the medical condition worsens or does not improve, it may be necessary for the patient to be admitted to the hospital as an inpatient. In this case, the medical condition which led to the hospital admission would be the principal diagnosis.

Admission for Palliative Care

Palliative care is an alternative to aggressive treatment for patients who are in the terminal phase of an illness. Care is focused on the management of pain and other symptoms of the disease, which is often more appropriate than aggressive care when a patient is dying of an incurable illness. Code **V66.7, Encounter for palliative care,** is used to classify admissions or encounters for end-of-life care, hospice care, and terminal care. It may be used in any health care setting. It cannot be used as the principal diagnosis or reason for encounter; instead, the code for the underlying disease is sequenced first.

Special Investigations and Examinations

When a patient receives only diagnostic services during an episode of care, a code for the condition or problem that was chiefly responsible for the encounter is assigned first. A code from category **V72, Special investigative examinations,** is assigned as the reason for encounter only when no problem, diagnosis, or condition is identified as the reason for the examination. Codes from category V72 are rarely appropriate for inpatient coding and are never assigned as additional codes. For example:

- A patient is referred to the radiology department for a chest X-ray, with the reason for the examination identified as cough and fever, which may rule out pneumonia. The radiologist's report indicates that the X-ray is normal. The code for the cough (786.2) or the fever (780.6) is listed as the reason for the encounter. A code for pneumonia is not assigned; neither is a code from category V72.
- A patient is referred to the radiology department for a chest X-ray with the reason for the examination identified as cough and fever, rule out pneumonia. The radiologist's report confirms a diagnosis of bronchopneumonia. Code **485, Bronchopneumonia, organism unspecified,** is listed as the reason for the visit. Codes are not assigned for the cough or fever because these symptoms are implicit in the diagnosis of bronchopneumonia. No code from category V72 is assigned.
- A patient is referred to the clinical laboratory for blood work, with the reason for the examination identified as vertigo with possibly the need to rule out hypothyroidism. Code **780.4, Vertigo,** is assigned as the reason for the visit. A code for hypothyroidism is not assigned because hypothyroidism is not an established diagnosis. Code **V72.6, Laboratory examination,** is not assigned.
- A patient is referred to the radiology department for a chest X-ray as part of a routine physical examination. Code **V72.5, Radiological examination, not elsewhere classified,** is listed as the reason for the encounter because there are no presenting symptoms and the X-ray was not performed to rule out any suspected disease.

Patients are often referred to hospital ancillary services for preoperative evaluations that involve a variety of tests performed in various departments. Patients may also be referred for preoperative blood typing. In this situation, one of the following codes is assigned, with additional codes for the condition for which surgery is planned and for any findings related to the preoperative evaluation:

- V72.81   Preoperative cardiovascular examination
- V72.82   Preoperative respiratory examination
- V72.83   Other specified preoperative examination
- V72.84   Preoperative examination, unspecified
- V72.86   Encounter for blood typing

For example:

- A patient with the diagnosis of cholelithiasis was referred to the radiology department for a preoperative chest X-ray. Code **V72.83, Other specified preoperative examination,** should be listed as the reason for the encounter, with an additional code for the cholelithiasis. Note that a preoperative chest X-ray is coded to V72.83, not V72.82, because the physician is not looking only at the lungs but also at the heart, bronchus and other structures in the patient's chest.

Screening Examinations

Codes from categories V73 through V82, Special screening examinations, are assigned to tests performed to identify a disease or disease precursors for the purpose of early detection and treatment for those who test positive. Screening is performed on apparently well individuals who present no signs or symptoms relative to the disease. Many V codes have been expanded to provide more specificity. For example, a screening mammogram may be performed because the patient falls into one of several high-risk categories, as stated by the physician (V76.11). However, if the physician has not documented that there is a high risk, code V76.12 would be used. If a screening examination identifies pathology, the code for the reason for the test (namely the screening code from categories V73 through V82) is assigned as the principal diagnosis or first-listed code followed by a code for the pathology or condition found during the screening exam. For example:

- A patient underwent routine mammography, which revealed no pathology. Code **V76.12, Other screening, mammogram,** is assigned.
- An asymptomatic patient undergoes a screening mammography. The radiologist reports the presence of microcalcifications. Assign code **V76.12, Other screening mammogram,** followed by code **793.81, Mammographic microcalcification.**
- A patient with a family history of breast cancer in her mother, aunt, and older sister presents for a screening mammogram because she is considered at high risk for the disease (V76.11, V16.3).

Codes Representing Patient History, Status, or Problems

Codes from categories V10 through V15 are used to indicate a personal history of a previous condition. When the condition mentioned is still present or still under treatment, or if a complication is present, a code from the series V10 through V15 is not assigned. Categories V16 through V19 indicate a family history and may be assigned when the family history is the reason for examination or treatment.

Categories V40 through V49 indicate that the patient has a continuing condition or health status that may influence care, such as the fact that a tracheostomy (V44.0), colostomy (V44.3), cardiac pacemaker (V45.01), or aortocoronary bypass graft (V45.81) is in place. V codes indicating status are redundant when the diagnosis code itself indicates that the status exists. For example, in the case of an acute rejection crisis of a transplanted kidney, Code **996.81, Complications of transplanted organ, kidney,** is used. As the patient's transplant status is implicit in that diagnosis, an additional Code V42.0, indicating kidney-transplant status, is not meaningful and should not be assigned.

A diagnostic statement expressed as "status post" most often refers to an earlier surgery, injury, or previous illness and usually has no significance for the episode of care. No code for the condition is assigned in this case. A personal history code can be assigned if desired. Note the important distinction between history and status codes. History codes indicate that the problem no longer exists. Status codes indicate that the condition is present.

Codes from categories V60 through V63 are used to indicate certain problems that may affect the patient's care or prevent satisfactory compliance with the recommended regimen. Housing problems, social maladjustment, and economic or job concerns are examples of situations that can affect a patient's compliance.

History, status, and problem codes cannot be used as the principal diagnosis or reason for encounter except for codes from category V10, V12, V13 (except V13.4 and V13.69) and V16–V19, which can be used when the history is the reason for admission. They can be used as additional codes for any patient regardless of the reason for the encounter, but they are ordinarily assigned only when the history, status, or problem has some significance for the episode of care. For example, a history of previously treated carcinoma or a family history of malignant neoplasm may be useful in explaining why certain tests are performed. Status code V43.6x indicates that the patient has had a joint replacement, but this fact would probably be significant only if it limits the patient's movement to the extent that additional nursing care is required or when it prevents full participation in a rehabilitation program.

Genetic Susceptibility to Disease

Codes from category V84 are used to report genetic susceptibility to disease. Genetic susceptibility refers to a genetic predisposition for contracting a disease. Patients with a genetic susceptibility to disease may request prophylactic removal of an organ to prevent the disease from occurring. It is important to distinguish susceptibility from carrier state. An individual who is a carrier of a disease is able to pass it on to an offspring. Subcategory V84.0, Genetic susceptibility to malignant neoplasm, is further subdivided to identify the potential body site, such as breast (V84.01), ovary (V84.02), prostate (V84.03), endometrium (V84.04), and other (V84.09).

Codes from category V84 should not be used as principal or first-listed codes. Sequencing of category V84 codes would depend on the circumstances of the encounter as follows:

- If the patient has the condition to which he/she is susceptible, and that condition is the reason for the encounter, the code for the current condition is sequenced first, followed by the V84 code.
- If the patient is being seen for follow-up after completed treatment for this condition, and the condition no longer exists, a follow-up code should be sequenced first, followed by the appropriate personal history (V10.x–V13.x) and genetic susceptibility codes (V84.x).
- If the purpose of the encounter is genetic counseling associated with procreative management, assign first a code from subcategory V26.3, Genetic counseling and testing, followed by a code from category V84.

V Code Table: *Effective December 1, 2005*

(A revised V code table, with the new V codes going into effect on October 1, 2006, was not available at the time this handbook went to press and was not available for inclusion in this edition. The revised V code table is expected in the next revision of the *ICD-9-CM Official Guidelines for Coding and Reporting*. To obtain the guidelines when they are updated, visit www.ahacentraloffice.org or www.cdc.gov.)

Certain V codes can be used only as a principal diagnosis or reason for encounter; others can be assigned only as additional codes, as shown in the lists below. V codes not listed may be used as principal diagnoses, as reasons for encounter, or as additional codes.

FIRST LISTED: The following V codes and categories are acceptable only as the first listed code for either admission or outpatient encounter:

- V20   Health supervision of infant or child
- V22.0   Supervision of normal first pregnancy
- V22.1   Supervision of other normal pregnancy
- V24   Postpartum care and examination
- V29   Observation and evaluation of newborn for suspected conditions not found

Exception: a code from the V30–V39 may be sequenced before the V29 if it is the newborn record

- V30–V39   Live born infants according to type of birth
- V46.12   Encounter for respirator dependence during power failure
- V46.13   Encounter for weaning from respirator [ventilator]
- V56.0   Extracorporeal dialysis
- V58.0   Radiotherapy

When both radiotherapy and chemotherapy are used during the same episode of care, both codes V58.0 and V58.11 may be assigned with either one being sequenced first.

- V58.11   Encounter for antineoplastic chemotherapy

When both radiotherapy and chemotherapy are used during the same episode of care, both codes V58.0 and V58.11 may be assigned with either one being sequenced first.

- V58.12   Encounter for antineoplastic immunotherapy
- V57   Care involving use of rehabilitation procedures
- V59.x   Donors
- V66.x   Convalescence and palliative care
  Exception: V66.7 Palliative care
- V68.x   Encounters for administrative purposes
- V70.x   General medical examination
  Exception: V70.7 Examination of participant in clinical trial
- V71.x   Observation and evaluation for suspected conditions not found
- V72.x   Special investigations and examinations
  Exceptions: V72.4   Pregnancy examinaton or test
                        V72.5   Radiological examination, NEC
                        V72.6   Laboratory examination
                        V72.86 Encounter for blood typing

ADDITIONAL ONLY: Categories and subcategories that may be used only as additional codes; cannot be the first listed.

- V09.x   Infection with drug-resistant microorganisms
- V14.x   Personal history of allergy to medicinal agents
- V15.x   Other personal history presenting hazards to health
  Exception: V15.7   Personal history of contraception
                        V15.88 History of fall
- V21.x   Constitutional states in development
- V22.2   Pregnant state, incidental
- V26.5   Sterilization status
- V27.x   Outcome of delivery
- V42.x   Organ or tissue replaced by transplant
- V43.x   Organ or tissue replaced by other means
  Exception: V43.22 Fully implantable artifical heart status
- V44.x   Artificial opening status
- V45.x   Other postsurgical states
  Exception: Subcategory V45.7 Acquired absence of organ
- V46.x   Other dependence on machines
  Exception: V46.12 Encounter for respirator dependence during power failure
                        V46.13 Encounter for weaning from respirator [ventilator]
- V49.82   Dental sealant status
- V49.83   Awaiting organ transplant status
- V58.6x   Long-term (current) drug use
- V60.x   Housing, household, and economic circumstances
- V62.x   Other psychosocial circumstances
- V64.x   Persons encountering health services for specified procedure, not carried out
- V66.7   Palliative care
- V84   Genetic susceptibility to disease
- V85   Body mass index

FIRST OR ADDITIONAL: Categories or subcategories that may be used either as first or additional codes:

- V01.x   Contact with or exposure to communicable disease
- V02.x   Carrier or suspected carrier of infectious diseases
- V03.x–V06.x Need for prophylactic vaccination and inoculations
- V07.x   Need for isolation and other prophylactic measures
- V08.x   Asymptomatic HIV infection status

- V10.x   Personal history of malignant neoplasm
- V12.x   Personal history of certain other diseases
- V13.x   Personal history of other diseases
  Exceptions: V13.4   Personal history of arthritis
                 V13.69 Personal history of other congenital malformations
- V15.88   History of fall
- V16.x–V19.x   Family history of disease
- V23.x   Supervision of high-risk pregnancy
- V25.x   Encounter for contraceptive management
- V26.x   Procreative management
  Exception: V26.5 Sterilization
- V28.x   Antenatal screening
- V43.22   Fully implantable artifical heart status
- V45.7   Acquired absence of organ
- V46.14   Mechanical complication of respirator [ventilator]
- V49.6x   Upper limb amputation status
- V49.7x   Lower limb amputation status
- V49.81   Postmenopausal status (age-related) (natural)
- V49.84   Bed confinement status
- V49.89   Other specified conditions influencing health status
- V50.x   Elective surgery for purposes other than remedying health states
- V52.x   Fitting and adjustment of prosthetic device and implant of devices
- V53.x   Fitting and adjustment of other device
- V54.x   Other orthopedic aftercare
- V55.x   Attention to artificial openings
- V56.x   Encounter for dialysis and dialysis catheter care
  Exception: V56.0 Extracorporeal dialysis
- V58.3   Attention to surgical dressings and sutures
- V58.4   Other aftercare following surgery
- V58.7   Aftercare following surgery to specified body systems,
                 not elsewhere classified
- V58.8   Other specified procedures and aftercare
- V61.x   After family circumstances
- V63.x   Unavailability of other medical facilities for care
- V65.x   Other persons seeking consultation without complaint or sickness
- V67.x   Follow-up examination
- V69.x   Problems related to style
- V70.7   Examination of participant in clinical trial
- V72.4   Pregnancy examination or test
- V72.5   Radiological examination NEC
- V72.6   Laboratory examination
- V72.86   Encounter for blood typing
- V73.x–V82.x   Special screening examinations
- V83.x   Genetic carrier status

Nonspecific V Codes

The following V codes are so nonspecific, or potentially redundant with other codes, that there is little justification for their use in the inpatient setting. In the outpatient setting their use should be limited to those situations where there is no documentation to permit assignment of a more precise code. Any sign or symptom or other reason for the visit that can be captured in another code should be used.

- V11.x   Personal history of mental disorder
- V13.4   Personal history of arthritis
- V13.69   Personal history of other congenital malformations

- V15.7   Personal history of contraception
- V40.x   Mental and behavioral problems
- V41.x   Problems with special senses and other special functions
- V47.x   Other problems with internal organs
- V48.x   Problems with head, neck and trunk
- V49.0   Deficiencies of limbs
- V49.1   Mechanical problems with limbs
- V49.2   Motor problems with limbs
- V49.3   Sensory problems with limbs
- V49.4   Disfigurements in limbs
- V49.5   Other problems with limbs
- V49.9   Unspecified condition influencing health status
- V51   Aftercare involving the use of plastic surgery
- V58.2   Blood transfusion, without reported diagnosis
- V58.5   Orthodontics
- V58.9   Unspecified aftercare
- V72.5   Radiological examination, NEC
- V72.6   Laboratory examination

Review Exercise 8.1

Code the following diagnoses.

	Code(s)
1. Visit to change surgical dressing	V58.31
2. Family history of polyps of the colon	V18.51
3. Status post aortocoronary bypass procedure	V45.81
4. Encounter for occupational therapy rehabilitation	V57.21
5. Adjustment of cardiac pacemaker	V53.31
6. Long-term use of anticoagulant therapy	V58.61
7. Encounter for weaning from respirator	V46.13
8. Aftercare for healing traumatic fracture of arm	V54.10
9. Screening mammogram, high-risk patient	V76.11
10. Encounter for radiation therapy	V58.0

Coding of Signs and Symptoms

9 Symptoms, Signs, and Ill-Defined Conditions

A sign is defined as objective evidence of disease that can be observed by the examining physician. A symptom, on the other hand, is a subjective observation reported by the patient but not confirmed objectively by the physician.

Symptoms and signs are classified in two ways in *ICD-9-CM*. Those that are indicative of a condition that ordinarily affects only one body system are classified to the relevant chapter of *ICD-9-CM*. Those that can point to more than one disease or system, or that are of unexplained etiology, are classified to chapter 16 of *ICD-9-CM*.

SIGNS AND SYMPTOMS AS PRINCIPAL DIAGNOSES

Codes for symptoms, signs, and ill-defined conditions from chapter 16 of *ICD-9-CM* cannot be used as principal diagnoses or reasons for outpatient encounters when related diagnoses have been established. For example:

- Coma due to poisoning by heroin   965.01 + 780.01 + E980.0
- Syncope due to third-degree atrioventricular block   426.0 + 780.2

If the patient is an inpatient, a diagnosis described as possible, probable, and so on is considered to be an established diagnosis. For example, a patient is admitted with severe generalized abdominal pain. The physician's diagnostic statement is abdominal pain, probably due to acute gastritis (535.00). Only the code for the gastritis is assigned, as the abdominal pain is integral to the probable gastritis. The words such as possible, probable, and so on are not considered to be established for outpatient visits or encounters. If there is not an established diagnosis, only whatever symptoms or signs that are available at the highest level of certainty are assigned.

There are only a few situations in which a symptom code from chapter 16 can be correctly designated the principal diagnosis:

1. When the diagnostic statement lists the symptom first, followed by two or more contrasting/comparative conditions. In this case a symptom code may be assigned as the principal diagnosis. More detail was offered in chapter 3 of this handbook.
2. When no related condition is identified and the symptom is the reason for the encounter a code from chapter 16 of *ICD-9-CM* is assigned as the principal diagnosis even though other unrelated diagnoses may be listed. For example: A patient was admitted with tachycardia. An EKG did not provide any conclusive evidence of the type of tachycardia or of any underlying cardiac condition. The patient is also an insulin-dependent diabetic; blood sugars were monitored daily during the hospital stay. The reason for admission was tachycardia; therefore; code **785.0, Tachycardia** is the principal diagnosis. Because the diabetes was treated during the hospital stay, an additional code was assigned for the diabetes mellitus.

3. This guideline does not apply if the diagnosis is stated as a symptom due to two conditions, rather than as two contrasting diagnoses. In this case, both conditions would be coded, and the symptom code would be assigned as an additional code only if it met criteria for the reporting of additional diagnoses. For cxample, if a diagnosis was stated as chest pain due to costochondritis and possible hiatal hernia, both the costochondritis and the hiatal hernia would be coded according to the guideline governing coding of contrasting/comparative conditions. No code for chest pain would be assigned because it is integral to both diagnoses.

4. Other situations in which codes from chapter 16 of the *ICD-9-CM* manual can be appropriately used as the principal diagnosis for an inpatient admission include the following:

   ■ Presenting signs or symptoms are transient, and no definitive diagnosis can be made.
   ■ The patient is referred elsewhere for further study or treatment before a diagnosis is made.
   ■ A more precise diagnosis cannot be made for any other reason.
   ■ The symptom is treated in an outpatient setting without the additional workup required to arrive at a more definitive diagnosis.
   ■ Provisional diagnosis of a sign or symptom is made for a patient who fails to return for further investigation or care.
   ■ A residual late effect is the reason for admission, and the Alphabetic Index directs the coder to an alternative sequencing.

Generally speaking, symptom codes classified to other chapters are not designated as principal diagnoses when a related condition has been identified. The symptom can be designated as principal diagnosis, however, when the patient is admitted for the sole purpose of treating the symptom and there is no treatment or further evaluation of the underlying disease. For example, patients with dehydration secondary to gastroenteritis are sometimes admitted for the purpose of rehydration when the gastroenteritis itself could be managed on an outpatient basis. In this case, the code for the dehydration can be designated as the principal diagnosis even though the cause of the dehydration is stated.

Note that these guidelines do not apply when coding and reporting hospital outpatient care or physician services. Outpatient encounters do not ordinarily permit the type of study that results in an established diagnosis, and treatment is often directed at relieving symptoms rather than treating the underlying condition. The highest level of certainty is reported as the reason for encounter for outpatients. This often means that a symptom code is assigned as the reason for the encounter.

SIGNS AND SYMPTOMS AS ADDITIONAL DIAGNOSES

Codes from chapter 16 are assigned as secondary codes only when the symptom or sign is not integral to the underlying condition and when its presence makes a difference in the severity of the patient's condition and/or the care given. For example, many but not all patients with cirrhosis of the liver have ascites. When ascites is present, it makes a difference in the care given, and so the chapter 16 code for ascites (789.5) should be assigned as an additional code. Codes from chapter 16 are not assigned when they are implicit in the diagnosis or when the symptom is included in the condition code. Such redundant coding is inappropriate. For example:

- Abdominal pain due to gastric ulcer: No symptom code is assigned to the abdominal pain because it is integral to the ulcer.
- Coma due to diabetes mellitus: The symptom code for coma is not assigned because combination codes are provided for diabetes with associated coma.
- Patient admitted with chest pain, initially thought to be angina: Diagnostic studies did not support this and the physician's diagnosis is chest pain, probable costochondritis (733.6). The chest pain is not coded because it is implicit in the costochondritis.

ABNORMAL FINDINGS

Although categories 790 through 796 in chapter 16 are provided for coding nonspecific abnormal findings, it is rarely appropriate to assign one of these codes for acute inpatient hospital care. They are assigned only when (1) the physician has not been able to arrive at a definitive related diagnosis and lists the abnormal finding itself as a diagnosis and (2) the condition meets the Uniform Hospital Discharge Data Set (UHDDS) criteria for reporting of other diagnoses.

For example, if the physician lists a diagnosis of abnormal electrocardiographic findings without any mention of associated disease, assigning code **794.31, Abnormal electrocardiogram (ECG) (EKG)** would be appropriate if there was evidence of further evaluation for a possible cardiac condition. On the other hand, a coder might note an elevated blood pressure reading in the medical record, but the physician has not listed it as a diagnosis, and there is no evidence of any follow-up or treatment. In this situation, assigning a code for this abnormal finding would be inappropriate.

If the coder notes clinical findings outside the normal range but no related diagnosis is stated, the coder should review the medical record to determine whether additional tests and/or consultations were carried out related to these findings, or whether specific related care was given. If such documentation is present, it is appropriate to ask the physician whether a code should be assigned.

For example, a patient with a low potassium level treated with oral or intravenous potassium has a clinically significant condition that probably should be reported; the physician should be asked whether a diagnosis should be added. On the other hand, a finding of degenerative arthritis on a routine postoperative chest X-ray of an elderly patient when no treatment or further diagnostic evaluation has been carried out would not warrant a code assignment.

ILL-DEFINED CONDITIONS

The final section of chapter 16 of *ICD-9-CM* contains codes for ill-defined conditions or unknown causes of morbidity and mortality, such as senility without psychosis, asphyxia, nervousness, and sudden unexplained death. These codes should never be used when a more definitive diagnosis is available.

Review Exercise 9.1

Code the following diagnoses and procedures as statements given at the time of discharge. Do not assign E codes.

	Code(s)
1. Dysuria	788.1
Transurethral biopsy of bladder	57.33
2. Acute chest pain due to influenzal pleurisy	487.1
3. Gross, painless hematuria, cause undetermined	599.7
Intravenous pyelogram	57.93
Cystoscopy with control of bladder hemorrhage	87.73
4. Pyuria, intermittent, cause undetermined	791.9
5. Hyperplastic lymph node, left axilla	785.6
Biopsy, axillary lymph node	40.11

Review Exercise 9.1 *(continued)*

6. Elevated glucose tolerance test   790.22

7. Severe vertigo, left temporal headache, and nausea   780.4
                                                                    784.0
                                                                    787.02

8. Syncope, cause undetermined   780.2

9. Chest pain, probably angina pectoris   413.9

10. Psychogenic dysuria   306.53

11. Arteriosclerotic gangrene, left foot   440.24

12. Chronic epistaxis, severe, recurrent   784.7

    Anterior and posterior nasal packing   21.02

Review Exercise 9.1 *(continued)*

13. Severe epistaxis due to hypertension   401.9
                                                                  784.7

     Nasal packing   21.01

14. Hereditary epistaxis   448.0

15. Generalized abdominal pain due to pancreatitis   789.07
    versus cholecystitis   577.0
                                                                     575.10

16. Chronic fatigue syndrome   780.71

Coding of Infectious and Parasitic Diseases, Endocrine Diseases and Immunity Disorders, and Mental Disorders

10 Infectious and Parasitic Diseases

Chapter 1 of *ICD-9-CM* classifies infectious and parasitic diseases that are easily transmissible (communicable). The primary axis for this chapter is the organism responsible for the condition. Infectious and parasitic conditions are classified in one of several ways, making careful use of the index imperative. For example:

- A single code from chapter 1 is assigned to indicate the organism. For example, code 072.x is assigned for mumps. Some codes of this type use a fourth digit to indicate a site or an associated condition. For example, code 112.4 is assigned for Candidiasis of the lung.
- Combination codes frequently identify both the condition and the organism. For example:
  —Pneumonia due to Staphylococcus aureus   482.41
  —Orchitis due to mumps   072.0

Dual classification is also used extensively for chapter 1. For example:

- Meningitis due to actinomycosis   039.8 + 320.7
- Pneumonia in whooping cough (Bordetella pertussis)   033.0 + 484.3

Codes from chapter 1 take precedence over codes from other chapters for the same condition. For example, urinary tract infection due to candidiasis is classified to code **112.2, Candidiasis of other urogenital sites,** rather than to code **599.0, Urinary tract infection, unspecified site.** Conditions that are not considered to be easily transmissible or communicable are classified in the appropriate body-system chapter with an additional code from category 041 or 079 to assign to indicate the responsible is organism. For example, codes **601.0, Acute prostatitis, and 041.01, Streptococcus, group A,** are assigned for acute prostatitis due to group A Streptococcus.

ORGANISM VS. SITE OR OTHER SUBTERM

A thorough index search is required in coding infection. When the main term for the condition has been located, a subterm for the organism always takes precedence over a more general subterm (such as acute or chronic) when both subterms occur at the same indention level in the Alphabetic Index. For example, for a diagnosis of chronic cystitis due to Monilia, the Alphabetic Index provides subterms for both chronic and monilial:

> **Cystitis** (bacillary) . . .
> chronic   595.2 . . .
> monilial   112.2

In this case, only code 112.2 is assigned because the subterm for the organism takes precedence over the subterm "chronic."

When the organism is specified but is not indexed under the main term for the condition, the coder should refer to the main term **Infection** or to the main term for the organism. For example, consider a diagnosis of cryptococcal cystitis. No subterm for cryptococcal is located under the main term **Cystitis,** but there is a main term entry **Infection,** followed by a subterm for Cryptococcus as well as a main term **Cryptococcus.** Code 117.5 is therefore assigned for this diagnosis rather than the code for cystitis.

CYCLOSPORIASIS

A specific code has been provided for cyclosporiasis (007.5). This is a condition that is spread by ingesting contaminated wood or water and usually has watery diarrhea movements. It infects the small intestine.

SEVERE ACUTE RESPIRATORY SYNDROME (SARS)

There are specific codes provided for severe acute respiratory syndrome (SARS). This is a respiratory illness caused by a new, previously unrecognized coronavirus. SARS begins with a fever and may include chills, headache, and malaise. In some patients, there are also mild respiratory symptoms, dry cough, and trouble breathing. The codes are as follows:

- Contact with or exposure to SARS-associated coronavirus   V01.82
- SARS-associated coronavirus infection   079.82
- Pneumonia due to SARS-associated coronavirus   480.3

TICK-BORNE RICKETTSIOSIS

Three codes have been developed to code Ehrlichiosis. This condition ranges from an infection to a mild virus-like illness to a severe life-threatening disease. Symptoms develop between 3–16 days after the patient has been bitten by an infected tick. There is a wide variety of symptoms, as well as mental abnormalities, breathing difficulties, kidney problems, seizures, coma, or sensitivity to light. The codes are as follows:

- Ehrlichiosis, unspecified   082.40
- Ehrlichiosis, chafeensis (E.Chafeensis)   082.41
- Other Ehrlichiosis   082.49

WEST NILE VIRUS FEVER

Category 066.4 is used to report West Nile fever. The virus is transmitted to humans by the bite of a mosquito that has bitten an infected bird. Most healthy people infected by the virus have few symptoms or have a mild illness consisting of fever, headache and body aches prior to recovering. In elderly patients or those with a weakened immune system, the virus may cause encephalitis, meningitis or permanent neurological damage and be life-threatening. Category 066.4 has been expanded to distinguish between West Nile Fever unspecified (066.40), with encephalitis (066.41), with other neurologic manifestation (066.42), and with other complications (066.49). This expansion will allow differentiation between the milder cases of the disease and those with more serious complications and neurological manifestations.

LATE EFFECTS

Chapter 1 provides three late effect codes for use when there is a residual condition due to previous infection or parasitic infestation:

- Late effects of tuberculosis   137
- Late effects of acute poliomyelitis   138
- Late effects of other infectious and parasitic diseases   139

As discussed earlier, the code for the residual effect is sequenced first, followed by the appropriate late effect code, except in a few instances where the Alphabetic Index instructs otherwise. A code for the infection itself is not assigned because it is no longer present. For example:

- Brain damage resulting from previous viral encephalitis (three years ago)   <u>348.9</u> + 139.0
- Scoliosis due to poliomyelitis   <u>138</u> + 737.43

TUBERCULOSIS

Tuberculosis is classified to categories 010 through 018, with the primary axis the site or type of tuberculosis. A fifth-digit subclassification is provided to indicate the method by which the diagnosis was determined. The fifth digit 1 should be used only when there is a specific statement in the record that no histological or bacteriological examination was performed. Fifth digit 2 indicates that an examination was performed but the method was unknown. The remaining fifth digits 3, 4, 5, and 6 identify various methods for establishing a diagnosis of tuberculosis. The use of these fifth digits is more germane to coding outpatient diagnostic workups; such information is generally present in outpatient records, but is often not documented in inpatient records. Fifth digit 0, unspecified, should be assigned when the information is not available in the medical record. Two examples of fifth-digit subclassification for tuberculosis follow:

- Tuberculosis of lung, with capitation (bacilli by microscopy)   011.23
- Tuberculosis of hip (confirmed histological)   015.15

Care should be taken to differentiate between a diagnosis of tuberculosis and a positive tuberculin skin test without a diagnosis of active tuberculosis. Code 795.5 classifies the following:

- Nonspecific reaction to tuberculin skin test without active tuberculosis
- Positive tuberculin skin test without active tuberculosis
- Positive PPD

BACTEREMIA, SEPTICEMIA, SIRS, SEPSIS, SEVERE SEPSIS, AND SEPTIC SHOCK

It is important for coders to understand the differences between bacteremia, septicemia, SIRS, sepsis, and severe sepsis in order to assign the proper codes.

At press time, a revised set of *Official Guidelines for Coding and Reporting* was under development. Guideline changes may affect sequencing of codes in this section. Please refer to www.ahacentraloffice.org for a copy of the updated guidelines expected for October 1, 2006, implementation.

Definitions

Bacteremia (790.7) refers to the presence of bacteria in the bloodstream after a trauma or mild infection. This condition is usually transient and ordinarily clears promptly through the action of the body's own immune system.

Septicemia is now defined as a systemic disease associated with the presence of pathological microorganisms or toxins in the blood. These toxins can include bacteria, viruses, fungi, and other organisms. Septicemia and sepsis have often been used interchangeably by physicians and by the *ICD-9-CM* classification. Code titles in the *ICD-9-CM* use the term *septicemia*. That is in keeping with the international version of the *ICD-9*, on which the *ICD-9-CM* is based. So as not to confuse existing statistics, the term *septicemia* will continue to be used in the *ICD-9-CM*. However, more current terminology makes a distinction between sepsis and septicemia.

Most septicemia is classified to category 038, with fourth and fifth digits indicating the responsible organism. Staphylococcal septicemia uses the fifth digit to indicate that the infection is due to either Staphylococal aureus (038.11) or other specified type of staphylococcus (038.19). Other types of septicemia are classified to another organism, such as disseminated candidiasis (112.5) or herpetic septicemia (054.5). Organisms are sometimes transferred to other tissue, where they may seed infection in another site and lead to such conditions as arteritis, meningitis, and pyelonephritis. Additional codes are assigned for these manifestations when they are present.

A diagnosis of septicemia can neither be assumed nor ruled out on the basis of laboratory values alone. Negative or inconclusive blood cultures do not preclude a diagnosis of septicemia in patients with clinical evidence of the condition. A code for septicemia is assigned only when the physician makes a diagnosis of septicemia.

Systemic inflammatory response syndrome, or **SIRS,** is the systemic response to infection or trauma. SIRS includes systemic inflammation, elevated or reduced temperature, elevated white blood count, and rapid heart rate and respiration. SIRS is classified to subcategory 995.9, Systemic inflammatory response syndrome (SIRS).

Sepsis is defined as SIRS due to infection. **Severe sepsis** is defined as sepsis with associated acute organ dysfunction.

Septic shock is defined as sepsis with hypotension, a failure of the cardiovascular system. However, it would be inappropriate to automatically assign septic shock when sepsis and hypotension are both documented together in the health record. The physician must specifically record "septic shock" in the diagnostic statement in order to code it as such. Septic shock is a form of organ dysfunction associated with severe sepsis.

The unusual or imprecise diagnostic reference to a site-specific or organ-specific sepsis, such as urosepsis, may require further clarification for coding purposes. For instance, the term **urosepsis** refers to pyuria or bacteria in the urine, not the blood. Unfortunately, urosepsis is sometimes stated as the diagnosis even though the condition has progressed to a septicemia in which a localized urinary tract infection has entered the bloodstream and become a generalized sepsis. Although the Alphabetic Index assigns urosepsis to code **599.0, Urinary tract infection, site unspecified,** this may or may not be what the physician intended by this diagnosis, and the coder should consult the physician if his intention is not clear.

When there is an equivocal diagnosis of this type, the coder should review the medical record to see whether there is any documentation that suggests the possibility of sepsis. If there is, the physician should be asked whether the diagnosis of urosepsis is intended to mean (1) generalized sepsis caused by leakage of urine or toxic urine by-products into the general vascular circulation or (2) urine contaminated by bacteria, bacterial by-products, or other toxic material but without other findings (599.0). A diagnostic statement of urinary tract infection followed by a diagnosis of septicemia, for example, usually indicates that the condition has progressed to septicemia. In such cases, it is the septicemia that should be coded.

Coders should be guided by the following instructions when coding sepsis, septicemia, SIRS, or septic shock. The coding of these conditions is dependent on the documentation available.

- When sepsis is present on admission, sepsis is assigned as the principal diagnosis following the UHDDS definition of principal diagnosis—that is, the condition after study that necessitated the admission. Assign first the code for the underlying systemic infection (e.g., 038.xx, 112.5, etc.) followed by code **995.91, Sepsis.** When there is an underlying localized infection (e.g., pneumonia, cellulitis, or nonspecific urinary tract infection) with sepsis, severe sepsis, or SIRS: Assign code 038.xx first, followed by code 995.91, followed by the code for the initial localized infection (e.g., pneumonia, cellulitis, etc.).
- When sepsis develops after admission, sepsis codes are assigned as secondary diagnoses according to the sequencing rules in the Tabular List. When the documentation is not clear as to whether sepsis was present on admission, the physician must be queried for clarification to properly select the principal diagnosis.
- Subcategory 995.9 may **not** be assigned if the term *sepsis* or *SIRS* is not documented. A code from subcategory 995.9 can never be assigned as a principal diagnosis.
- Sepsis and septic shock associated with abortion, ectopic pregnancy, or molar pregnancy are classified to category codes in chapter 11 (630–639). If the infection occurs during labor, code 659.3x, Generalized infection during labor, is assigned; if the infection occurs during the puerperal period, code 670.0x, Major puerperal infection, is assigned.

Note carefully in the following cases the different codes that would be assigned based on the information available:

1. Streptococcal septicemia: Assign code **038.0, Streptococcal septicemia.** Code 995.91 is not assigned in this case if there is no documentation of sepsis or SIRS. Query the provider to determine whether the patient has sepsis—an infection with SIRS.
2. Streptococcal sepsis: Assign code 038.0 first, followed by code 995.91.
3. Severe sepsis: Assign first the code for the systemic infection (038.xx, 112.5, etc.), followed by code 995.92. Additional codes are also assigned to identify the specific acute organ dysfunction (e.g., renal, respiratory, hepatic, etc.).
4. Septic shock: Assign first the code for the initiating systemic infection (e.g., 038.xx, 112.5, etc.), followed by the codes for severe sepsis (995.92) and septic shock (785.52).
5. Sepsis due to a postoperative infection: This is considered a complication of care. Assign code **998.59, Other postoperative infections,** followed by the codes for sepsis (038.xx, 995.91).

TOXIC SHOCK SYNDROME

Toxic shock syndrome (040.82) is caused by a bacterial infection. The symptoms include high fever of sudden onset, vomiting, watery diarrhea and myalgia, followed by hypotension and sometimes shock. It was originally reported almost exclusively in menstruating women using high-absorbency tampons. The organism isolated was Staphylococcus Aureus. A similar syndrome has been identified in children and males infected with Group A Streptococcus. An additional code from chapter 1 is reported to identify the responsible organism.

GRAM-NEGATIVE BACTERIAL INFECTION

Gram-negative bacteria are a specific group of organisms with particular staining characteristics. They are clinically similar, as is the case with Klebsiella and Pseudomonas, and are thought of as a group even when the specific organism cannot be determined. Occasionally, several gram-negative organisms may be seen, but no single organism is identified as the causative agent, resulting in a diagnosis of gram-negative infection. Gram-negative infections are ordinarily more severe and require more intensive care than gram-positive infections. Again, a code is never assigned solely on the basis of gram-stain results; the assignment is based on the physician's clinical evaluation of the condition.

When the infectious organism has been identified, a specific code is often provided, such as **482.0, Pneumonia due to Klebsiella pneumoniae.** When a more general code is provided, such as that for urinary tract infection, an additional code from category 041 or 079 is assigned to indicate the responsible organism. Two examples follow:

- Pneumonia, due to anaerobic gram-negative bacteria   482.81
- Chronic pyelonephritis due to gram-negative bacteria   <u>590.00</u> + 041.85

Table 10.1 provides a sampling of gram-negative and gram-positive organisms. A more complete list can be obtained from the health care organization's clinical laboratory director.

TABLE 10.1   Gram-Negative and Gram-Positive Bacteria

Gram-Negative Bacteria		Gram-Positive Bacteria
Bacteroides (anaerobic)	Hemophilus	Actinomyces
Bordetella	Klebsiella	Corynebacterium
Branhamella	Legionella	Lactobacillus
Brucella	Morganella	Listeria
Campylobacter	Neisseria	Mycobacterium
Citrobacter	Proteus	Nocardia
E. coli	Pseudomonas	Peptococcus
Enterobacter	Salmonella	Peptostreptococcus
Francisella	Shigella	Staphylococcus
Fusobacterium (anaerobic)	Trichinella vaginalis	Streptococcus
Gardnerella	Vellonella (anaerobic)	
Helicobacter	Yersinia	

DRUG-RESISTANT INFECTIONS

ICD-9-CM provides category V09 to identify infections that have become resistant to the drugs commonly used to treat them. The fourth digit indicates the type of drug to which the organism has become resistant; when more than one drug is specified, codes are assigned for each. Codes can be located in the Alphabetic Index by referring to the main term **Resistance.** For several drug types (V09.5, V09.7–V09.9), a fifth digit indicates whether multiple drugs of those particular types are affected.

Codes from category **V09, Infection with drug-resistant organisms,** are assigned only as additional codes and only when the physician specifically documents an infection that has become drug resistant. Such statements as "multi-drug resistant" or "(specified drug) resistant condition" or similar terminology indicate this condition. If no more specificity as to the type of drug can be obtained, code V09.9x should be assigned. For example:

- Resistant to penicillin   V09.0
- Staphylococcal pneumonia resistant to penicillin and bacitracin
  482.40 + V09.0 + V09.81

Exercise 10.1

Code the following diagnoses.

	Code(s)
1. Viral hepatitis (Australian antigen) with hepatitis delta and hepatic coma	070.21
2. Chronic gonococcal cystitis	098.31
3. Infectious mononucleosis with hepatitis B	075 070.30
4. Postmeasles otitis media	055.2
5. Acute scarlet fever	034.1

Exercise 10.1 *(continued)*

6. Gram-negative septicemia due to Bacteroides   038.3

7. Chronic pulmonary coccidioidomycosis   114.4

8. Chronic moniliasis of vulva   112.1

9. Pulmonary tuberculosis, infiltrative, moderately
   advanced, confirmed by bacterial culture   011.04

10. Late, latent syphilis   096

11. Herpes zoster of conjunctiva   053.21

12. Anthrax pneumonia   022.1
                                                              484.5

13. Acute empyema due to group B streptococcal infection   510.9
                                                              041.02

Exercise 10.1 *(continued)*

---

14. Encephalitis due to typhus   081.9
                                                                  323.1

---

15. Acute respiratory distress due to sin nombre virus   518.82
                                                                  079.81

---

16. Adenoviral pneumonia   480.0

---

17. Chronic gonococcal urethritis   098.2

---

18. Chronic vulvitis due to Monilia with microorganisms   112.1
    resistant to cephalosporin   V09.1

---

19. Amebic abscess of brain and lung   006.5
    Long-term use of antibiotic   V58.62

AIDS AND OTHER HIV INFECTIONS

Because the human immunodeficiency virus (HIV) infection has become a major health care concern, the collection of accurate and complete data on conditions associated with HIV infection is important for health care resource planning. Code 042 is assigned for all types of HIV infections, which are described by a variety of terms, such as the following:

- AIDS
- Acquired immune deficiency syndrome
- Acquired immunodeficiency syndrome
- AIDS-like syndrome
- AIDS-like disease (illness)
- AIDS-related complex (ARC)
- AIDS-related conditions

- Pre-AIDS
- Prodromal-AIDS
- HIV disease

Unconfirmed Diagnosis of HIV Infection

Code 042 is not assigned when the diagnostic statement indicates that the infection is "suspected," "possible," "likely," or "?". This is an exception to the general guideline that directs the coder to assign a code for a diagnosis qualified as suspected or possible as if it were established. Confirmation in this case does not require documentation of a positive serology or culture for HIV; the physician's diagnostic statement that the patient is HIV-positive or has an HIV-related illness is sufficient. The physician should be asked to state the diagnosis in positive terms.

Serologic Testing for HIV Infection

When an asymptomatic patient with no prior diagnosis of HIV infection or positive-HIV status requests testing to determine his or her HIV status, use code **V73.89, Screening for other specified viral disease.** When the patient shows signs or symptoms of illness or has been diagnosed with a condition related to HIV infection, code the signs and symptoms or the diagnosis rather than the screening code.

When the patient makes a return visit to learn the result of the serology test, code **V65.44, HIV counseling,** should be assigned as the reason for the encounter when the test result is either negative or inconclusive (795.71) or positive. Code V65.44 can be assigned as an additional code when counseling is provided for patients who test HIV positive. When a patient is known to be in a high-risk group for HIV infection, code **V69.8, Other problems related to lifestyle,** can be assigned as an additional code. When the test result is positive but the patient displays no symptoms and has no related complications and no established diagnosis of HIV infection, code **V08, Asymptomatic human immunodeficiency (HIV) infection status,** is assigned. Code V08 is not assigned when the term AIDS is used, when the patient is under treatment for an HIV-related illness, or when the patient is described as having any active HIV-related condition; code 042 is assigned instead.

When a patient has had contact with, or been exposed to, the HIV virus but shows no signs or symptoms of illness and has not been diagnosed with a condition related to HIV, assign code **V01.79, Contact with or exposure to communicable diseases, other viral diseases.**

There are federal and state laws with stringent regulations prohibiting the release of information. Therefore, the facility should have a reporting policy that conforms to federal law as well as the laws of the state in which it operates.

Newborns with HIV-positive mothers often test positive on ELISA and/or western blot HIV tests. This finding usually indicates the antibody status of the mother rather than the status of the newborn; antibodies can cross the placenta and remain for as long as 18 months after birth without the newborn ever having been infected. Such inconclusive test results are also coded 795.71. (See chapter 23 of this handbook for further information on coding HIV infection in the newborn.)

Sequencing of HIV-Related Diagnoses

When a patient is admitted for treatment of an HIV infection or any related complications, code **042, Human Immunodeficiency Virus (HIV) disease,** is sequenced as the principal diagnosis, with additional codes for the related conditions. When a patient with an HIV infection is admitted for treatment of an entirely unrelated condition, such as an injury, that condition is designated as the principal diagnosis, with code 042 and codes for any associated conditions assigned as additional codes.

When an obstetric patient is identified as having any HIV infection, a code from sub-category **647.6** for **Other viral diseases** is assigned, with code 042 assigned as an additional code. If an obstetric patient tests positive for HIV but has no symptoms and no history of an HIV infection, code **V08, Asymptomatic Human Immunodeficiency Virus (HIV) infection status** would be assigned rather than 042.

Exercise 10.2

Code the following diagnoses.

	Code(s)
1. Candidiasis, of esophagus, opportunistic, secondary to AIDS-like disease	042
	112.84
2. Pneumocystis carinii	042
AIDS	136.3
3. Positive HIV test in patient who is asymptomatic, presents no related symptoms, and has no history of HIV infection	V08
4. Acute lymphadenitis due to ARC	042
	683
5. Acute appendicitis (admitted for appendectomy)	540.9
Kaposi's sarcoma of skin of chest, due to HIV infection	042
	176.0
6. Kaposi's sarcoma of oral cavity	042
AIDS	176.8

Exercise 10.2 *(continued)*

7. Agranulocytosis due to HIV infection   042
                                                                        288.04

8. Burkitt's tumor of inguinal region associated with AIDS   042
                                                                         200.25

9. Background retinopathy due to AIDS-like disease   042
                                                                         362.10

10. Inconclusive HIV test   795.71

11 Endocrine, Metabolic and Nutritional Diseases and Immune–System Disorders

This chapter covers a variety of conditions that are related in a general way. Because diabetes mellitus is a common medical problem, it is the condition coders encounter most often when working with chapter 3 of *ICD-9-CM*.

DIABETES MELLITUS

Diabetes mellitus, classified in category 250, is a chronic disorder of impaired carbohydrate, protein, and fat metabolism. The disorder is caused by either an absolute decrease in the amount of insulin secreted by the pancreas, or a reduction in the biologic effectiveness of the insulin secreted. Other conditions include the term diabetes, such as bronze diabetes and diabetes insipidus, but a diagnosis of diabetes without further qualification should be interpreted as diabetes mellitus.

Diabetes mellitus has two classification axes. The fourth digit identifies the presence of any associated complication, and the fifth-digit subclassification indicates both the type of diabetes and whether or not it is considered to be out of control. The terms "out of control" and "uncontrolled" are synonymous in this context. Sometimes the physician may indicate "poorly controlled" or "poor control." These are vague terms and do not necessarily indicate uncontrolled blood glucose levels. Obtain clarification from the physician to determine if the patient's diabetes is uncontrolled. Diabetes is classified as uncontrolled only when the physician specifically identifies it as such; this determination is not based on blood glucose levels documented in the medical record. Uncontrolled diabetes mellitus is a nonspecific term indicating that the patient's blood sugar level is not kept within acceptable levels by his or her current treatment regimen. Causes of uncontrolled diabetes mellitus may be noncompliance, insulin resistance, dietary indiscretion, and intercurrent illness.

Types of Diabetes Mellitus

There are two major types of diabetes mellitus: type I (or type 1) and type II (or type 2).

Type 1 diabetes mellitus may also be described as ketosis-prone, juvenile type, juvenile onset, or juvenile diabetes. It is characterized by the body's failure to produce insulin at all, or by an absolute decrease in such production. These patients require regular insulin injections to sustain life, and experience significant health problems when they do not follow the prescribed regimen for medication and diet. Careful monitoring is required in order to avoid serious complications. Code **V58.67, Long-term (current) use of insulin,** is not required for type 1 diabetics because these patients require insulin. However, this code may be assigned, if desired, to provide additional information. This textbook has followed this principle based on the advice published in *Coding Clinic*, Fourth Quarter 2004, p. 55.

Type 2 diabetes mellitus may also be described as ketosis resistant. Insulin is produced but either it is produced in insufficient quantity or the body is unable to utilize it adequately. Type 2 diabetic patients usually do not require insulin; they are ordinarily managed with oral hypoglycemic agents, diet, and exercise. For some patients, however, these measures are not effective, and insulin therapy may be required to control persistent hyperglycemia.

Category 250 has a fourth digit that identifies the presence of any associated complication and a fifth digit that indicates both the type of diabetes and whether the patient's status is controlled or uncontrolled. Nonessential modifiers related to "insulin dependent," "noninsulin dependent," and "adult onset" have been removed and are no longer considered for selection of the fifth digit. This change has been implemented to clarify that the type of diabetes (1 or 2) is the essential element in the selection of the fifth digit, rather than whether the patient is on insulin. Note that the uncontrolled status is classified only when the physician specifically documents this status. If the medical record documentation is not clear with regard to the type of diabetes, query the physician, or select the fifth digit of "0" for "unspecified." When the type of diabetes is not documented, but does indicate that the patient uses insulin, the default is type 2. The fact that a patient is receiving insulin does not indicate that the diabetes is type 1.

When a type 2 diabetic patient routinely uses insulin, assign code **V58.67, Long-term (current) use of insulin.** However, code V58.67 should not be used if insulin is given temporarily to bring the patient's blood sugar under control during the encounter.

Some diabetic patients require the use of an insulin pump to receive insulin therapy. An insulin pump is a small, computerized device attached to the body that delivers insulin via a catheter. The pump may provide a continuous drip of insulin all day long, or it may also allow the patient to self-administer an insulin bolus by pushing a button. Failure or malfunction of the pump may result in underdosing or overdosing of insulin. Both of these situations are considered mechanical complications and are assigned code **996.57, Mechanical complication due to insulin pump.** When there is an overdose of insulin as a result of pump malfunction, code **962.3, Poisoning by insulins and antidiabetic agents,** is assigned as an additional code.

Complications and Manifestations of Diabetes Mellitus

Both type 1 and type 2 diabetes mellitus can lead to a variety of complications that involve either acute metabolic derangements (250.1x–253.3x) or long-term complications (250.4x–250.8x). The code for the diabetes mellitus (category 250) is ordinarily assigned first, with an additional code for the complication or manifestation, unless the manifestation is included in the basic code. Assign as many codes from category 250 as necessary to identify all the associated diabetic conditions the patient may have.

Acute Metabolic Complications

Acute metabolic complications include ketoacidosis (250.1x), hyperosmolarity with or without associated coma (250.2x), and other coma (250.3x). Typical findings for patients with diabetic ketoacidosis (DKA) are glycosuria, strong ketonuria, hyperglycemia, ketonemia (blood ketone), acidosis (low arterial blood pH), and low plasma bicarbonate. Type 2 diabetics seldom develop ketoacidosis. A diagnosis of diabetic ketoacidosis should be classified as type 1 diabetes mellitus unless the physician specifically identifies it as type 2.

Diabetes with hyperosmolarity (250.2x) is a condition in which there is hyperosmolarity and dehydration without significant ketosis. This condition most often occurs in patients with type 2 diabetes. Coma may or may not be present.

Diabetes with other coma (250.3x) includes patients with ketoacidosis who have progressed to a comatose state. This code includes hypoglycemic coma in a patient with diabetes and insulin coma, not otherwise specified.

Chronic Complications

Patients with diabetes mellitus are susceptible to one or more chronic conditions that affect the renal, nervous, and peripheral vascular systems, particularly the feet and the eyes. Onset may occur early or late in the course of the diabetes and may occur in both insulin-dependent and non-insulin-dependent patients.

Dual coding is required for this type of complication, with a code for the diabetes assigned first, followed by a code for the associated manifestation code indicating the complication. Diabetic patients often suffer several complications concurrently, in which case multiple codes from subcategories 250.4 through 250.8 are assigned, with a manifestation code assigned for each.

Renal Complications.   Patients with diabetes are particularly prone to developing complications that affect the kidneys, such as nephritis, nephrosis, or chronic renal failure. Nephritis is an inflammation of the kidney that develops slowly, over a long period of time. Nephrosis is an advanced stage of disease characterized by massive edema and marked proteinuria. Chronic renal failure is often the ultimate progression of such conditions.

Diabetic nephropathy is coded as 250.4x and **583.81,** *Nephritis and nephropathy, not specified as acute or chronic, in diseases classified elsewhere,* or as 250.4x and 582.8x when the renal condition is described as "chronic glomerulonephritis." Diabetes with nephrosis or nephrotic syndrome is coded 250.4x and **581.81,** *Nephrotic syndrome in diseases classified elsewhere.* When the renal condition has progressed to chronic kidney disease, the diagnosis is sometimes stated in a way that appears to require three codes, one for the diabetes (250.4x), one for an interim manifestation (581.81), and one for the final or current problem (**585.x, Chronic kidney disease**). It is not necessary to code the intermediate condition, but all three codes may be assigned if the hospital prefers.

Patients who have both diabetes and hypertension may develop renal failure as a result. In this case, three codes are required: one code for the diabetes with renal manifestation, 250.4x; a second code from category 403 (or 404), with a fifth digit of (0) with chronic kidney disease stage I through stage IV, or unspecified, or a fifth digit of (1) with chronic kidney disease stage V or end-stage renal disease; and a third code from category 585 to indicate the specific stage of the chronic kidney disease. No other manifestation code is assigned. For example:

- Progressive diabetic nephropathy with hypertensive renal disease and chronic kidney disease stage V   250.40 + 403.91 + 585.5

Diabetic Eye Disease.   Retinopathy is a common complication of diabetes. Any disease of the retina said to be due to diabetes requires a code of 250.5x and an additional code for the retinal complication. Nonproliferative diabetic retinopathy may be specified as mild (362.04), moderate (362.05), or severe (362.06). If the degree of severity of the diabetic retinopathy is not specified, code 362.03 should be assigned. Diabetic macular edema is only present with diabetic retinopathy; therefore, if the documentation refers to diabetic macular edema, code 362.07 must be used with a code for the diabetic retinopathy (362.01–362.06).

Senile cataracts develop more frequently in patients with diabetes, but they are not true diabetic cataracts and are not classified as ocular manifestations of the disease. A code from subcategories **366.1x, Senile cataract,** and **250, Diabetes mellitus,** should be assigned for senile cataracts in a diabetic patient, with sequencing depending on the circumstances of admission. Diabetic cataract (snowflake cataract, true diabetic cataract) is relatively rare. Assign codes for diabetic cataract only when the physician specifically describes the condition as such. For example:

- Diabetes mellitus with diabetic cataract   250.50 + 366.41
- Diabetes mellitus with mature senile cataract   250.00 + 366.17

Diabetic Neuropathy.   Peripheral, cranial, and autonomic neuropathy are chronic manifestations of diabetes mellitus. The codes for peripheral polyneuropathy are 250.6x and **357.2,** *Polyneuropathy in diabetes,* and the codes for autonomic neuropathy are 250.6x and **337.1,** *Peripheral autonomic neuropathy in disorders classified elsewhere.* Do not use the code for autonomic neuropathy unless the diagnosis is stated as such by the physician. When the neurological condition is specified, the more specific manifestation code should be assigned. For example:

- Diabetic third (cranial) nerve palsy   250.6x + 378.51
- Mononeuropathy of the lower limb due to type 2 diabetes   250.60 + 355.8

Diabetic Peripheral Vascular Disease.   Peripheral vascular disease is a frequent complication of diabetes mellitus. Diabetic peripheral vascular disease is coded as 250.7x and **443.81, Peripheral circulatory disease in diseases classified elsewhere.** Although arteriosclerosis occurs earlier and more extensively in diabetic patients, coronary artery disease, cardiomyopathy, and cerebrovascular disease are not complications of diabetes and are not included in code 250.7x. These conditions are coded separately unless the physician documents a causal relationship.

Other Manifestations of Diabetes Mellitus.   Ulcers of the lower extremities, particularly the feet, are common complications of diabetes. They may result from either diabetic neuropathy (250.6x) or diabetic peripheral vascular disease (250.7x). The code for the diabetes is assigned first, with an additional code of 707.1x with the fifth digit indicating the specific site of the ulcer. If gangrene is present, code **785.4, Gangrene,** should be assigned as an additional code, with or without the intervening code for the ulcer. It is important to recognize that not all ulcers in diabetic patients are diabetic ulcers; if there is a question as to the relationship, the physician should be consulted.

Organic impotence is often the result of either diabetic peripheral neuropathy or diabetic peripheral vascular disease. It is coded first to either 250.6x or 250.7x, with an additional code of **607.84, Impotence of organic origin.**

Either of the preceding conditions specified as diabetic but without an indication as to whether the condition is due to neuropathy or peripheral vascular disease is coded as **250.8x, Diabetes with other specified manifestations,** with an additional code for the complications. Any other specified chronic manifestation that cannot be assigned to codes 250.0 through 250.7x is also assigned to code 250.8x. For example:

- Diabetes mellitus, type 1, with ulcer of great toe of right foot   250.81 + 707.15

DIABETES MELLITUS COMPLICATING PREGNANCY

Diabetes mellitus complicating pregnancy, delivery, or the puerperium is classified in chapter 11 of *ICD-9-CM.* Code 648.0x is sequenced first, with an additional code from category 250 to indicate the type of diabetes involved. Because diabetes mellitus inevitably complicates the pregnant state, is aggravated by the pregnancy, or is a main reason for obstetric care, it is appropriate to assign these codes for a pregnant diabetic patient. Assign also code **V58.67, Long-term (current) use of insulin,** if the diabetes mellitus is routinely treated with insulin.

Gestational Diabetes

A diagnosis of gestational diabetes refers to abnormal glucose tolerance that appears during pregnancy in previously nondiabetic women; it is not a true diabetes mellitus. It is thought to be due to metabolic or hormonal changes that occur during pregnancy. Patients with gestational diabetes are usually placed on a diabetic diet and sometimes require insulin therapy to maintain normal blood glucose levels during pregnancy, but the condition usually resolves during the postpartum period. Code **648.8x, Abnormal glucose tolerance,** is assigned for this condition. Assign also code **V58.67, Long-term (current) use of insulin,** if the diabetes mellitus is routinely treated with insulin. Codes 648.0x (diabetes mellitus complicating pregnancy) and 648.8x (abnormal glucose tolerance complicating pregnancy) should never be used together on the same record.

Neonatal Conditions Associated with Maternal Diabetes

Newborns with diabetic mothers sometimes experience either a transient decrease in blood sugar (**775.0, Syndrome of infant of diabetic mother**) or a transient hyperglycemia (**775.1, Neonatal diabetes mellitus**). The latter condition is sometimes referred to as pseudodiabetes and occasionally requires a short course of insulin therapy. Note, however, that these codes are assigned only when the maternal condition has actually had such an effect; the fact that the mother has diabetes in itself does not warrant the assignment of one of these codes for the newborn. When laboratory reports seem to indicate either condition, it is appropriate to check with the attending physician.

When a normal infant is born to a diabetic mother, and the infant presents no manifestations of the syndrome, assign code **V30.00, Single liveborn, born in hospital, delivered without mention of cesarean delivery,** as the principal diagnosis. Code **V18.0, Family history of certain other specific conditions, Diabetes mellitus,** should be assigned as an additional diagnosis. In addition, assign code **V29.3, Observation and evaluation of newborns and infants for suspected condition not found, Observation for suspected genetic or metabolic condition,** as an additional diagnosis for a newborn infant who requires special surveillance after being born to a diabetic mother, but who lacks manifestations of infant of a diabetic mother syndrome.

Exercise 11.1

Code the following diagnoses. Do not assign E codes.

	Code(s)
1. Diabetes mellitus, type 1	250.41
Diabetic nephrosis	581.81
2. Uncontrolled type 1 diabetes mellitus	250.53
Snowflake cataract	366.41
3. Type 1 diabetes with ketoacidosis	250.11
4. Diabetes mellitus, type 2, out of control, with hyperosmotic, nonketotic coma	250.22
5. Diabetic Kimmelstiel-Wilson disease	250.40
	581.81
6. Chronic kidney disease, stage IV due to type 1 diabetic nephrotic syndrome (Optional)	250.41
	581.81
	585.4
7. Impotence due to diabetic peripheral neuropathy	250.60
	607.84

SECONDARY DIABETES

Secondary diabetes is usually the result of therapy such as the surgical removal of the pancreas or the use of certain medications. For example, steroid-induced diabetes mellitus due to the prolonged use of corticosteroids for an unrelated condition is coded as **251.8, Other specified disorder of pancreatic internal secretion,** with an additional code of **E932.0, Adverse effect of therapeutic use of adrenal cortical steroids.** Code **251.3, Postsurgical hypoinsulinemia,** is assigned for a diagnosis of postpancreatectomy diabetes mellitus (lack of insulin due to the surgical removal of all or part of the pancreas). Codes from category 250 are not assigned for secondary diabetes.

HYPOGLYCEMIC AND INSULIN REACTIONS

Hypoglycemic reactions can occur in both diabetic and nondiabetic patients. In a diabetic patient, hypoglycemia is coded as **250.3x, Diabetes mellitus with other coma,** or **250.8x, Diabetes with other specified complication,** if there is no mention of coma. Such reactions may occur when there is an imbalance between eating or exercise patterns and the dosage of insulin or oral hypoglycemic drugs. Hypoglycemia due to insulin may also occur in a newly diagnosed, type 1 diabetic during the initial phase of therapy while the dosage is being adjusted.

In a patient who does not have diabetes, code 251.0 is assigned for hypoglycemic coma and code 251.1 is assigned for other specified hypoglycemia if no coma is present. Code 251.2 is assigned for hypoglycemia not otherwise specified.

Hypoglycemia due to a drug used as prescribed requires an E code to indicate the responsible drug. Hypoglycemic coma or shock resulting from the incorrect use of insulin or other antidiabetic agent is coded as poisoning (962.3 + E858.0).

Exercise 11.2

Code the following diagnoses. Do not assign E codes.

	Code(s)
1. Neonatal hypoglycemia	775.6
2. Hypoglycemic coma in patient without diabetes	251.0
3. Patient with type 2 diabetes mellitus participated in a strenuous game of racquetball without adjusting his insulin dosage; he is admitted with blood sugar of 35 and is diagnosed as being hypoglycemic Hypoglycemia	250.80 V58.67
4. Type 1 diabetic developed hypoglycemia even though she had taken only the prescribed dose of insulin and did not alter her exercise or eating regimen	250.81 V58.67

CODES FOR NUTRITIONAL DISORDERS

Nutritional disorders, such as deficiency of specific vitamins and minerals, are classified in categories 260 through 269, with the exception of deficiency anemias, which are classified in the 280 through 281.9 series.

Obesity due to a specified cause, such as a thyroid disorder (240–246), is coded to the underlying condition. These codes can be assigned as the principal diagnosis when the underlying cause has not been identified; otherwise, assign code **278.00, Obesity unspecified,** or code **278.01, Morbid obesity,** as an additional code. Morbid obesity is insufficient to prevent normal activity or physiologic function or to lead to the onset of an associated pathologic condition. These codes are assigned only on the basis of the physician's diagnostic statement. Subcategory 278.0, Overweight and obesity, require that an additional code (V85.0–V85.54) for the body mass index (BMI) be assigned, if known. BMI is a tool for indicating weight status in adults. It is a measure of weight for height. The BMI code assignment should be based on medical record documentation, which may be found in a dietitian's note. This is an exception to the guideline that requires that code assignment be based on the documentation by the physician or any qualified health care practitioner who is legally accountable for establishing the patient's diagnosis. While BMI may be reported on the basis of a dietitian's documentation, the codes for overweight and obesity should be based on the provider's documentation.

CYSTIC FIBROSIS

Cystic fibrosis (277.x), also known as mucoviscidosis or cystic fibrosis of the pancreas, is a disorder of the exocrine glands that causes the accumulation of thick, tenacious mucus. It is the primary cause of pancreatic deficiency and chronic malabsorption in children. Although cystic fibrosis affects the body in a number of ways, progressive respiratory insufficiency is the major cause of illness in patients with this disease. The symptoms primarily affect the digestive and respiratory systems. In some glands, like the pancreas, the thick mucus may obstruct the pancreas preventing digestive enzymes from reaching the intestines. The pulmonary manifestation results in mucus secretions that clog the airways and allow bacteria to multiply. Sometimes this progresses to complications such as acute and chronic bronchitis, bronchiectasis, pneumonia, atelectasis, peribronchial and parenchyma scarring, pneumothorax, and hemoptysis. Intra-abdominal complications such as meconium ileus, rectal prolapse, inguinal hernia, gallstones, ileocolic intussusception, and gastroesophageal reflux also occur.

New codes have been created to specify the site of manifestation involvement such as pulmonary involvement (277.02), gastrointestinal involvement (277.03), or other site involvement (277.09). These manifestation codes may be used together if different sites are involved.

If a patient is admitted due to a complication of cystic fibrosis with pulmonary involvement, such as acute bronchitis (466.0), code the complication as the principal diagnosis or first-listed code, followed by the cystic fibrosis code (277.02).

Because there is no known cure for cystic fibrosis, therapy is directed toward the complications of the disease, with the major focus on the maintenance of adequate nutritional and respiratory status. Admissions due to the cystic fibrosis itself most often occur when the patient is brought in for workup to confirm the diagnosis.

CODES FOR DISORDERS OF THE IMMUNE SYSTEM

Category 279 classifies various disorders of the immune system, with the exception of conditions associated with or due to the human immunodeficiency virus (HIV), which are classified to code 042.

Review Exercise 11.3

Code the following diagnoses and procedures. Do not assign E codes.

	Code(s)
1. Hypercholesterolemia and endogenous hyperglyceridemia	272.2
2. Cystic fibrosis with mild mental retardation	277.00
	317
3. Thymic dysplasia with immunodeficiency	279.2
4. Congenital myxedema	243
Inappropriate antidiuretic hormone secretion syndrome	253.6
5. Uninodular toxic nodular goiter with thyrotoxicosis	242.10
Unilateral thyroid lobectomy	06.2
6. Adenomatous goiter with thyrotoxicosis	242.30
Substernal thyroidectomy, complete	06.52

Review Exercise 11.3 *(continued)*

7. Toxic diffuse <u>goiter</u> with thyrotoxic crisis   242.01

8. <u>Hypothyroidism</u>, ablative, following total   244.0
   thyroidectomy performed three years ago

9. Cell-mediated immune <u>deficiency</u> with thrombocytopenia   279.12
   and eczema

10. <u>Hypopotassemia</u>   276.8

12 Mental Disorders

Mental disorders of all types are classified in chapter 5 of *ICD-9-CM*. Referring to the glossary of mental disorders located in appendix B of volume 1 can be helpful in understanding the psychiatric terms used in this chapter.

Psychiatrists ordinarily state diagnoses in accordance with the nomenclature used in the *Diagnostic and Statistical Manual of Mental Disorders,* published by the American Psychiatric Association. Most of these codes are the same as those used in *ICD-9-CM* but the terminology may be somewhat different. Coders working with mental health records may find it useful to become familiar with this manual, but actual coding assignment is made according to the classifications in *ICD-9-CM*.

ORGANIC BRAIN SYNDROME

Organic brain syndrome is a complex of mental symptoms related to impaired cerebral function. This impairment may be due to a wide variety of diseases, chronic alcoholism, or trauma. Organic brain syndrome may be either acute and reversible or chronic and irreversible.

When coding organic brain syndrome, the first step is to determine whether the condition is psychotic or nonpsychotic. Psychosis is characterized by personality derangement and loss of contact with reality. In addition it is frequently associated with delusions, illusions, or hallucinations. Neurosis, on the other hand, does not involve any gross distortion of reality or disorganization of the personality. When the diagnostic statement mentions "with dementia," "delirium," or "psychotic" or similar terms, the condition should be coded as psychotic. Unless there is clear documentation of psychosis in the medical record, however, codes indicating psychosis should not be assigned. For example:

- Organic brain syndrome psychosis associated with chronic alcoholism
  <u>291.2 + 303.90</u>
- Organic brain syndrome, nonpsychotic, due to old concussion   <u>310.2 + 907.0</u>

ORGANIC ANXIETY SYNDROME

Organic anxiety syndrome is a transient organic psychosis characterized by clinically significant anxiety. It is considered to be the direct physiological effect of a general medical condition. The code for the general condition is sequenced first, with an additional code of **293.84, Anxiety disorder in conditions classified elsewhere.**

DEMENTIA IN CONDITIONS CLASSIFIED ELSEWHERE

Code 294.1x has been expanded to specifically identify the presence or absence of behavioral disturbances such as aggressive behavior, violent behavior, wandering off, or combative behavior. The dementia classified in subcategory 294.1x is due to direct physiological effects of a general medical condition. Dementia is characterized by the development of multiple cognitive deficits such as memory impairment and cognitive disturbances such as aphasia, apraxia, or agnosis. When assigning codes 294.10 and 294.11, code first the underlying disease associated with the dementia, such as Alzheimer's disease or Huntington's.

ALZHEIMER'S DISEASE

Alzheimer's disease is a process of progressive atrophy involving the degeneration of nerve cells. This degeneration leads to mental changes that range from subtle intellectual impairment to dementia with loss of cognitive functions and failure of memory. **Alzheimer's disease is coded as 331.0.** When there is associated dementia, code **294.1x, Dementia in conditions classified elsewhere,** is assigned as an additional diagnosis. For example:

- Alzheimer's disease [without any mention of dementia]   331.0
- Dementia due to Alzheimer's disease   331.0 + 294.1x

METABOLIC ENCEPHALOPATHY

Encephalopathy is a general term used to describe any disorder of cerebral function. Metabolic encephalopathy refers to an altered state of consciousness, usually characterized as delirium. It is either hypoactive or hyperactive and transient in nature, and is essentially a reversible dysfunction of cerebral metabolism, although the delirium may be persistent. Some physicians use the term "acute confusional state" to describe this condition.

Metabolic encephalopathy can result from a wide variety of conditions, some of which affect the brain and some of which involve various body systems. Because it is a manifestation of such a variety of causes, there is no one code for this condition; code entries are located under the main term **Delirium** in the Alphabetic Index.

ALTERED MENTAL STATE

An alteration in level of consciousness not associated with delirium or with another identified condition is classified to subcategory 780.0 in chapter 16 of *ICD-9-CM*. Fifth digits are used to indicate whether it is identified as coma (780.01), transient alteration of awareness (780.02), or persistent vegetative state (780.03). Other altered mental states, such as somnolence, stupor, or states not further specified, are classified as 780.09. An altered mental status, or a change in mental status, of unknown etiology is coded to **780.97, Altered mental status.** If the condition causing the change in mental status is known, do not assign code 780.97; code the condition instead.

TRANSIENT GLOBAL AMNESIA

Transient global amnesia is a distinct form of amnesia of unknown etiology, characterized by a sudden loss of memory function. During an episode, the patient is unable to form memories or remember recent events and may ask the same question over and over because no memories of previous answers are formed. The episode usually lasts for a few hours, followed by total or near-total resolution of the memory loss, although the patient will remain amnesic for the event itself. Transient global amnesia is not psychotic in nature, and it is not considered to be due to ischemia; rather it is a distinct cerebrovascular condition with its own code, 437.7.

SCHIZOPHRENIC DISORDERS

Schizophrenic disorders are classified in category 295, with a fourth digit indicating the type of schizophrenia. A fifth-digit subclassification is used to indicate the course of the illness, as follows:

- 0   unspecified
- 1   subchronic (continuous illness for more than six months but less than two years)
- 2   chronic (continuous illness for more than two years)
- 3   subchronic with acute exacerbation (duration of illness same as subchronic but prominent psychotic features re-emergent in a patient who had been in the residual phase)
- 4   chronic with acute exacerbation (duration of illness same as chronic but prominent psychotic features re-emergent in a patient who had been in the residual phase)
- 5   in remission

Assignment of fifth digits 1 through 5 must be based on the physician's statement.

AFFECTIVE DISORDERS

Affective disorders are common mental diseases characterized by mood disturbance. Major depressive disorders are classified as episodic mood disorders under category 296 in *ICD-9-CM;* code 311 is assigned for other nonpsychotic depressive disorders.

Patients diagnosed as suffering from a major affective disorder are classified according to the type of symptoms they exhibit. Patients who experience sadness and withdrawal and lose interest in social activities or other aspects of life are classified as follows:

- 296.2x   Major depressive disorder, single episode
- 296.3x   Major depressive disorder, recurrent episode

Patients who exhibit symptoms of hypomania—for example, rapid speech, flight of ideas, grandiosity, and poor judgment—are classified as follows:

- 296.0x   Bipolar I disorder, single manic episode
- 296.1x   Manic disorder, recurrent episode

Many patients experience cyclic, recurring mood changes that result in periods of severe depression alternating with extreme elation that are beyond the normal range of mood swings. Such disorders are called bipolar or circular disorders and are classified as 296.4x through 296.6x, with the fourth digit indicating the current phase of the illness, as follows:

- 296.4x   Bipolar I disorder, most recent episode (or current) manic (patient is presently in manic phase but has experienced depression in the past)
- 296.5x   Bipolar I disorder, most recent episode (or current) depressed (patient is presently in depressive phase but has experienced hypomania in the past)
- 296.6x   Bipolar I disorder, most recent episode (or current) mixed (patient is presently exhibiting both depressive and manic behavior)

Fifth digits are used with subcategories 296.0 through 296.6 to provide information about the current severity of the disorder, as follows:

- 0   unspecified
- 1   mild
- 2   moderate
- 3   severe, without mention of psychotic behavior
- 4   severe, specified as with psychotic behavior
- 5   in partial or unspecific remission
- 6   in full remission

Again, fifth digits 1 through 6 are assigned only when documentation of severity is included in the medical record.

Exercise 12.1

Code the following diagnoses and procedures. Do not assign E codes.

	Code(s)
1. Schizo-affective psychosis, chronic, with acute exacerbation	295.74
2. Schizophrenia, catatonic type, subchronic	295.21
3. Schizophrenia, reactive, paranoid type	295.30
Electroshock treatment	94.27
4. Severe manic disorder, recurrent episode	296.13

Exercise 12.1 *(continued)*

5. Reactive depressive <u>psychosis</u>   298.0

6. Bipolar <u>disorder</u>, in manic phase, mild   296.41

7. Mixed bipolar affective <u>disorder</u>, in partial remission   296.65

NONPSYCHOTIC MENTAL DISORDERS

A variety of neurotic disorders, personality disorders, and other nonpsychotic mental disorders are classified in categories 300 through 316. These include such conditions as anxiety states, alcohol and drug dependence and abuse, adjustment to stress, and certain physiological disorders.

Reactions to Stress

ICD-9-CM provides two categories for coding transient reactions to physical or mental stress, one for an acute stress reaction and one for an adjustment or chronic stress reaction. Category 308 classifies acute reaction to stress. This condition represents a fairly severe reaction to exceptional or gross stress and may be characterized by panic, agitation, stupor, or fugue. It generally lasts for a short time, usually several hours, but occasionally can persist for days.

   Chronic reaction to stress is classified into category **309, Adjustment reaction.** These conditions are usually situation-specific and reversible. Adjustment reactions are usually less severe than acute stress reactions and last somewhat longer, although in most cases no more than a few months. The fourth-digit axis for this category is the nature of the reaction—for example, anxiety or depression. The following situations would fall into this category:

- Patient depressed over death of son (two years ago)   309.1
- Patient expresses severe anxiety over separation from husband   309.21
- Patient has just taken a new job and is having a severe anxiety adjustment to the work situation   309.23

Psychophysiologic Disorders

Two categories are provided for psychophysiologic disorders: 306 and 316. Category 306 classifies physiological malfunction arising from mental factors, with the fourth digit indicating the body system involved. For the most part, the four-digit code includes the associated symptom, and there is no need to assign an additional code. Examples of conditions that are classified in category 306 include the following:

- Psychogenic paralysis   306.0
- Psychogenic diarrhea   306.4
- Psychogenic dysmenorrhea   306.52

In assigning codes from category 306, it is important to make the distinction between these conditions and similar conditions that fall under the categories for neurotic disorders, psychoses, or organic disorders.

Category 316 classifies psychic factors associated with diseases classified elsewhere. Typical conditions that are often associated with code 316 include asthma, ulcerative colitis, and dermatitis. If such a condition is considered to be psychogenic in origin, code 316 is assigned first, followed by an additional code for the associated condition. For example:

- Psychogenic asthma   316 + 493.90
- Psychogenic paroxysmal tachycardia   316 + 427.2

Special Symptoms or Syndromes

Category 307 includes codes for a variety of special symptoms and syndromes of nonorganic origin, such as tics and specified nonorganic sleep disorders. These codes are not assigned when they are due to a mental disorder classified elsewhere or are of organic origin. Eating disorders such as bulimia nervosa (307.51) and anorexia nervosa (307.1) are included in this category. For some anorexic patients, the weight loss is so severe that it leads to malnutrition. Code 261, Nutritional marasmus, should be assigned as an additional diagnosis to further describe the severity of the patient's condition.

Exercise 12.2

Code the following diagnoses.

	Code(s)
1. Acute delirium resulting from pneumonia	482.2
due to Hemophilus influenzae	293.0
2. Passive-aggressive personality	301.84
3. Depression with anxiety	300.4
Conversion reaction (tremors)	300.11

Exercise 12.2 *(continued)*

4. Adolescent adjustment <u>reaction</u>, with severe
   disturbance of conduct   309.3

5. Severe <u>involutional depression</u>, recurrent   296.33

6. Stress <u>reaction</u>, psychomotor   308.2

SUBSTANCE ABUSE DISORDERS

Substance abuse and dependence are classified as mental disorders in *ICD-9-CM*. Alcohol dependence syndrome is classified in category 303, drug dependence is classified in category 304, and nondependent abuse of drugs, including both alcohol or drugs, is classified in category 305. Although the terms "abuse" and "dependence" may be used interchangeably in certain treatment programs, they are actually quite different conditions and are coded differently in *ICD-9-CM*. For both abuse and dependence codes, the fifth digit represents the pattern of use, as follows:

- 0 unspecified
- 1 continuous
  —alcohol: refers to daily intake of large amounts of alcohol or regular heavy drinking on weekends or days off from work
  —drugs: daily or almost daily use of drug
- 2 episodic
  —alcohol: refers to alcoholic binges lasting weeks or months, followed by long periods of sobriety
  —drugs: indicates short periods between drug use or use on weekends
- 3 remission: refers to either a complete cessation of alcohol or drug intake or to the period during which a decrease toward cessation is taking place

The coder should not attempt to apply these digits without documentation of the pattern of use in the medical record. It is common for technical and professional personnel other than the attending physician to provide much of the documentation in facilities dealing with detoxification and rehabilitation, however, and it is appropriate to accept such documentation for the purpose of assigning fifth digits.

Alcohol Dependence and Abuse

Alcoholism (alcohol dependence) is a chronic condition in which the patient has become dependent on alcohol, with increased tolerance, and is unable to stop its use even with such strong incentives as impairment of health, deteriorating social interactions, and interference with job performance. Such patients often experience physical signs of withdrawal when there is a sudden cessation of drinking.

Code 303.0x, Alcohol dependence syndrome, acute alcoholic intoxication, is assigned when a patient who is dependent on alcohol presents for care in a state of acute intoxication. If the patient presents when not acutely intoxicated, as for a rehabilitation program, the condition is classified as 303.9x, Other and unspecified alcoholism. Because alcoholism is by definition a chronic condition, both codes are not assigned; when the diagnosis is stated as "acute and chronic alcoholism," code 303.0x covers both conditions. Although there is a code for history of alcoholism (V11.3), it is very rare for a patient with alcoholism to experience a full recovery; alcoholism in remission is ordinarily the code that should be assigned.

Alcohol abuse represents problem drinking and includes those patients who drink to excess but have not reached a stage of physical dependence on alcohol. It may include such alcohol-related conditions as temporary mental disturbance, slurred speech, blackouts, difficulty in driving, arguments with family and friends, and difficulty in the work environment. Alcohol abuse is classified as code 305.0x, Alcohol abuse. This code is also assigned for a diagnosis of simple drunkenness.

Drug Dependence and Abuse

Drug dependence is a chronic mental and physical condition related to the patient's drug use. It is characterized by behavioral and psychological responses and also includes a compulsion to take the drug in order to experience its psychic effect or to avoid the discomfort that results from its absence. Such patients often experience physical signs of withdrawal when there is a sudden cessation of drug use. Category 304, Drug dependence, uses a fourth digit to indicate the class of drug involved. Certain codes indicate a combination of drugs; in particular, code 304.7x is assigned when an opioid drug is involved with other drugs and code 304.8x when no opioid drug is present.

Drug abuse represents problematic use of drugs by patients who take drugs to excess but have not reached a stage of dependence. It represents use of the drug in a maladaptive pattern that may adversely affect social functioning or physical and/or mental health. Nondependent abuse drugs are classified in category 305, with the fourth digit indicating the drug involved. For both alcohol and drug dependence and abuse, fifth digits provide the pattern of use:

- 0   unspecified
- 1   continuous
- 2   episodic
- 3   in remission

Substance-Related Conditions

Patients with substance abuse or dependence often develop related physical complications or psychotic symptoms. Mental disorders related to alcohol use are classified in category **291, Alcohol-induced mental disorders;** those related to drug use are classified in category **292, Drug-induced mental disorders.**

Patients dependent on either alcohol or drugs or on a combination of the two frequently experience withdrawal symptoms and require detoxification. Symptoms and signs of withdrawal include tremulousness, agitation, irritability, disturbed sleep, anorexia, autonomic hyperactivity, seizures, and hallucinations. A severe form of withdrawal known as delirium tremens is characterized by fever, tachycardia, hypertension or hypotension, hallucinations, agitation, confusion, fluctuating mental states, and seizures. Symptoms of withdrawal usually begin after a significant decline in the blood alcohol level.

Three subcategory codes—291.0, 291.3, and 291.81—are provided for alcoholic withdrawal. Only one of these codes should be assigned, with code 291.0 taking precedence over the other two and code 291.3 taking precedence over code 291.81, as indicated by the exclusion notes. Note that fifth digits have been added to subcategory 291.8 to provide separate codes for withdrawal (291.81) and alcoholic anxiety and alcoholic mood (291.89).

When the patient is admitted in withdrawal or when withdrawal develops after admission, the withdrawal code is designated as the principal diagnosis, with an additional code for alcoholism. For example:

- Alcoholic withdrawal delirium due to acute and chronic alcoholism
  <u>291.0</u> + 303.00
- Alcohol-induced psychotic disorder with hallucinations due to chronic alcoholism
  <u>291.3</u> + 303.90
- <u>Alcoholic withdrawal due to continuous chronic alcoholism</u>   <u>291.81</u> + 303.91

Drug withdrawal symptoms are coded as **292.0, Drug withdrawal.** Other mental disorders due to drug dependence or abuse are classified in the 292.1 through 292.9 series. A code should also be assigned for the dependence or abuse.

Selection of the Principal Diagnosis

The designation of the principal diagnosis for patients with either substance abuse or substance dependence depends on the circumstances of the admission, as defined in the following guidelines:

1. When a patient is admitted with a diagnosis of a substance-related psychosis, sequence the psychosis code first, followed by the alcohol or drug dependence or abuse code.
2. When a patient is admitted for the purpose of detoxification or rehabilitation or both, and there is no indication of withdrawal or other psychotic symptoms, sequence the substance abuse or dependence code as the principal diagnosis.
3. When a patient is admitted for detoxification or rehabilitation for both drug and alcohol abuse or dependence, and both are treated, either condition may be designated as the principal diagnosis.
4. When a patient with a diagnosis of substance abuse or dependence is admitted for treatment or evaluation of a physical complaint related to the substance use, follow the directions in the index for conditions described as alcoholic or due to drugs; sequence the physical condition first, followed by the code for abuse or dependence.
5. When a patient with a diagnosis of alcohol or drug abuse or dependence is admitted because of an unrelated condition, follow the usual guidelines for selecting a principal diagnosis.

Substance Abuse Therapy

Treatment for patients with a diagnosis of substance abuse or dependence consists of detoxification, rehabilitation, or both. The abuse or dependence is the principal diagnosis for a patient admitted for such programs.

Detoxification is the management of withdrawal symptoms for a patient who is physically dependent on alcohol or drugs. It is more than simple observation; it involves active management. Treatment may involve evaluation, observation and monitoring, and administration of thiamine and multivitamins for nutrition as well as other medications (such as methadone, long-acting barbiturates or benzodiazepines, or carbamazepine) as needed. The detoxification program for patients with alcohol dependence is usually continued over a four- or five-day period. Detoxification takes longer for opiates and sedatives/hypnotics, usually lasting from three weeks to a period of months, and may be carried out in either a residential or an outpatient setting. If the medical record documents detoxification as having been carried out, the code can be assigned even when no medications were actually administered.

Rehabilitation is a structured program carried out with the goal of establishing strict control of drinking and drug use. A variety of rehabilitation modalities may be utilized. These include methadone maintenance, therapeutic residential communities, and long-term outpatient drug- or alcohol-free treatments. A code for rehabilitation therapy is assigned for a patient who begins a program even when it is not completed. Category **V57, Care involving use of rehabilitation procedures,** is used for physical rehabilitation only and is not assigned for alcohol or drug rehabilitation programs.

Detoxification and rehabilitation for patients with alcohol dependence or abuse are coded as follows:

- 94.61   Alcohol rehabilitation
- 94.62   Alcohol detoxification
- 94.63   Alcohol rehabilitation and detoxification

Treatment for drug abuse or dependence is coded as follows:

- 94.64   Drug rehabilitation
- 94.65   Drug detoxification
- 94.66   Drug rehabilitation and detoxification

Many patients exhibit maladaptive use of both alcohol and drugs, and combined therapy may be used for these patients:

- 94.67   Combined alcohol and drug rehabilitation
- 94.68   Combined alcohol and drug detoxification
- 94.69   Combined alcohol and drug rehabilitation and detoxification

It is also possible to provide detoxification for either drugs or alcohol and rehabilitation for both, which would require assignment of either **94.62, Alcohol detoxification,** or **94.65, Drug detoxification,** along with **94.69** for **Combined alcohol and drug rehabilitation and detoxification.**

Psychiatric Therapy

Mental disorders other than substance abuse disorders are commonly treated with psychodynamic ("talk") therapy, drug therapy, electroconvulsive therapy, or a combination of therapeutic modes. Commonly used procedures include lithium therapy (94.22), play therapy (94.36), group therapy (94.44), and electroconvulsive therapy (ECT) (94.27). Because the diagnosis alone does not always explain the length of stay or the level of resource utilization for such patients, therapy codes are helpful in analyzing patterns of care.

Review Exercise 12.3

Code the following diagnoses and procedures.

	Code(s)
1. Paranoid alcoholic psychosis with chronic alcoholism, continuous	291.5
	303.91
2. Alcoholic cirrhosis of liver	571.2
Chronic alcoholism	303.90
3. Acute alcoholic intoxication, episodic	305.02
4. Marijuana dependence, used continuously	304.31
5. Acute intoxication and chronic alcoholism	303.00
Detoxification and rehabilitation	94.63
6. Episodic barbiturate abuse	305.42
7. Cocaine dependence, episodic	304.22

Review Exercise 12.3 *(continued)*

8. <u>Amphetamine abuse</u>, continuous   305.71

9. <u>Dependence</u> on barbiturate and heroin   304.70

10. Admitted because of syndrome of <u>inappropriate</u>   <u>253.6</u>
    secretion of antidiuretic hormone secondary   303.90
    to chronic <u>alcoholism</u>

Coding of Diseases of the Blood and Blood-Forming Organs and Diseases of the Nervous System

13 Diseases of the Blood and Blood-Forming Organs

Diseases of the blood and blood-forming organs—including bone marrow, lymphatic tissue, platelets, and coagulation factors—are classified in chapter 4 of *ICD-9-CM*. Neoplastic diseases, such as leukemia, are classified in chapter 2 of *ICD-9-CM* along with other neoplastic diseases. Diseases of the blood and blood-forming organs complicating pregnancy, childbirth, or the puerperium are reclassified in chapter 11 of *ICD-9-CM*. Anemia of pregnancy, for example, is coded 648.2x, with an additional code from chapter 4 assigned to indicate the specific type of anemia. Hematological disorders of the fetus and newborn are classified as perinatal conditions in chapter 15 of *ICD-9-CM*.

ANEMIA

The condition that coders must deal with most often in chapter 4 of *ICD-9-CM* is anemia. Anemia refers to either a reduction in the quantity of hemoglobin or a reduction in the volume of packed red cells, a condition which occurs whenever the equilibrium between red cell loss and red cell production is disturbed. A decrease in production can result from a variety of causes, including aging, bleeding, and cell destruction.

The use of precise terminology is important in classifying anemias. When a diagnostic statement of anemia is not qualified in any way, the coder should review the medical record to determine whether more information can be located in laboratory or pathology reports or in a hematology consultation before the code for an unspecified type of anemia is assigned. Remember, however, that a code should not be assigned on the basis of a diagnostic report alone; when it appears that a more specific type of anemia is present, the coder should check with the physician for concurrence.

Deficiency Anemias

Iron-deficiency anemias are classified in category 280. This type of anemia may be due to a chronic blood loss (280.0) from conditions such as chronic hemorrhagic gastrointestinal conditions or menorrhagia, or to inadequate intake of dietary iron (280.1). If the cause is unspecified, code 280.9 is assigned. Other deficiency anemias are coded in category 281, with a fourth digit indicating the specific type of deficiency such as pernicious anemia or B12 vitamin deficiency.

Code the following diagnoses and procedures. Do not assign E codes.

	Code(s)
1. Anemia, hypochromic, microcytic, with iron deficiency, cause unknown	280.9
2. Macrocytic anemia secondary to vitamin B-12 malabsorption with proteinuria	281.1

Anemia Due to Acute Blood Loss

It is important to distinguish between anemia due to chronic blood loss and anemia due to acute blood loss, because the two conditions have entirely different codes in *ICD-9-CM*. Acute blood-loss anemia results from a sudden, significant loss of blood over a brief period of time. It may occur due to trauma such as laceration, or a rupture of the spleen or other injury of abdominal viscera, where no external blood loss is noted. A diagnosis of acute blood-loss anemia should be supported by documented evidence of the condition, such as a sustained, significant lowering of the hemoglobin level and/or hematocrit.

Acute blood-loss anemia may occur following surgery, but it is not necessarily a complication of the procedure and should not be coded as a postoperative complication unless the physician identifies it as such. Many surgical procedures, such as hip replacement, routinely involve a considerable amount of bleeding as an expected part of the operation. This may or may not result in anemia; a code for anemia should be assigned only when the anemia is documented by the physician. If, in the physician's clinical judgment, surgery results in an expected amount of blood loss and the physician does not describe the patient as having anemia or a complication of surgery, do not assign a code for the blood loss. If a postoperative blood count is low enough to suggest anemia, it is appropriate to ask the physician whether a diagnosis of anemia should be added. The coder should not assume, however, that mention of blood loss and/or transfusion during surgery is an indication that anemia is present. Blood replacement is sometimes carried out as a preventive measure. When neither the diagnostic statement nor review of the medical record indicates whether a blood-loss anemia is acute or chronic, code 280.0 should be assigned.

Code the following diagnoses and procedures. Do not assign E codes.

	Code(s)
1. Anemia due to blood loss from chronic gastric ulcer	280.0
	531.40

Exercise 13.2 *(continued)*

2. Anemia, chronic, secondary to blood loss due to   280.0
   adenomyosis   617.0

3. Posthemorrhagic anemia due to acute blood loss   285.1
   following perforation of chronic duodenal ulcer   532.60

Anemia of Chronic Disease

Patients with chronic illnesses are often seen with anemia, which may be the cause of the health care admission or encounter. Treatment is often directed at the anemia, not the underlying condition. Codes for this type of anemia are classified as follows:

- Anemia in chronic kidney disease   285.21
- Anemia in neoplastic disease   285.22
- Anemia of other chronic disease   285.29

These codes may be used as the principal or first-listed diagnosis when the reason for the encounter is to deal with the anemia. On the other hand, they may be used as secondary diagnosis codes when the reason for the encounter is to deal with the underlying chronic disease or another condition. The code for the chronic condition causing the anemia should also be assigned. There is no effective therapy for anemia of chronic illness but very symptomatic patients may require a transfusion of packed blood cells.

Aplastic Anemia

Aplastic anemia (284.x) is caused by a failure of the bone marrow to produce red blood cells. The condition may be congenital, but it is usually idiopathic or acquired. It may be due to an underlying disease such as a malignant neoplasm or an infection (for example, viral hepatitis). It may also be caused by exposure to ionizing radiation, chemicals, or drugs, and it often results from treatment for malignancy. When the type of anemia is not specified but appears to be related to a diagnosis of malignancy or treatment for malignancy, the physician should be queried to determine whether the code for aplastic anemia may be appropriate.

Pancytopenia (284.1) is a type of aplastic anemia that represents a deficiency of all three elements of the blood. When a patient has anemia (deficiency of red cells), neutropenia (deficiency of white cells) and thrombocytopenia (deficiency of platelets), only the code for pancytopenia (284.1) should be assigned. Code **284.01, Constitutional red blood cell aplasia,** would be assigned if the pancytopenia was congenital rather than due to chronic disease. Do not assign code 284.1 if the pancytopenia is due to bone marrow infiltration (284.2), hairy cell leukemia (202.4), human immunodeficiency virus disease (042), leukoerythroblastic anemia (284.2), malformations (284.09), myelodysplastic syndromes (238.72–238.75), myeloproliferative disease (238.79), or other constitutional aplastic anemia (284.09), or if it is drug induced (284.8).

Exercise 13.3.

Code the following diagnoses and procedures. Do not assign E codes.

	Code(s)
1. Aplastic anemia due to ionizing radiation	284.8
2. Myelophthisic anemia	284.2

Sickle-Cell Anemia

In coding sickle-cell disorders, it is important to understand the difference between sickle-cell anemia or disease (282.6x) and sickle-cell trait (282.5). Sickle-cell disease is a hereditary disease of the red blood cells; the disease is passed to a child when both parents carry the genetic trait. Sickle-cell trait occurs when a child receives the genetic trait from only one parent. Patients with sickle-cell trait do not generally develop sickle-cell disease; they are carriers of the trait. When a medical record contains both the terms sickle-cell trait and sickle-cell disease, only the code for the sickle-cell disease is assigned.

Code **282.62, Hb-SS disease with crisis,** is assigned when vaso-occlusive crises or other crises are present. An additional code is assigned to report the type of crisis, such as acute chest syndrome (517.3) or splenic sequestration (289.52). If a condition such as cerebrovascular embolism occurs, a code should also be assigned to indicate its presence.

Another possible type of sickle-cell disease is sickle-cell thalassemia. Specific codes are available for sickle-cell thalassemia with crisis (282.42) or without crisis (282.41). Additional codes are assigned when the type of crisis is specified.

Exercise 13.4

Code the following diagnoses. Do not assign E codes.

	Code(s)
1. Classical hemophilia	286.0
2. Hemolytic anemia, sickle-cell Hb-SS disease	282.61
3. Hereditary spherocytic, hemolytic anemia	282.0

Exercise 13.4 *(continued)*

4. Thalassemia   282.49

5. Sickle-cell crisis   282.62

COAGULATION DEFECTS

Coagulation defects are characterized by prolonged clotting time. Some are congenital in origin; others are acquired. **Hemorrhagic disorder due to intrinsic circulating anticoagulants, 286.5,** is essentially the only condition that presents any problem to the coder. This condition results from the presence of circulating anticoagulants in the blood that interfere with normal clotting. These anticoagulants are usually inherent or intrinsic in the blood, like other coagulation defects, but occasionally may be augmented by long-term anticoagulant therapy. This condition is a relatively rare disorder, even more so when it occurs as a result of anticoagulant therapy.

Bleeding in a patient who is being treated with Coumadin, heparin, or another anticoagulant does not indicate that a hemorrhagic disorder due to intrinsic circulating anticoagulant is present. In this situation, a code for the condition and associated hemorrhage is assigned, with an additional code of **E934.2, Anticoagulants,** to indicate the responsible medication. Code 286.5 is not assigned unless the physician specifically documents a diagnosis of hemorrhagic disorder due to circulating anticoagulants.

Hypercoagulable state refers to a condition caused by increased thrombin generation. There is an increased tendency for blood clotting and there may be fibrin deposition in the small blood vessels. Hypercoagulable state may be due to several etiologies, including genetic predisposition to clotting, medications, pregnancy, malignancy, or inherited protein antibodies. Primary hypercoagulable state is coded to 289.81, while secondary hypercoagulable state is coded to 289.82.

Prolonged prothrombin time or other abnormal coagulation profiles are no longer coded as a coagulation defect. Code **790.92, Abnormal coagulation profile,** is assigned for this abnormal laboratory finding. If the patient is receiving Coumadin therapy, however, a prolonged bleeding time is an expected result, and therefore code 790.92 is not assigned. Note also that Coumadin is not a circulating anticoagulant; it induces anticoagulation through other mechanisms. Examples of appropriate code assignments include the following:

- Duodenal ulcer with hemorrhage due to Coumadin therapy   532.40 + E934.2
- Acute gastritis with hemorrhage due to anticoagulant therapy   535.01 + E934.2

Here are some additional case examples:

- A 50-year-old man receiving Coumadin therapy is admitted with hematemesis secondary to acute gastritis. A prolonged prothrombin time is reported, secondary to the anticoagulant effects of the Coumadin therapy. Code **535.01, Acute gastritis with hemorrhage,** is assigned; code 286.5 is not reported because no hemorrhagic disorder was identified. No code is assigned for the prolonged bleeding time because this is an expected result of Coumadin therapy. Note again that Coumadin is not a circulating anticoagulant; it induces anticoagulation through other mechanisms.

■ A patient is admitted following multiple episodes of hematemesis secondary to Coumadin therapy. No significant pathology was discovered. The Coumadin is discontinued, and no recurrence of the bleeding occurs. Code 578.0, **Hematemesis,** is assigned with an additional code of E934.2 to indicate Coumadin as the responsible external agent. Code 286.5 is not assigned.

DISEASES OF WHITE BLOOD CELLS

White blood cells (leukocytes) play an important role in the body's immune system by fighting off infection. Many different diseases can affect white blood cells. There are several different types of normal white blood cells (WBCs), including neutrophils, lymphocytes, monocytes, eosinophils, and basophils.

Diseases that may decrease production of WBCs include drug toxicity, vitamin deficiencies, blood diseases, infections (viral diseases, tuberculosis, typhoid), or abnormalities of the bone marrow; or the decrease could be cyclic (varying in severity possibly due to biorhythms). Antibodies may attack WBCs as a result of a disease or because of medications stimulating the immune system. Pooling of WBCs occurs with some overwhelming infections, heart-lung bypass during heart surgery, and hemodialysis.

Some diseases increase the production of WBCs. If all types of WBCs are affected, leukocytosis occurs. Leukocytosis can be caused by infection, inflammation, allergic reaction, malignancy, hereditary disorders, or other miscellaneous causes—for example, medications such as cortisone-like drugs (prednisone), lithium, and nonsteroidal anti-inflammatory drugs. Other illnesses target specific types of WBCs, such as neutrophilia, lymphocytosis, and granulocytosis.

Diseases of the WBCs are primarily classified on the basis of whether the WBC count is low or elevated. In addition, more specific codes are available depending on the type of blood cell affected. For example:

■ Low neutrophil count or neutropenia (subcategory 288.0) is further subdivided as follows: unspecified (288.00), congenital (288.01), cyclic or periodic (288.02), drug-induced (288.03) (for example, due to chemotherapy), neutropenia due to infection (288.04), or other reasons such as immune or toxic (288.09).

■ Decreased WBC counts (subcategory 288.5) are classified as follows: unspecified leukocytopenia (288.50); decreased lymphocytes or lymphocytopenia (288.51); or other decreased WBC count including basophils, eosinophils, monocytes, or plasmacytes (288.59).

■ Elevated WBC counts (subcategory 288.6), on the other hand, are classified as: unspecified leukocytosis (288.60); elevated lymphocytes or lymphocytosis (288.61); leukemoid reaction including basophilic, lymphocytic, monocytic, myelocytic, or neutrophilic leukemoid reaction (288.62); monocytosis (288.63); plasmacytosis (288.64); basophilia (288.65); or other elevated WBC count (288.69).

It is important to remember that these codes should not be assigned on the basis of laboratory findings alone. Physician concurrence regarding the significance of the laboratory results should be confirmed before assigning these codes.

Review Exercise 13.5

Code the following diagnoses.

	Code(s)
1. Pancytopenia, congenital	284.01
2. Cyclic neutropenia	288.02
3. Hereditary thrombocytopenia	287.33

4. Anemia
   Neutropenia
   Thrombocytopenia
	284.1

Pancytopenia	
5. Cervical adenitis due to Staphylococcus aureus	289.3 041.11
6. Autoerythrocyte sensitization purpura	287.2
7. Pernicious anemia, Addison type	281.0
8. Acute gastritis with hemorrhage, exacerbated by heparin therapy	535.01 E934.2
Table: heparin	

14 Diseases of the Nervous System and Sense Organs

Diseases of the nervous system and sense organs are classified in chapter 6 of *ICD-9-CM*. Because the nervous system is complex and difficult to comprehend, thinking of it as a two-level system may help to simplify the coding process:

- 320–349   central nervous system (brain and spinal cord)
- 350–359   peripheral nervous system (all other neural elements)

Cerebral degeneration, Parkinson's disease, and meningitis are conditions affecting the central nervous system. Polyneuropathy, myasthenia gravis, and muscular dystrophies affect the peripheral nerves. The peripheral nervous system includes the autonomic nervous system, which regulates the activity of the cardiac muscle, smooth muscle, and glands.

INFECTIOUS DISEASES OF THE CENTRAL NERVOUS SYSTEM

Infectious diseases of the central nervous system are classified in several ways, and it is imperative that the coder carefully follows the directions provided by the Alphabetic Index and Tabular List. Dual coding is frequently required, with the code for the underlying condition sequenced first, followed by a manifestation code. For example, meningitis sarcoidosis is classified as **135, Sarcoidosis**, with a manifestation of **321.4, Meningitis in sarcoidosis**. Bacterial meningitis due to certain organisms such as Pneumococcus, Streptococcus, and Staphylococcus is classified in categories 320 and 321, with a fourth digit indicating the responsible organism.

Exercise 14.1

Code the following diagnoses and procedures.

	Code(s)
1. Candidal meningitis	112.83
2. Influenzal encephalitis	487.8
	323.41
3. Encephalitis due to rubella	056.01

Exercise 14.1 *(continued)*

4. Chronic serous <u>otitis</u> media, left ear   381.10

   <u>Myringotomy</u> with insertion of drainage tube   20.01

5. Herpes zoster with <u>meningitis</u>   053.0

6. Staphylococcal <u>meningitis</u>   320.3

EPILEPSY

Epilepsy is a paroxysmal disorder of cerebral function characterized by recurrent seizures. Coders must not assume, however, that any diagnostic statement describing convulsions or seizures should be coded to epilepsy; these conditions also occur in a number of other diseases, such as brain tumor, cerebrovascular accident, alcoholism, electrolyte imbalance, and febrile conditions. Grand mal seizures, for example, can be due to causes other than epilepsy. Because a diagnosis of epilepsy can have serious legal and personal implications for the patient, such as the inability to obtain a driver's license, a code for epilepsy must not be assigned unless the physician clearly identifies the condition as such in the diagnostic statement. When the diagnosis is stated only in terms of convulsion or seizure without any further identification of the cause, code 780.39 should be assigned. When the physician mentions a history of seizure in the workup but does not include any mention of seizures in the diagnostic statement, no code should be assigned unless there is clear documentation that the criteria for reporting the condition have been met and the physician agrees that a code should be added.

ICD-9-CM provides a fifth-digit subclassification for category **345, Epilepsy and recurrent seizures,** that permits identification of epilepsy as intractable when so described by the physician. In the absence of a specific statement to this effect, fifth digit 0 is assigned. The coder should not assume that the condition is intractable from general statements in the medical record.

Exercise 14.2

Code the following diagnoses and procedures. Do not assign E codes.

	Code(s)
1. Intractable epilepsy, grand mal type	345.11
Electroencephalogram	89.14
2. Psychomotor epilepsy	345.40
3. Intractable Jacksonian epilepsy	345.51
4. Intractable temporal lobe epilepsy	345.41
5. Febrile convulsions, recurrent	780.31
6. Psychosensory epilepsy, partial	345.40

HEMIPLEGIA/HEMIPARESIS

Hemiplegia is paralysis of one side of the body. It is classified to category 342, with a fifth digit to indicate whether the dominant or nondominant side is affected. Hemiplegia occurring in connection with a cerebrovascular accident (CVA) often clears quickly and is sometimes called a transient hemiplegia; no code is assigned when the paralysis clears before discharge. When hemiplegia is still present at the time of discharge, however, a code from category 342, Hemiplegia, is assigned as an additional code. When the patient is admitted at a later time with hemiplegia, code 438.2x is assigned to indicate that the condition is a late effect of a cerebrovascular accident. (See chapter 24 of this handbook for more discussion of cerebrovascular disease.)

Examples of appropriate coding for hemiplegia follow:

- Cerebral thrombosis with transient hemiplegia that has cleared by discharge 434.00
- Cerebral thrombosis with hemiplegia still present at discharge   434.00 + 342.90
- Hemiplegia of dominant side due to previous CVA   438.21
- Hemiparesis due to old spinal cord injury   342.90 + 907.2

PARKINSON'S DISEASE

Parkinson's disease, also known as Parkinsonism, is a chronic, progressive disorder of the central nervous system characterized by a fine, slowly spreading involuntary tremor, postural instability, and muscle weakness and rigidity. The fourth-digit axis for category **332, Parkinson's disease,** is based on whether the disease is primary (332.0) or secondary (332.1). Secondary Parkinson's disease is often an adverse effect of the therapeutic use of medication, in which case an E code to indicate the responsible drug is assigned as an additional code. Parkinson's disease is sometimes due to syphilis and in that case is coded to **094.82, Syphilitic Parkinsonism.**

AUTONOMIC DYSREFLEXIA

Autonomic dysreflexia is a syndrome characterized by an abrupt onset of excessively high blood pressure caused by an uncontrolled sympathetic nervous system discharge in persons with spinal cord injury, usually at or above the T6 level. Anything that would ordinarily cause pain below this level may trigger a parasympathetic response resulting in bradycardia, blurred vision, and sweating. True autonomic dysreflexia is potentially life-threatening and is considered a medical emergency. Code **337.3, Autonomic dysreflexia,** is used to report this condition. It is not necessary to code each manifestation or symptom separately. Unlike most dual coding where the underlying condition is listed first, in this case the code for the dysreflexia is sequenced first, with an additional code for the underlying chronic condition that has precipitated this life-threatening condition.

NARCOLEPSY

Narcolepsy is a chronic neurological disorder with inability to regulate sleep and wakefulness normally. Symptoms are excessive daytime sleepiness, sleep paralysis (paralysis upon falling asleep or waking up), cataplexy (sudden, brief episodes of paralysis or muscle weakness), and vivid hallucinations (vivid dream-like images that occur at sleep onset). Other possible symptoms are disturbed nighttime sleep, leg jerks, nightmares, and frequent awakenings. Irresistible sleep attacks may occur throughout the day regardless of the amount or quality of prior nighttime sleep. Affected individuals may fall asleep at work or school, or while eating, talking, or driving.

In about 10 percent of the cases, cataplexy is the first symptom to be recognized and may be misdiagnosed as a seizure disorder. The duration and intensity of cataplexy attacks vary. The milder attacks may be barely noticeable, such as a mild drooping of the eyelids, while the more severe attacks may result in total physical collapse. Cataplexy can occur spontaneously, but it is more often brought on by strong emotions such as laughter, anger, fear, or excitement.

The pathogenesis of narcolepsy is unclear, although recent gene research has discovered genes strongly associated with this disorder. It is currently believed that narcolepsy involves multiple factors interacting to cause neurological dysfunction and rapid eye movement (REM) sleep disturbances. *ICD-9-CM* distinguishes between subcategory 347.0 (narcolepsy) and 347.1 (narcolepsy in conditions classified elsewhere). When reporting subcategory 347.1, the underlying condition is coded first. In addition, fifth digits distinguish between narcolepsy with cataplexy (347.01, 347.11) and without cataplexy (347.00, 347.10).

Exercise 14.3

Code the following diagnoses.

	Code(s)
1. Parkinson's disease	332.0
2. Secondary Parkinsonism due to prescribed drug (Thorazine)	332.1 E939.1
3. Severe hypertension and pounding headache due to autonomic dysreflexia due to fecal impaction	337.3 + 560.39

DISORDERS OF THE PERIPHERAL NERVOUS SYSTEM

Disorders of the peripheral nervous system are classified to categories 350 through 359 according to the condition and the nerves involved. Many codes in this section are manifestations of other disease and are assigned as additional codes, with the underlying condition listed first.

CRITICAL ILLNESS POLYNEUROPATHY

Critical illness polyneuropathy is commonly associated with complications of sepsis and multiple organ failure. It is considered to be secondary to Systemic Inflammatory Response Syndrome (SIRS). Synonyms for critical illness polyneuropathy include: neuropathy of critical illness, intensive care unit (ICU) neuropathy, and intensive care polyneuropathy. Patients with this condition show abnormal electrophysiologic changes consistent with primary axonal degeneration of motor fibers. They also demonstrate severe weakness making it difficult to wean them from mechanical ventilation. Assign code **357.82, Critical illness polyneuropathy,** for this condition.

CRITICAL ILLNESS MYOPATHY

Critical illness myopathy is also associated with sepsis. It is a cause of difficulty in weaning patients from mechanical ventilation and prolonged recovery after illness. It is also associated with neuromuscular blocking agents and corticosteroids (in asthma and organ transplant patients), and neuropathy. Code **359.81, Critical illness myopathy,** is used to report this condition.

Exercise 14.4

Code the following diagnoses and procedures.

	Code(s)
1. Nephropathic amyloidosis	277.31
	583.81
2. Interdigital neuroma, 3–4 and 4–5 interspaces, left foot	355.6
Excision of Morton's neuroma, left foot	04.07
3. Tardy palsy due to entrapment of ulnar nerve	354.2
4. Peripheral polyneuritis, severe, due to chronic alcoholism	357.5
	303.90
5. Polyneuropathy in sarcoidosis	135
	357.4
6. Tic douloureux	350.1

DISORDERS OF THE EYE AND ADNEXAE

The classification for diseases of the eye is very detailed, and understanding the terminology used is especially important for the coder. Terms that seem similar may have entirely different meanings. The coder should be sure to fully understand the diagnostic statement in the medical record before assigning a code.

Visual impairment (369) is classified according to severity, with the status of the better eye listed first and the lesser eye listed second in the code title. Legal blindness in the United States is defined as severe or profound impairment of both eyes. Sample codes include the following:

- Better eye, profound impairment; lesser eye, near-total impairment   369.07
- Better eye, severe impairment; lesser eye, near-total impairment   369.13

Occasionally, visual problems can cause tilting of the head resulting in ocular torticollis or ocular-induced torticollis. Torticollis refers to abnormal head posture. Palsy of the superior or inferior oblique muscles will cause the patient to hold the head at an angle to compensate for the visual disturbance. Ocular torticollis is coded by assigning first the appropriate code for the ocular condition causing the torticollis, e.g. nystagmus (379.50), strabismus (378.9), fourth nerve palsy (378.53), etc., followed by code **781.93, Ocular torticollis.**

Corneal Injury

Code **370.24, Photokeratitis,** is assigned for a corneal flash burn, generally referred to as ultraviolet keratitis. This type of burn results from unprotected exposure to the sun or ultraviolet light, for example, the light from a welder's torch. It is always an injury; code **E926.2, Visible and ultraviolet light sources,** is assigned as an additional code.

Corneal or corneoscleral lacerations are classified in category **871, Open wound of the eyeball.** The fourth digits are assigned to indicate whether there is associated prolapse of intraocular tissue, whether it is a penetrating injury, whether it is with or without a magnetic foreign body, and whether it is related to other conditions. An E code is assigned for the external cause. Repair is classified as **11.51, Suture of corneal laceration.**

Conjunctivitis

Conjunctivitis is an inflammation of the conjunctiva that may be due to infection, allergy, or other cause. Giant papillary conjunctivitis (372.14) is an inflammation resulting from an allergic reaction to contact lenses. **Vernal conjunctivitis (372.13)** is due to an allergic reaction to pollen. Conjunctivitis due to Chlamydia is classified to 077.x or to 076.x when designated as trachoma.

Disorders of conjunctivochalasis are reported using code 372.81. This is a situation in which redundant conjunctiva lies over the lower eyelid margin and covers the lower punctum. It can create a variety of symptoms from aggravation of a dry eye at the mind stage, disruption of the normal flow of tears at the moderate state, and exposure problems of the severe stage. Treatment consists of a simple local surgical excision to relieve the symptoms. Code **370.34, Exposure keratoconjunctivitis,** is assigned for dry eye related to Bell's palsy. Code **375.15, Tear film insufficiency, unspecified,** is provided by the index for dry eye syndrome, a disorder of the lacrimal gland. Code 375.15, however, is inappropriate for the dry eye associated with Bell's palsy, which does not involve the lacrimal gland but is due to exposure to the air resulting from the inability to close the eye as a result of the acute severe facial paralysis of Bell's palsy.

Operations on Extraocular Muscles

Recession of an extraocular muscle involves temporary detachment of the muscle from the globe, followed by posterior movement along the surface of the eye and consequent lengthening of the muscle. During a resection, a piece of the muscle is taken out to shorten the muscle, which is then reattached at the original site.

The first axis for coding procedures involving recession and resection of the extraocular muscles is the number of muscles involved. When only one muscle is involved, code **15.11, Recession of one extraocular muscle,** or code **15.13, Resection of one extraocular muscle,** is assigned. When the procedure involves two or more muscles or when both resection and recession are carried out, code **15.3, Operations on two or more extraocular muscles,** is assigned. When either procedure is performed bilaterally, the code should be assigned twice.

Exercise 14.5

Code the following diagnoses and procedures. Do not assign E codes.

	Code(s)
1. Intermittent monocular esotropia	378.21
Recession of medial rectus muscle	15.11
2. Senile entropion, left	374.01
Repair entropion by suture technique	08.42
3. Blepharoptosis, congenital	743.61
Repair blepharoptosis, tarsal technique	08.35
4. Ectropion due to cicatrix	374.14

Exercise 14.5 *(continued)*

Blepharoplasty with extensive repair	08.44

5. Conjunctivochalasis	372.81

Cataracts

In coding cataracts the coder must avoid making assumptions about the type of cataract based on the patient's age or other conditions. A cataract in an older patient is not necessarily senile or mature; the coder should be alert to the terminology used in the diagnostic statement. Cataracts in patients with diabetes are most often senile; a true diabetic cataract is rare and its code should not be assigned unless the physician clearly identifies it as such.

Cataract extraction is coded according to the technique used. If an artificial lens is implanted at the same time the cataract is removed, codes are assigned for both procedures, with the cataract extraction sequenced first.

Exercise 14.6

Code the following diagnoses and procedures. Do not assign E codes.

	Code(s)
1. True diabetic cataract in type 1 diabetes mellitus	250.51 366.41
2. Incipient senile cataract, right eye Diabetes mellitus, type 2	366.12 250.00
Extracapsular cataract extraction, OD Intraocular lens implant insertion	13.59 13.71
3. Myotonic cataract with Thomsen's disease	359.2 366.43

Glaucoma

Glaucoma is an eye disease characterized by increased intraocular pressure that causes pathological changes in the optic disk and defects in the field of vision. Category **365, Glaucoma,** uses a fourth digit to classify glaucoma by type and a fifth digit to provide more specificity.

Aqueous misdirection was formerly known as malignant glaucoma. There is no true malignancy associated with this type of glaucoma. It is associated with fluid build up in the back of the eye, pushing the lens and iris forward, blocking off the drain and thereby increasing the intraocular pressure. This condition is extremely difficult to treat and often requires surgical intervention. Code **365.83, Aqueous misdirection,** is used to report this condition.

Exercise 14.7

Code the following diagnoses and procedures. Do not assign E codes.

	Code(s)
1. Glaucoma secondary to posterior dislocation of lens	379.34
	365.59
2. Exophthalmos secondary to thyrotoxicosis	242.00
	376.21
3. Acute narrow-angle glaucoma, OD	365.22
Chronic narrow-angle glaucoma, OS	365.23
Iridectomy with scleral fistulization	12.65
4. Primary open-angle glaucoma	365.11

DEAFNESS AND HEARING LOSS

Most hearing loss is classified in one of three ways:

- Conductive, with decrease due to a defect in the conductive apparatus of the ear (also called conduction deafness)

- Sensorineural, with the loss due to a defect in the sensory mechanism of the ear or nerves
- Mixed conductive and sensorineural hearing loss

Hearing Devices

Three major types of hearing devices are used to overcome hearing deficits:

- Externally worn battery-powered hearing aids
- Implantable bone conduction (electromagnetic) hearing devices
- Implantable cochlear prosthetic devices

The most widely used and least expensive of these is the externally worn battery-powered hearing aid, which includes a microphone, amplifier, and controls. It is commonly used to correct mild to moderate conductive hearing loss. Fitting of the hearing aid does not require surgical intervention and is coded 95.48.

The implantable bone conduction hearing device is implanted surgically on the surface of the mastoid bone. Although its circuitry is similar to the hearing aid in that it also contains a microphone, amplifier, and controls, it produces an electromagnetic inductive coil-energy transmission rather than a battery-powered amplification of sound. This device is used primarily for patients with a conductive hearing impairment (389.0x) who cannot use the battery-powered hearing aid and for whom a cochlear implant is not a viable option.

The cochlear implant is used for persons with profound sensorineural deafness (389.1x) that cannot be mitigated by the use of a modern, powerful hearing aid. Speech and sound information are transformed into electrical signals that create a perception of sound when they act on the fibers of the auditory nerve within the cochlea. The cochlear prosthesis is designed to stimulate the auditory nerve in a manner that exploits the ability of the cochlea and the central nervous system to discriminate the frequency, tempo, and intensity of ambient sound in ways that help the patient to recognize source and information content.

Cochlear implants incorporate a single channel (20.97) or multiple channels (20.98) of electrical information that is transmitted to the auditory nerve via one or more electrodes within the cochlea. The codes for this procedure include implantation of a complete device, with the receiver implanted into the skull and the electrodes into the cochlea. Replacement of the complete device is also assigned to codes 20.96 through 20.98. If only the internal coils and/or electrodes are replaced, code **20.99, Other operations on middle and inner ear**, should be assigned. Repair or removal of prosthetic device or electrodes without replacement is also classified as 20.99.

Review Exercise 14.8

Code the following diagnoses and procedures. Do not assign E codes.

	Code(s)
1. Congenital external canal <u>atresia</u>	744.02
2. Sudden hearing <u>loss</u> due to chlamydial <u>infection</u>	388.2 079.98

Review Exercise 14.8 *(continued)*

Implant of electromagnetic hearing device   20.95

---

3. Sensory hearing loss, bilateral   389.11

---

4. Sensorineural deafness, combined types, bilateral   389.18

Implant of multiple-channel cochlear device   20.98

---

5. Perforation of tympanic membrane due to acute   382.01
   suppurative otitis media

Coding Diseases of the Respiratory, Digestive, and Genitourinary Systems

15 Diseases of the Respiratory System

Except for neoplastic diseases and some major infectious diseases, respiratory diseases are classified in categories 460 through 519 in chapter 8 of *ICD-9-CM*. Note that Streptococcus and Neisseria are normal flora for the respiratory system; therefore, their presence does not indicate an infection unless they are seriously out of control. A respiratory infection cannot be assumed from a laboratory report alone; physician concurrence and documentation are necessary. Remember also that infectious organisms are not always identified by laboratory examination, particularly when antibiotic therapy has been started; an infection code may be assigned without laboratory evidence when it is supported by clinical documentation.

PNEUMONIA

Pneumonia is a common respiratory infection that is coded in several ways in *ICD-9-CM*. Combination codes that account for both pneumonia and the responsible organism are included in chapters 1 and 8 of *ICD-9-CM*. Examples of appropriate codes for pneumonia include the following:

- Pneumonia due to Klebsiella   482.0
- Pneumonia due to Staphylococcus aureus   482.41
- Salmonella pneumonia   003.22
- Postmeasles pneumonia   055.1
- Pneumonia with influenza   487.0

Other pneumonias are coded as manifestations of underlying infections classified in chapter 1, and two codes are required in such cases. Examples of this dual classification coding include the following:

- Pneumonia in anthrax   022.1 + 484.5
- Bronchial pneumonia in typhoid fever   002.0 + 484.8

When the diagnostic statement is pneumonia without any further specification, the coder should review laboratory reports for mention of the causative organism and check with the physician to determine whether there appears to be support for a more definitive diagnosis. When the organism is not identified, code **486, Pneumonia, organism unspecified,** is assigned.

Lobar Pneumonia

A diagnosis of pneumonia that mentions the affected lobe is not classified as lobar pneumonia unless specifically documented as such by the physician. A diagnosis of lobar pneumonia (481) does not refer to the lobe involved but to a particular type of pneumonia, which is usually caused by Streptococcus pneumoniae.

Interstitial Pneumonia

Interstitial pneumonia is characterized by interstitial fibrosis and the shedding of mononuclear cells within the alveolar spaces. If not more specifically identified, it is classified in *ICD-9-CM* as **516.8, Other specified alveolar and parietoalveolar pneumonopathies.** Bronchiolitis obliterans with organizing pneumonia (BOOP) is an interstitial lung disease that is diagnosed by pathological examination; it is also coded as 516.8.

Plasma cell interstitial pneumonia is an acute and highly contagious pneumonia caused by Pneumocystis carinii. It is coded as **136.3, Pneumocystosis.** This condition is frequently seen in patients with acquired immunodeficiency syndrome (AIDS) and is a major cause of death among AIDS patients. When associated with AIDS, code 042 is sequenced first with an additional code of 136.3. This type of pneumonia is not limited to patients with AIDS, however; it may develop in patients with immunocompromised states due to other causes, such as cancer, severe malnutrition, and debility. It may also occur in patients treated with certain types of immunosuppressive drugs after undergoing organ transplantation or cancer treatment. Never assume that this code should be assigned because the patient's condition is severe enough to warrant admission to the hospital. Interstitial pneumonia is classified as 136.3 only when specifically diagnosed by the physician as plasma cell pneumonia, pneumocystosis, or pneumonia caused by Pneumocystis carinii.

Legionnaires Disease

Legionnaires disease (482.84) is a type of pneumonia that is almost always caused by inhalation of aerosols that come from a contaminated water source. Legionnaires disease is often difficult to distinguish from other types of pneumonia. It is usually identified by the presence of bacteria in the sputum, by the presence of Legionella antigens in the urine, or by comparing Legionella antibody levels in two blood samples taken several weeks apart. Legionnaires disease accounts for about four percent of lethal nosocomial pneumonia, and about five to fifteen percent of known cases have been fatal. Because of the serious nature and frequent incidence of this disease, a separate code is provided for greater specificity—code **482.84, Other bacterial pneumonia, Legionnaires disease.** An additional code should be assigned for the responsible organism.

Gram–Negative Pneumonia

Gram-negative pneumonia NEC is classified as **482.83, Pneumonia due to other gram-negative bacteria;** or to 482.81 when it is specified as anaerobic. When the organism has been identified, the index may provide a more specific code. As discussed earlier, a gram-negative organism is one that develops a particular type of stain on testing and is considered part of a group of organisms that require careful management. Gram-positive pneumonia, not otherwise qualified, is classified as **482.9, Bacterial pneumonia unspecified.** This type of pneumonia is far easier to treat and requires the expenditure of fewer resources than the treatment of gram-negative pneumonia.

Gram-negative pneumonia usually appears as a complication of surgery, trauma, or chronic illness such as advanced carcinoma, cardiac failure, or alcoholism. It also is a common complication of chronic obstructive pulmonary disease and frequently follows treatment with immunosuppressive drugs or use of inhalation therapy apparatus.

Findings in a debilitated, chronically ill, or aged patient that might suggest a complicating gram-negative pneumonia include the following:

- Worsening of cough, dyspnea and reduction of oxygen level
- Fever

- Purulent sputum
- Patchy infiltrate on chest X-ray (in addition to previously noted densities caused by a primary underlying disease)
- Elevated leukocyte count

Note, however, that a diagnosis of gram-negative or other bacterial pneumonia cannot be assumed on the basis of the presence of any or all such findings; only the physician can determine the diagnosis. Such findings can, however, help document a diagnosis or could serve as the basis for a query to the doctor.

Aspergillosis

Pneumonia due to infectious aspergillosis is classified as code **117.3, Aspergillosis,** with an additional code of **484.6, Pneumonia in aspergillosis.** Allergic bronchopulmonary aspergillosis, however, occurs as an eosinophilic pneumonia caused by an allergic reaction to the aspergillosis fungus, commonly found on dead leaves, bird droppings, compost stacks, or other decaying vegetation. Code 518.6 is assigned for this allergic condition.

Aspiration Pneumonia

Aspiration pneumonia is a severe type of pneumonia resulting from the inhalation of foods, liquids, oils, vomitus, or micro-organisms from the upper respiratory tract or the oropharyngeal area. Pneumonitis due to inhalation of foods or vomitus is coded 507.0, with that due to inhalation of oils and essences as 507.1, and that due to inhalation of other solids or liquids to 507.8. Pneumonia due to aspiration of micro-organisms is classified as bacterial pneumonia in categories 480 through 483. Although aspiration pneumonia usually develops from one type of aspirated material, it is possible for both the type of pneumonia coded to category 507 and that coded to the 480 through 483 series to be present concurrently. Patients transferred from a nursing home to an acute-care hospital because of pneumonia are often suffering from aspiration pneumonia due to aspirated organisms, usually gram-negative bacteria.

Exercise 15.1

Code the following diagnoses. Do not assign E codes.

	Code(s)
1. Lobar pneumonia with influenza	487.0
2. Pneumonia, left upper lobe	486

Exercise 15.1 *(continued)*

3. Klebsiella pneumonia	482.0
4. Pneumonia due to fungus	117.9
	484.7
5. Acute lobar pneumonia	481
6. Perihilar viral pneumonia	480.9
7. Pneumonia due to Chlamydia	483.1
Intermittent positive-pressure breathing (IPPB)	93.91
8. Aspiration pneumonia due to aspiration of vomitus	507.0
9. Plasma cell interstitial pneumonia due to AIDS	042
	136.3
10. Pneumonia due to pulmonary coccidioidomycosis	114.0

SUPRAGLOTTITIS

Supraglottitis, which is also called epiglottitis, is an acute life-threatening upper respiratory infection. It seems to occur primarily in children but can be rapidly fatal in all ages. This fatal event appears to result from an edematous epiglottis that is obstructing the airway. It is an infection of the supraglottic structures that affects the lingual tonsillar areas, epiglottic folds, false vocal cords, and the epiglottis. Because the infection covers all the supraglottic structures, the term supraglottitis is nonspecific. Categories of 464, acute laryngitis and tracheitis, the larynx, the trachea, and the epiglottis have unique subcategories; the exception of acute laryngitis, with and without obstruction, is identified at the code level. The diagnosis supraglottitis may represent any of the codes within 464. A unique code for supraglottitis is provided for cases when the term is used and a specific site of infection is not identified. These codes are as follows:

- 464.0 Acute laryngitis
     464.00 without mention of obstruction
     464.01 with obstruction
- 464.5 Supraglottitis, unspecified
     464.50 without mention of obstruction
     464.51 with obstruction

CHRONIC OBSTRUCTIVE PULMONARY DISEASE

Chronic obstructive pulmonary disease (COPD) is a general term used to describe a variety of conditions that result in obstruction of the airway. The conditions that comprise COPD are:

- Chronic obstructive asthma   493.2x
- Chronic obstructive bronchitis   491.2x
- Emphysema   492.8
- Chronic bronchitis with emphysema   491.20

The correct coding of COPD depends on the accurate identification of the specific condition responsible for the airway obstruction, as well as on whether an acute condition, such as respiratory failure, is associated with it. When the diagnosis is stated only as COPD, the coder should review the medical record to determine whether a more definitive diagnosis is documented. Code **496, Chronic airway obstruction, not elsewhere classified,** is assigned only when the medical record documentation does not specify the type of COPD being treated and a more specific code cannot be assigned.

The conditions that make up COPD and asthma may sometimes overlap. Careful review of the conditions documented is necessary for accurate code selection. It is essential to review first the index and then verify the code selection in the Tabular List. Many instructional notes under the different COPD subcategories and codes provide guidance for code selection.

The medical record documentation may reveal varying degrees of severity of COPD. All of the following terms are coded to **491.21, Obstructive chronic bronchitis, With acute exacerbation:** COPD in exacerbation; severe COPD in exacerbation; endstage COPD in exacerbation; decompensated COPD; exacerbation of COPD; and acute exacerbation of chronic obstructive bronchitis.

Acute Bronchitis with Chronic Obstructive Bronchitis

A diagnosis of acute bronchitis with chronic obstructive bronchitis is assigned to code **491.22, Obstructive chronic bronchitis with acute bronchitis.** Code **466.0, Acute bronchitis,** is not assigned as an additional code. If the documentation indicates acute bronchitis with COPD with acute exacerbation, only code 491.22 is assigned. The acute bronchitis included in code 491.22 supersedes the acute exacerbation.

Asthma

Asthma is a bronchial hypersensitivity characterized by mucosal edema, constriction of bronchial musculature, and excessive viscid edema. Manifestations of asthma are wheezing, dyspnea out of proportion to exertion, and cough. A diagnosis of wheezing alone is not classified as asthma; code 786.07 would be assigned in such a case. Asthma is classified into category 493, with a fourth digit indicating the type of asthma and a fifth digit indicating whether status asthmaticus or exacerbation is present.

Status asthmaticus is defined in slightly different ways by different authorities, but in general it represents a patient who continues extreme wheezing in spite of conventional therapy or who has suffered from an acute asthmatic attack in which the degree of obstruction is not relieved by the usual therapeutic measures. Early status asthmaticus represents patients who are refractory to treatment or who fail to respond to the usual therapies; advanced status asthmaticus represents patients who show full development of an asthma attack that could result in respiratory failure, with signs and symptoms of hypercapnia (excess carbon dioxide in the blood). Fifth digit 1 is assigned for both types of status asthmaticus. Use of this fifth digit usually indicates a medical emergency for treatment of acute, severe asthma. Other terms used to describe status asthmaticus include the following:

- Intractable asthma attack
- Refractory asthma
- Severe, intractable wheezing
- Airway obstruction not relieved by bronchodilators
- Severe, prolonged asthmatic attack

The coder should never assume that status asthmaticus is present without a specific statement from the physician. However, asthma described as acute, characterized by prolonged or severe intractable wheezing, or asthma being treated by the administration of adrenal corticosteroids should alert the coder that status asthmaticus may exist and that the physician should be asked whether the diagnosis should be added.

Acute exacerbation of asthma refers to increased severity of the asthma symptoms, such as wheezing and shortness of breath. The fifth digit of "2" is used for asthma referred to as "exacerbated" or in "acute exacerbation."

Asthma characterized as obstructive or diagnosed in conjunction with COPD is classified as chronic obstructive asthma 493.2x. Other asthma is coded as 493.0x, 493.1x, 493.8x, or 493.9x. Fifth digits "0" for unspecified, "1" for status asthmaticus, and "2" indicating the asthma is in exacerbation or acute exacerbation, apply only to codes 493.0x, 493.1x and 493.9x. An asthma code with a fifth digit of "2," with acute exacerbation, may *not* be assigned with an asthma code with a fifth digit of "1," with status asthmaticus. Only the code with the fifth digit of "1" should be assigned.

A diagnosis of acute asthmatic bronchitis or asthmatic bronchitis without further specification is coded as 493.9x. If the diagnosis is stated as acute bronchitis with chronic obstructive asthma, code 493.2x is assigned. A diagnosis of chronic asthmatic bronchitis or asthmatic bronchitis with COPD is coded **493.2x, Chronic obstructive asthma.** Examples of coding for asthma include the following:

- Acute asthmatic bronchitis with status asthmaticus   493.91
- Childhood asthma   493.00
- Asthma with COPD   493.20
- Chronic asthmatic bronchitis with acute exacerbation   493.22
- Psychogenic asthma   <u>316</u> + 493.90

Bronchospasm

Bronchospasm is an integral part of asthma or any other type of chronic airway obstruction, but no additional code is assigned to indicate its presence. Code **519.11, Acute bronchospasm,** is assigned only when the underlying cause has not been identified.

Exercise 15.2

Code the following diagnoses. Do not assign E codes.

	Code(s)
1. Bronchial asthma, allergic, due to house dust	493.00
2. Chronic bronchitis with decompensated COPD	491.21
3. Acute exacerbation of chronic asthmatic bronchitis	493.22
4. Acute asthmatic bronchitis	493.90
5. Chronic obstructive lung disease with acute exacerbation	491.21
6. Chronic asthmatic bronchitis	493.20
7. Obstructive asthma with status asthmaticus	493.21
8. Acute bronchitis with acute bronchiectasis	494.1

ATELECTASIS

Atelectasis reduces the ventilatory function. Minor atelectasis is an integral part of pulmonary disease and is included in the code for associated lung disease. Pulmonary collapse can be a severe problem, but mild atelectasis usually has little effect on the patient's condition or the therapy provided. Slight strands of atelectasis are often noted on X-ray reports, but this finding is generally of little clinical importance and is usually not further evaluated or treated. Code **518.0, Pulmonary collapse,** should not be assigned on the basis of an X-ray finding alone; it should be coded only when the physician identifies it as a clinical condition that meets the criteria for a reportable diagnosis.

PLEURAL EFFUSION

Pleural effusion is an abnormal accumulation of fluid within the pleural spaces. It occurs in association with pulmonary disease and certain cardiac conditions, such as congestive heart failure, or certain diseases involving other organs. It is almost always integral to the underlying disease and is usually addressed only by treatment of that condition. In this situation, only the code for the underlying disease is assigned. However, occasionally the effusion is addressed separately, with additional diagnostic studies such as decubitus X-ray or diagnostic thoracentesis. The effusion may be treated by therapeutic thoracentesis, or chest-tube drainage. When treatment is addressed only to the pleural effusion, it can be designated as the principal diagnosis; otherwise, it can be assigned as an additional code when it is further evaluated or treated. Pleural effusion noted only on an X-ray report is not reported.

Pleural effusion due to tuberculosis is classified to 012.0x unless it is due to primary progressive tuberculosis (010.1x). When pleural effusion is due to another bacterial infection, code 511.1 is assigned, with an additional code for the responsible organism. Malignant pleural effusion (197.2) is classified as a secondary neoplasm of the pleura. Traumatic effusion is classified to code 862.39 if open wound; otherwise code 862.29 is assigned.

RESPIRATORY FAILURE

Respiratory failure is a life-threatening condition that is always due to an underlying condition. It may be the final pathway of a disease process, or a combination of different processes. Respiratory failure can result from either acute or chronic diseases that cause airway obstruction, parenchymal infiltration, or pulmonary edema. It can arise from an abnormality in any of the components of the respiratory system, central nervous system, peripheral nervous system, respiratory muscles, and chest wall muscles. The diagnosis is based largely on arterial blood gas analysis findings, which vary from individual to individual, depending on several factors. The coder should never assume a diagnosis of respiratory failure without a documented diagnosis by the physician. Respiratory failure is classified as acute (518.81), chronic (518.83), or acute and chronic combined (518.84). When respiratory failure follows surgery or trauma, code 518.5 is assigned.

Careful review of the medical record is required for the coding and sequencing of respiratory failure. The coder must review the circumstances of admission to determine the principal diagnosis. Code **518.81, Acute respiratory failure,** may be assigned as a principal diagnosis when it is the condition established after study to be chiefly responsible for occasioning the admission to the hospital, and the selection is supported by the Alphabetic Index and Tabular List. Respiratory failure may be listed as a secondary diagnosis if it develops after admission.

When a patient is admitted with respiratory failure and another acute condition, the principal diagnosis will depend on the individual patient's situation and what caused the admission of the patient to the hospital. The physician should be queried for clarification if the documentation is unclear as to which one of the two conditions was the reason for the admission. The guideline regarding two or more diagnoses' equally meeting the definition of principal diagnosis (Section II, C) may be applied in situations when both the respiratory failure and the other acute condition are equally responsible for occasioning the admission to the hospital.

Example 1:   A patient with chronic myasthenia gravis goes into acute exacerbation and develops acute respiratory failure. The patient is admitted due to the respiratory failure.

Principal diagnosis:	518.81	Acute respiratory failure
Secondary diagnosis:	358.01	Myasthenia gravis with (acute) exacerbation

Example 2:   A patient with emphysema develops acute respiratory failure. The patient is admitted through the emergency department for treatment of the respiratory failure.

Principal diagnosis:	518.81	Acute respiratory failure
Secondary diagnosis:	492.8	Other emphysema

Example 3:   A patient arrived in the hospital in acute respiratory failure. The patient was intubated, and the physician documents that the patient is being admitted to the hospital for treatment of the acute respiratory failure. The patient also has congestive heart failure.

Principal diagnosis:	518.81	Acute respiratory failure
Secondary diagnosis:	428.0	Congestive heart failure, unspecified

Some chapter-specific coding guidelines (e.g., obstetrics, poisoning, HIV, and newborn) provide sequencing direction. These guidelines would take precedence over code 518.81 when coding respiratory failure associated with a condition from one of these chapters.

Example 1:   A patient is admitted to the hospital postpartum as a result of developing pulmonary embolism leading to respiratory failure.

Principal diagnosis:	673.24	Obstetrical blood-clot embolism, postpartum condition or complication
Secondary diagnosis:	518.81	Acute respiratory failure

In this example, the obstetrical code is sequenced first because there is a chapter-specific guideline (Section I, C, 11, a, 1) that provides sequencing directions specifying that chapter 11 codes have sequencing priority over codes from other chapters.

Example 2:   A patient who is diagnosed as overdosing on crack is admitted to the hospital with respiratory failure.

Principal diagnosis:	970.8	Poisoning by other specified central nervous system stimulant
Secondary diagnosis:	518.81	Acute respiratory failure
	305.60	Nondependent abuse of drugs, Cocaine abuse, unspecified

In this example, poisoning is sequenced first because there is a chapter-specific guideline (Section I, C, 17, e, 2, d) that provides sequencing directions specifying that the poisoning code is sequenced first, followed by a code for the manifestation. The acute respiratory failure is a manifestation of the poisoning. This advice is consistent with information previously published in *Coding Clinic,* First Quarter 1993, page 25.

Example 3:   A patient is admitted with respiratory failure due to Pneumocystis carinii, which is due to AIDS.

Principal diagnosis:	042	Human immunodeficiency virus [HIV]
Secondary diagnosis:	518.81	Acute respiratory failure
	136.3	Pneumocystosis

In this example, the HIV is sequenced first because there is a chapter-specific guideline (Section I, C, 1, a, 2, a) that provides sequencing directions specifying that if a patient is admitted for an HIV-related condition (in this case the pneumocystis carinii), the principal diagnosis should be 042, followed by additional diagnosis codes for all reported HIV-related conditions.

In the event that instructional notes in the Tabular List provide sequencing direction, the sequencing of respiratory failure is dependent on these notes.

Example: A patient is admitted to the hospital with severe staphylococcus aureus sepsis and acute respiratory failure.

Principal diagnosis:	038.11	Staphylococcus aureus septicemia
Secondary diagnosis:	995.92	Severe sepsis
	518.81	Acute respiratory failure

Sepsis is sequenced first in this case because there is an instructional note under code 995.92 indicating to code first the underlying systemic infection. In addition, code 995.92 has a "use additional code" note to specify acute organ dysfunction and lists acute respiratory failure (518.81). This instruction means that respiratory failure would be a secondary diagnosis.

ADULT RESPIRATORY DISTRESS SYNDROME

Adult respiratory distress syndrome (ARDS) is an acute clinical-pathological state characterized by severe dyspnea, diffuse infiltrative lung lesions, and hypoxemia, with tachypnea and tachycardia present on physical examination. Treatment includes maintaining fluid balance, providing oxygen or ventilatory support, and treating the underlying condition. The condition is ordinarily a manifestation of an associated disease process and may occur following shock, surgery, or trauma. When it is due to infection, an additional code for the responsible organism should be assigned.

Adult respiratory distress syndrome following shock, surgery, or trauma is assigned to code 518.5. When neither trauma nor surgery is involved, it is classified as **518.82, Pulmonary insufficiency not elsewhere classified.** It is sometimes described as respiratory failure due to shock or trauma that occurs in lungs that were previously normal. It differs from respiratory failure in that pulmonary insufficiency does not imply that the respiratory system is completely unable to supply adequate oxygen to maintain metabolism and/or eliminate sufficient carbon dioxide to avoid respiratory failure. Terms such as shock lung, traumatic wet lung, white lung syndrome, and postperfusion lung also describe this condition.

Pulmonary insufficiency is implicit in asthma and various types of chronic obstructive pulmonary disease. In these conditions, it reflects the body's inability to excrete carbon dioxide rather than its failure to provide oxygen. It is included in the codes for those conditions; no additional code is assigned.

OTHER PULMONARY INSUFFICIENCY, NEC

Pulmonary insufficiency, not elsewhere classified, is a manifestation of another disease process, somewhat like respiratory failure. Unlike respiratory failure, however, it does not imply a complete inability of the respiratory system to supply adequate oxygen to maintain metabolism and/or eliminate sufficient carbon dioxide to avoid respiratory failure. It is an integral part of any COPD code, including such specific types as chronic obstructive bronchitis (491.2x), emphysema (492.x), chronic obstructive asthma (493.2x) or COPD not elsewhere classified (496). Code 518.82 is not assigned as an additional code.

ACUTE PULMONARY EDEMA

Acute pulmonary edema is a pathological state in which there is excessive, diffuse accumulation of fluid in the tissues and the alveolar spaces of the lung. It is broadly divided into two categories that reflect the origin of the condition: cardiogenic and noncardiogenic.

Cardiogenic

Acute pulmonary edema of cardiac origin is a manifestation of heart failure and as such is included in the following code assignments:

- Left ventricular failure   428.1
- Congestive heart failure   428.0
- Hypertensive heart disease   402.9x
- Rheumatic heart disease, acute   391.x
- Rheumatic heart failure (congestive)   398.91

Pulmonary edema is not included in the codes for acute myocardial infarction (410.10–410.92), acute or subacute ischemic heart disease (411.0–411.89), or coronary atherosclerosis (414.0x or 414.8). When pulmonary edema is present along with one of these conditions, the pulmonary edema is assumed to be associated with left ventricular failure (428.1) unless the heart failure is described as congestive or decompensated, in which case code **428.0, Congestive heart failure,** is assigned. Pulmonary edema is included in codes 428.x; no additional code is assigned.

Noncardiogenic

Noncardiogenic acute pulmonary edema occurs in the absence of heart failure or other heart disease. It is coded in a variety of ways, depending on the cause. When the cause is not specified, code **518.4, Acute edema of lung, unspecified,** is assigned. Postoperative pulmonary edema is also coded as 518.4.

Postradiation pulmonary edema (postradiation pneumonia) is an inflammation of the lungs due to the adverse effects of radiation. It is coded as **508.0, Acute pulmonary manifestations due to radiation.**

Acute pulmonary edema due to fumes and vapors is coded as 506.1. Acute pulmonary edema due to aspiration of water in a near-drowning is coded to **994.1, Drowning and nonfatal submersion;** other and unspecified effects of high altitude is coded as 993.2. Acute pulmonary edema in cases of drug overdose is classified as poisoning, with code 518.4 assigned as an additional code. Any mention of drug dependence or abuse should also be coded. E codes should be assigned with any of these codes to indicate the external circumstances involved.

Chronic pulmonary edema or pulmonary edema NOS that is not of cardiac origin is coded as **514, Pulmonary congestion and hypostasis,** unless the Alphabetic Index or the Tabular List instructs otherwise.

Pulmonary edema caused by congestive overloads, such as pulmonary fibrosis (515), congenital stenosis of the pulmonary veins (747.49), or pulmonary venous embolism (415.1x), is noncardiogenic. Such conditions are assigned to code 518.4 when described as acute or to code 514 when described as chronic or not otherwise specified. Be careful not to confuse this condition with edema associated with heart disease.

BIOPSIES OF BRONCHUS AND LUNG

An endoscopic biopsy of the bronchus (33.24) involves passing an endoscope into the lumen of the trachea and bronchus, where a bit of tissue is removed for pathological study. An endoscopic biopsy of the lung (33.27) goes through the main bronchus into the smaller bronchi and lung alveoli to perform a lung biopsy. Either type of biopsy can be performed independently, or both may be performed in the same operative episode, in which case both codes are assigned. Another type of lung biopsy is the thoracic wedge biopsy. In this procedure, small incisions are made into the chest wall and a thoracoscope is inserted through the incision in order to remove specimens for pathologic examination. This is coded as open biopsy of the lung (33.28); no code is assigned for the thoracoscopic approach.

Bronchoalveolar lavage (BAL), also called "liquid biopsy," should not be confused with whole lung lavage. BAL is a diagnostic procedure performed via a bronchoscope under local anesthesia. It involves washing out alveoli tissue and peripheral airways to obtain a small sampling of tissue. BAL is coded to **33.24, Closed [endoscopic] biopsy of bronchus.** Whole lung lavage is a therapeutic procedure performed for pulmonary alveolar proteinosis. The procedure is performed under general anesthesia and mechanical ventilation. The lungs are lavaged by filling and emptying one lung at a time with saline solution. The second lung is usually lavaged 3–7 days after the first lung. Report whole lung lavage using code **33.99, Other operations on lung.**

ABLATION OF LUNG

Tumor ablation is an alternative to surgical removal of lung lesions. Ablation can be achieved using extreme heat, freezing chemicals (cryoablation), focused ultrasound, microwaves, or radiofrequency. These procedures are typically performed by interventional radiologists using imaging guidance—such as computed tomography (CT), ultrasound, or fluoroscopy—and inserting a probe directly to the lesion.

ICD-9-CM procedure codes for ablation do not distinguish between the different energy sources used to ablate the tumor. Instead, the classification of ablation is arranged by the operative approach used, such as open (32.23), percutaneous (32.24), thoracoscopic (32.25), and other and unspecified (32.26).

MECHANICAL VENTILATION

Mechanical ventilation is a process by which the patient's own effort to breathe is augmented or replaced by the use of a mechanical device. With this kind of ventilatory assistance the patient either is intubated or undergoes a tracheostomy and receives assistance in an uninterrupted fashion. An endotracheal tube can be placed orally or nasally. If either intubation or tracheostomy is performed after admission, or in the emergency department of the same hospital immediately before admission, it should be reported. Intubation or tracheostomy carried out elsewhere prior to admission, or in an ambulance prior to arrival at the hospital, cannot be reported even though the ambulance may be operated by the same facility.

Codes for mechanical ventilation indicate whether the patient was on the ventilator for less than 96 consecutive hours (96.71) or more than 96 consecutive hours (96.72). The starting time for calculating the duration begins with one of these events:

- Endotracheal intubation performed in the hospital or hospital emergency room, followed by initiation of mechanical ventilation
- Initiation of mechanical ventilation through tracheostomy performed in the hospital or emergency room
- Admission of a patient who is already on mechanical ventilation after previous intubation or tracheostomy

A tracheal tube is often inserted to keep the tracheostomy open for attachment to the mechanical ventilator. Start counting hours on ventilation only after mechanical ventilation has actually been initiated.

It is occasionally necessary to replace an endotracheal tube because of a problem such as a leak; removal with immediate replacement is considered part of the duration and counting should continue. Patients who are started on mechanical ventilation by means of an endotracheal tube may later receive a tracheostomy through which the ventilation continues. Continue counting the number of hours the patient is on ventilation from the time the original intubation was initiated.

Once a patient's condition has stabilized and the patient no longer needs continuous ventilatory assistance, various weaning methods may be employed to allow the patient to gradually resume the work of breathing. During weaning, the patient is monitored for any evidence of cardiopulmonary instability. The period during which the weaning process takes place is counted as part of the duration time. Note that some patients do not require this weaning process.

Duration of mechanical ventilation ends with one of the following events:

- Removal of the endotracheal tube (extubation)
- Discontinuance of ventilation for patients with tracheostomy after any weaning period is completed
- Discharge or transfer while still on mechanical ventilation

Occasionally the condition of a patient who has been on ventilation earlier in the hospital stay deteriorates and a subsequent period of mechanical ventilation may be required. Use the guidelines above to calculate this additional period. In such cases, two codes from category 96.7x should be assigned.

When mechanical ventilation is utilized during surgery, it is not normally coded. However, if the patient requires mechanical ventilation for an extended period of time postoperatively, it may be coded. If the postoperative mechanical ventilation continues for more than two days, or if the physician has clearly documented an unexpected extended period of mechanical ventilation, the mechanical ventilation may be reported separately. The hours of mechanical ventilation should be counted starting from the point of intubation.

Other types of respiratory assistance not considered mechanical ventilation are continuous positive airway pressure (CPAP, 93.90), bilevel positive airway pressure (BiPAP,

93.90), intermittent positive-pressure breathing (IPPB, 93.91), noninvasive positive pressure ventilation (NIPPV, 93.90), and continuous negative-pressure ventilation (CNP, 93.99). The duration of treatment with these modalities does not affect code assignment.

Tracheostomy Complications

Complications of a tracheostomy are classified to subcategory 519.0 in chapter 8. Infection of a tracheostomy is classified to code 519.01, with an additional code to identify the type of infection and/or a code from category 041 to identify the organism. Mechanical complications are coded to 519.02; other complications, such as hemorrhage of tracheo-esophageal fistula due to the tracheostomy, are coded to 519.09.

Review Exercise 15.3

The following exercise provides examples of conditions classified in chapter 8 of *ICD-9-CM*. Code the following diagnoses and procedures. Do not assign E codes.

	Code(s)
1. Chronic left maxillary sinusitis	473.0
Left Caldwell-Luc sinusectomy	22.61
2. Acute upper respiratory infection due to Pneumococcus	465.9
Febrile convulsions	041.2
	780.31
3. Deviated nasal septum	470
Allergic rhinitis	477.9
Ethmoidal sinusitis	473.2
Submucous resection of nasal septum	21.5
4. Chronic pulmonary edema	514

Review Exercise 15.3 *(continued)*

5. Allergic rhinitis due to tree pollen   477.0

6. Congestive heart failure with pleural effusion   428.0

7. Acute respiratory failure due to intracerebral hemorrhage   431
                                                                            518.81

8. Acute pharyngitis due to Staphylococcus aureus   462
                                                                            041.11
                              Infection

9. Chronic chemical bronchitis due to inhalation of
   chlorine fumes   506.4

   Bronchoscopy with brush biopsy of bronchus   33.24

10. Total tension pneumothorax, spontaneous, left   512.0

Review Exercise 15.3 *(continued)*

11. Admitted in acute respiratory failure due to acute   518.81
    exacerbation of chronic obstructive bronchitis   491.21

12. Acute tracheobronchitis due to respiratory syncytial   466.0
    virus infection   079.6

13. Gram-negative pneumonia, anaerobic   482.81

14. Adult respiratory distress syndrome, due to shock   518.5

15. Acute respiratory distress syndrome due to   518.82
    hantavirus infection   079.81

16. Infected tracheostomy due to staphlyococcal   519.01
    abscess of the neck   682.1
                                                               041.10

16 Diseases of the Digestive System

Diseases of the digestive system are classified in chapter 9 of *ICD-9-CM*. The coding principles presented in previous chapters of this handbook apply throughout chapter 9. In addition, particular attention should be given to the use of combination codes and to the many exclusion notes in this chapter.

GASTROINTESTINAL HEMORRHAGE

Gastrointestinal (GI) bleeding manifests itself in several ways:

- Hematemesis (vomiting of blood), which indicates acute upper gastrointestinal hemorrhage
- Melena (presence of dark-colored blood in stool), which indicates upper or lower GI hemorrhage
- Occult bleeding (presence of blood in stool that can be seen only on laboratory examination), which indicates upper or lower GI bleeding
- Hematochezia (presence of bright-colored blood in stool), which indicates lower GI bleeding

The most common causes of GI bleeding are gastric and intestinal ulcers and diverticular disease of the intestine. A diverticular hemorrhage stops spontaneously in approximately 80 percent of cases, with the other 20 percent experiencing a second or third bleeding episode. *ICD-9-CM* provides fifth digits for gastrointestinal ulcers, gastritis, angiodysplasia, duodenitis, diverticulosis, and diverticulitis to indicate whether there is associated hemorrhage. For example:

- Acute gastritis with hemorrhage   535.01
- Diverticulitis with hemorrhage   562.13
- Angiodysplasia of duodenum with hemorrhage   537.83

Codes from category **578, Gastrointestinal hemorrhage,** are not assigned when codes for bleeding of any of the sites mentioned above are available. This category is acceptable only when the physician's diagnostic statement clearly states that the bleeding is due to another condition. Patients with a recent history of GI bleeding are sometimes seen for an endoscopy to determine the site of the bleeding, but do not demonstrate any bleeding during the examination. If the physician documents a clinical diagnosis based on the history or other evidence, the fact that no bleeding occurs during the episode of care does not preclude the assignment of a code that includes mention of hemorrhage, or a code from category 578 when the cause of bleeding could not be determined.

Occasionally, physician documentation may refer to GI bleeding and multiple GI-related endoscopic findings such as gastritis, duodenitis, esophagitis, diverticulosis (of colon), colon polyp, and so forth. If the physician does not link the GI bleeding with any specific condition, nor states that the GI bleeding is not due to these conditions, the physician needs to be queried to determine whether the GI bleeding was caused by any of the endoscopic findings. If the physician does not establish a causal relationship between the GI bleeding and the multiple findings, code **578.9, Hemorrhage of gastrointestinal tract, unspecified,** should be reported. In addition, codes for the multiple GI endoscopic findings without hemorrhage should be assigned as additional diagnoses. The combination codes describing hemorrhage should not be assigned unless the physician identifies a causal relationship. If the documentation provides more specific information and the bleeding is linked to a specific condition, assign the appropriate combination code with bleeding.

Patients may present for a colonoscopy because of rectal bleeding. If the findings include internal and external hemorrhoids with no statement as to whether the rectal bleeding is due to the hemorrhoids, the physician should be queried to determine whether the rectal bleeding is secondary to the hemorrhoids or if the hemorrhoids are an incidental finding. If the hemorrhoids are incidental findings and unrelated to the rectal bleeding, code **569.3, Hemorrhage of rectum and anus,** should be assigned followed by codes for the hemorrhoids without mention of complication. If, however, the physician establishes a causal relationship between the bleeding and the hemorrhoids, assign code **455.2, Internal hemorrhoids with other complication,** as the first-listed diagnosis. Code **455.5, External hemorrhoids with other complication,** should be assigned as a secondary diagnosis. Do not assign the combination code for hemorrhoids with bleeding unless the physician explicitly states a causal relationship.

ESOPHAGITIS

Esophagitis is classified to category code 530, with a variety of specific conditions. Acute esophagitis is classified to 530.12 and reflux esophagitis to 530.11. Ulcer of the esophagus without bleeding is classified to 530.20, while ulcer of the esophagus with bleeding is coded to 530.21, and dyskinesia of esophagus to 530.5.

Barrett's esophagus is a precancerous condition in which the normal cells of the lining of the esophagus are replaced by columnar cells. Code **530.85, Barrett's esophagus,** is used to uniquely report this condition.

Bleeding of the esophagus is coded as **530.82, Esophageal hemorrhage,** unless the bleeding is due to esophageal varices. Esophageal varices are not classified as a disease of the digestive system but as a disease of the circulatory system. They are coded as follows:

- Esophageal varices with bleeding   456.0
- Esophageal varices without mention of bleeding   456.1

When esophageal varices are associated with cirrhosis of the liver or portal hypertension, dual coding is required, with the underlying condition coded first. For example:

- Bleeding esophageal varices with cirrhosis of liver $\underline{571.5}$ + 456.20
- Bleeding esophageal varices in portal hypertension $\underline{572.3}$ + 456.20

Therapy for esophageal varices consists primarily of ligation (42.91) or endoscopic injection of a sclerosing agent (42.33). Diagnostic tests include esophageal motility studies classified as code **89.32, Esophageal manometry,** a test that is performed to rule out motor dysfunction of the esophagus, with particular attention to the competency of the gastroesophageal valve. Code 89.39, Other nonoperative measurements, is assigned for the pH esophageal monitoring test.

ULCERS OF THE STOMACH AND SMALL INTESTINE

Combination codes are provided for gastric, gastrojejunal and duodenal ulcers that indicate whether there is associated bleeding, associated perforation, or both. A fifth-digit subclassification indicates the presence or absence of obstruction that limits the ability of food or fluid to pass through the outlet of the stomach or the intestinal lumen. Such obstruction may be due to spasm, swelling, edema, and/or scarring.

Ulcers of the stomach and the small intestine are often described as peptic without any further identification of the site. The coder should review the medical record for any indication of the site involved; codes from category **533, Peptic ulcer, site unspecified,** should not be used when a more specific code can be assigned. Examples of appropriate coding include the following:

- Chronic gastric ulcer with obstruction   531.71
- Acute duodenal ulcer   532.30
- Gastric ulcer with hemorrhage and perforation   531.60

DIEULAFOY LESIONS

Dieulafoy lesions are a rare cause of major gastrointestinal bleeding. When gastrointestinal bleeding is present with Dieulafoy lesions, a separate code for the gastrointestinal bleeding would not be assigned because it is an integral part of the disease. Assign code 537.84 for Dieulafoy lesion of the stomach and duodenum and code 569.86 for Dieulafoy lesion of the intestine.

Code 530.82 would be assigned for Dieulafoy lesions of the esophagus. Dieulafoy lesions of the esophagus typically cause severe bleeding. Endoscopic adrenaline injections can be used to control the bleeding.

Exercise 16.1

Code the following diagnoses and procedures. Do not assign E codes.

	Code(s)
1. Acute gastric ulcer with massive gastrointestinal hemorrhage	531.00
Exploratory laparotomy with gastric resection, partial, with Billroth I anastomosis	43.6
2. Duodenal ulcer, with obstruction, perforation, and hemorrhage	532.61
3. Penetrating gastric ulcer	531.50
Subtotal gastrectomy with esophageal anastomosis Vagotomy	43.5 44.00
4. Bleeding gastric ulcer	531.40
Billroth II gastrectomy	43.7

COMPLICATIONS OF ESOPHAGOSTOMY AND GASTROSTOMY

Complications of an esophagostomy and gastrostomy are classified in chapter 9 rather than in the 996–999 series. Code 530.86 is assigned for an infection of the esophagostomy. An additional code would be assigned to specify the infection. Code 530.87 is assigned for a mechanical complication of the esophagostomy, such as malfunction.

The mechanical complication of a gastrostomy is assigned code 536.42. Code 536.41 is assigned for an infection of the gastrostomy. Additional codes would be assigned to specify the type of infection and the responsible organism if that information is available in the medical record.

COMPLICATIONS OF COLOSTOMY AND ENTEROSTOMY

Complications of colostomy or enterostomy procedures are classified as 569.6x. Codes from postoperative complication categories 996 through 999 are not assigned. For example:

- Malfunction of colostomy   569.62
- Cellulitis of abdominal wall due to complication of enterostomy   569.61 + 682.2

DIVERTICULOSIS AND DIVERTICULITIS

A diverticulum is a small pouch or sac opening from a tubular or saccular organ, such as the esophagus, intestine, or urinary bladder. Diverticulosis indicates the presence of one or more diverticula of the designated site; diverticulitis is the inflammation of existing diverticula. A diagnosis of diverticulitis assumes the presence of diverticula; only the code for diverticulitis is assigned, as indicated in the Alphabetic Index, even when both conditions are mentioned in the physician's diagnostic statement. Examples of appropriate coding include the following:

- Diverticulosis of duodenum   562.00
- Diverticulosis and diverticulitis of duodenum   562.01
- Diverticulitis of jejunum with hemorrhage   562.03
- Diverticulitis of cecum with abscess   562.11 + 569.5

ICD-9-CM assumes diverticulosis, not otherwise specified, to be a condition of the colon.

Congenital vs. Acquired Diverticula

Diverticula may be either acquired or congenital. For certain sites, *ICD-9-CM* assumes that the condition is congenital unless specified otherwise; in other sites, the presumption is that the diverticula are acquired. For example, diverticula of the colon are assumed to be acquired unless specified as congenital; but diverticula of the esophagus are assumed to be congenital unless otherwise specified. The Alphabetic Index (Volume 2) lists the following entries for diverticula of the colon and the esophagus:

Diverticula . . .   562.10 . . .
    colon (acquired)   562.10 . . .
        congenital   751.5 . . .
    esophagus (congenital)   750.4
        acquired   530.6 . . .
    Meckel's (displaced) (hypertrophic)   751.0

Acquired diverticula of the esophagus are often described by the type of diverticulum (pulsion or traction) or by the portion of the esophagus involved (pharyngoesophageal, midesophageal, or epiphrenic). These qualifications do not affect the code assignment; all are coded **530.6, Diverticulum of esophagus, acquired.** For example:

- Epiphrenic diverticula of esophagus   530.6
- Midesophageal traction diverticula of esophagus   530.6

DISEASES OF THE BILIARY SYSTEM

Acute and chronic cholecystitis without associated calculus is classified into category 575, with additional digits indicating whether it is acute (575.0), chronic (575.11), or both acute and chronic (575.12). Combination codes are assigned for cholecystitis, cholelithiasis, and choledocholithiasis to permit reporting these related conditions with a single code. These codes are presented in three groups: calculus of gallbladder (574.0–574.2), calculus of bile duct (574.3–574.5), and calculus of both gallbladder and bile ducts (574.6–574.9). Within each group, the fourth digit indicates whether there is associated cholecystitis and whether it is acute. Code 574.8 combines calculus of gallbladder and bile duct with both acute and chronic cholecystitis. Fifth digits indicate whether there is associated obstruction.

Codes **575.2, Obstruction of gallbladder,** and **576.2, Obstruction of bile duct,** are assigned only when there is obstruction but no calculi are present.

Cholesterolosis

Cholesterolosis is a condition characterized by abnormal deposits of cholesterol and other lipids in the lining of the gallbladder. In its diffuse form, it is known as strawberry gallbladder. This diagnosis is usually made by the pathologist on the basis of tissue examination and is ordinarily an incidental finding without clinical significance. It should not be coded when other gallbladder pathology is present.

Postcholecystectomy Syndrome

Postcholecystectomy syndrome (576.0) is a condition in which symptoms suggestive of biliary tract disease either persist or develop following cholecystectomy with no demonstrable cause or abnormality found on workup. A postoperative complication code from the 996 through 999 series is not assigned with code 576.0.

Cholecystectomy

A cholecystectomy (excision of the gallbladder) can be total or partial and can be performed either as an open procedure (51.21–51.22) or through a small, less-invasive laparoscopic incision (51.23–51.24). When coding a cholecystectomy, the coder should review the operative report to determine whether exploration or incision of the bile ducts was also performed for removal of stones (51.41) or for other relief of obstruction (51.42) as well as whether an intraoperative cholangiogram (87.53) was performed. Incision of the cystic duct is included in the basic procedure code.

Removal of Biliary Calculi

Biliary stones are removed in several ways. A cholecystectomy automatically removes any gallbladder calculus. Alternatively, a cholecystotomy (51.04) can be carried out for the removal of gallbladder stones without removing the gallbladder. Stones in the common duct can be removed percutaneously (51.96), by endoscopy (51.88), or by common duct exploration in connection with a cholecystectomy (51.41). Other biliary stones can also be removed percutaneously (51.98) or endoscopically (51.88).

Extracorporeal shock wave lithotripsy (98.52) destroys biliary stones without invasive surgery. The advantages of lithotripsy over conventional surgery for removal of stones include a shorter hospital stay and avoidance of the potential complications associated with surgical intervention.

Exercise 16.2

Code the following diagnoses and procedures. Do not assign E codes.

	Code(s)
1. Acute cholecystitis with calculus of gallbladder and bile duct	574.60
Laparoscopic cholecystectomy	51.23
2. Chronic cholecystitis with calculus in common duct	574.40
Cholecystectomy	51.22
Common bile duct exploration with removal of	51.41
common bile duct stone	87.53
Intraoperative cholangiogram	47.19
Incidental appendectomy	
3. Biliary obstruction, extrahepatic	576.2

Exercise 16.2 *(continued)*

4. Cholecystitis, acute and chronic, with cholesterolosis   575.12

   Total cholecystectomy   51.22

5. Acute cholecystitis with choledocholithiasis   574.30

6. Acute and chronic cholelithiasis with calculi in   574.90
   gallbladder and bile duct

7. Acute and chronic cholecystitis with gallbladder   574.81
   and bile duct calculus and obstruction

ADHESIONS

Intestinal and peritoneal adhesions are classified as code **568.0, Peritoneal adhesions** or as **560.81, Intestinal or peritoneal adhesions,** when obstruction is also present. These codes do not include pelvic peritoneal adhesions; such adhesions are classified as code **614.6, Pelvic peritoneal adhesion, female,** which also includes postoperative and postinfection adhesions.

Usually, minor adhesions do not cause symptoms or increase the difficulty of performing an operative procedure. When minor adhesions are easily lysed as part of another procedure, coding a diagnosis of adhesions and a lysis procedure is inappropriate. For example, there are often minor adhesions around the gallbladder that can be pushed aside easily without cutting during gallbladder surgery; coding of adhesions and/or lysis is not appropriate in such situations. Sometimes, however, a strong band of adhesions prevents the surgeon from gaining access to the organ to be removed, and a surgical lysis is required before the operation can proceed. In such cases, coding both the adhesions and lysis would be appropriate. If there is any question, the determination of whether the adhesions and the lysis are significant enough to merit coding must be made by the physician. Lysis of peritoneal adhesions can be performed by laparoscopy (54.51) or by an open procedure (54.59).

HERNIAS OF THE ABDOMINAL CAVITY

Hernias are classified by type and site, with combination codes used to indicate any associated gangrene or obstruction. With inguinal and femoral hernias, a fifth-digit subclassification indicates whether the hernia is unilateral or bilateral and whether it is specified as recurrent; that is, whether it had been repaired during a previous surgery. An incisional ventral hernia is classified as recurrent. Hernias described as incarcerated or strangulated are classified as obstructed. Careful review of the medical record and attention to instructional notes are important steps in coding these conditions. Coding examples include the following:

- Bilateral inguinal hernia with obstruction (no mention of gangrene)   550.12
- Unilateral recurrent inguinal hernia with gangrene   550.01
- Gangrenous femoral hernia, recurrent, bilateral   551.03
- Diaphragmatic hernia with gangrene   551.3
- Umbilical hernia with obstruction   552.1
- Incarcerated femoral hernia   552.00

When coding hernia repair, the coder should be careful not to use a bilateral repair code when the hernia itself is described as unilateral. A unilateral repair may be done even though bilateral hernias are present, but, obviously, it is impossible to repair bilateral hernias when only one hernia exists. Repair of inguinal hernias is further subdivided according to whether the hernia is direct or indirect, even though the diagnosis codes do not make this distinction. A direct hernia is one with protrusion through the abdominal wall; an indirect hernia protrudes through the inguinal ring only. Hernia repair codes also make a distinction between simple repairs and those repairs in which a graft or prosthesis (for example, mesh) is used to reinforce the repair. In coding repair of a diaphragmatic (esophageal or hiatal) hernia, the axis for the code is whether an abdominal or thoracic approach was used.

Coding examples include:

- Repair of unilateral direct inguinal hernia   53.01
- Repair of unilateral direct inguinal hernia with mesh prosthesis   53.03
- Repair of bilateral indirect inguinal hernias   53.12

Exercise 16.3

Code the following diagnoses and procedures. Do not assign E codes.

	Code(s)
1. Right direct inguinal hernia and left indirect sliding inguinal hernia	550.92
Repair of right direct and left indirect inguinal hernias	53.13

Exercise 16.3 *(continued)*

2. Incarcerated left inguinal hernia   550.10

Left indirect inguinal herniorrhaphy with mesh prosthesis   53.04

3. Recurrent left inguinal hernia   550.91

Repair of indirect inguinal hernia, left   53.02

4. Gangrenous umbilical hernia   551.1

Repair of umbilical hernia   53.49

5. Strangulated umbilical hernia   552.1

Repair of umbilical hernia with mesh prosthesis   53.41

Exercise 16.3 *(continued)*

---

6. Reflux <u>esophagitis</u> secondary to sliding   530.11
   esophageal hiatal <u>hernia</u>   553.3

   <u>Repair</u> of esophageal hiatus hernia, abdominal approach   53.7

---

7. Recurrent ventral incisional <u>hernia</u> with obstruction   551.21
   and gangrene

APPENDICITIS

Category **540, Acute appendicitis,** uses a fourth digit to indicate the presence of either generalized peritonitis (540.0) or peritoneal abscess (540.1). If both are listed in the diagnostic statement, only code 540.1 is assigned, as acute appendicitis often progresses to peritoneal abscess. Occasionally, an appendix ruptures during an appendectomy; this is not classified as a complication of surgery.

Category **541, Appendicitis, unqualified,** is a vague code that should not be used in an acute care facility. Additional information is almost always available in the medical record.

Surgical removal of a diseased appendix is coded **47.0x, Appendectomy.** Code **47.1x, Incidental appendectomy,** is used when the appendix is removed as a routine prophylactic measure in the course of other abdominal surgery. It should not be assigned when there is a diagnosis of significant appendiceal pathology. If the appendix is removed by means of exploratory laparotomy and no other therapeutic procedure is performed, code 47.09 should be assigned even though the appendix may not demonstrate any pathology on tissue examination. No code is assigned for the approach.

DIARRHEA

A code from categories 001 through 008 is assigned for infectious diarrhea when the organism has been identified. Code 009.2 is assigned for infectious diarrhea not otherwise specified, or described only as dysenteric diarrhea or epidemic diarrhea. Code 009.3 is provided for diarrhea presumed to be of infectious origin, but it does not apply in the United States and would be assigned only on the basis of the physician's specific statement. Check the Alphabetic Index carefully before coding, because diarrhea can be related to a variety of conditions. Symptom code 787.91 is assigned for diarrhea for which no appropriate subterm can be located. Note that the main term for diarrhea is followed by a long list of nonessential modifiers. Examples of appropriate code assignments include the following:

- Diarrhea due to Giardia   007.1
- Acute diarrhea   787.91
- Coccidian diarrhea   007.2
- Chronic ulcerative diarrhea   556.9
- Infantile diarrhea   787.91
- Functional diarrhea   564.5

CONSTIPATION

There is a single code for constipation (564.00), but there are two distinct subtypes recognized: slow transit constipation (564.01) and outlet dysfunction constipation (564.02). The slow transit results from a delay in transit of fecal material throughout the colon secondary to smooth muscle. The latter results from difficulty evacuating the rectum during attempts at defecation. Treatment for these two types is very different. The slow transit type is treated with either laxatives or surgery. Biofeedback is taught for relaxation for the outlet dysfunction constipation.

REDUCTION OF INTUSSUSCEPTION

Intussusception, primarily a disease of young children, is the prolapse of one part of the intestine into the lumen of an immediately adjacent part, resulting in intestinal obstruction. The most common therapy is reduction by using a fluoroscopically controlled hydrostatic barium enema. Air has recently become an alternative to barium as the contrast agent of choice and ionizing radiation enemas may also be used. An ultrasound-guided reduction is now being used in some institutions. In this type of reduction the condition is first diagnosed sonographically with the reduction carried out by means of a normal saline enema under ultrasound guidance. Code 96.29 is assigned for all these reductions; no additional code is assigned for either the fluoroscopic or ultrasound guidance. If these noninvasive procedures are not effective, surgical intervention may be required.

Review Exercise 16.4

Code the following diagnoses and procedures. Do not assign E codes.

	Code(s)
1. Acute ruptured appendicitis with postoperative paralytic ileus	540.0 997.4 560.1
Appendectomy	47.09

Review Exercise 16.4 *(continued)*

---

2. Acute hepatitis and early cirrhosis of the liver   571.1
        due to chronic alcoholism   571.2

                                                                303.90

---

3. Anorectal cryptitis, chronic   569.49

    Cryptectomy   49.39

---

4. Perirectal abscess   566
    Atony of colon   564.89

    Incision and drainage of perirectal abscess   48.81

---

5. Hepatic coma with massive ascites secondary to   572.2
    Laennec's cirrhosis   571.2

                                                        789.5

---

6. Intestinal obstruction due to peritoneal adhesive band   560.81

    Lysis of adhesive band   54.59

---

7. Diverticulosis and diverticulitis of right colon   562.11

Review Exercise 16.4 *(continued)*

Right <u>hemicolectomy</u> with end-to-end anastomosis	45.73

8. <u>Infection</u> of <u>gastrostomy</u> with abscess of abdominal wall due to Streptococcus B	<u>536.41</u> 682.2 041.02

9. <u>Polyp</u> of rectum	569.0

Colonoscopy with <u>polypectomy</u>	48.36

10. Neurogenic <u>bowel</u>	564.81

17 Diseases of the Genitourinary System

Diseases of the genitourinary system are classified in chapter 10 of *ICD-9-CM*, except those that are classified by etiology, such as certain easily transmissible infections, neoplastic diseases, and conditions complicating pregnancy, childbirth, and the puerperium. Subterms should be checked carefully in the Alphabetic Index, and special attention should be given to the terms "urethra" and "ureter," which are often confused by coders.

INFECTIONS OF THE GENITOURINARY TRACT

Physicians often use the term "urinary tract infection (UTI)" when referring to conditions such as urethritis, cystitis, or pyelonephritis. Urethritis and cystitis are lower urinary tract infections; pyelonephritis is an infection of the upper urinary tract infection. The main term for the specific condition should be referred to the Alphabetic Index before referring to the main term **Infection.** For example, under the main term cystitis, subterms are located for diphtheritis (032.840) and chlamydial (099.53) infection. There is also a subterm for amebic cystitis that indicates dual coding (006.8 + 595.4).

When there is no subterm for the organism the code for the condition is assigned, with an additional code from category 041 or 079 to indicate the organism. For example, there is no subterm for E. coli under the main term for cystitis; therefore codes 595.0 and 041.4 are assigned for cystitis due to E. coli.

The following examples indicate complete coding for such infections:

- Cystitis due to Trichomonas   131.09
- Acute cystitis due to Proteus infection   595.0 + 041.6
- Chronic pyelonephritis due to E. coli   590.00 + 041.4

Urinary tract infections that develop following surgery are rarely true postoperative infections and are not usually classified as such. When the operative procedure involves the urinary tract, however, it may be appropriate for the coder to ask the physician whether the infection is related to the procedure. When the infection is related to the presence of an implant, graft, or device (such as an indwelling catheter), code 996.6x is assigned. In the absence of documentation indicating that the infection is due to the surgical procedure, code **599.0, Urinary tract infection,** not otherwise specified, should be assigned.

Exercise 17.1

Code the following diagnoses and procedures. Do not assign E codes.

	Code(s)
1. Urethral stricture due to gonorrheal infection	098.2
	598.01

Exercise 17.1 *(continued)*

Urethral dilation	58.6

2. Abscess of right scrotum due to group B	608.4
Streptococcus	041.02

Incision and drainage of scrotal abscess	61.0

3. Acute pyelonephritis due to Helicobacter pylori	590.10
Infection	041.86

4. Chronic cystitis	595.2
Pseudomonas infection	041.7

5. Chronic cystitis due to Monilia infection	112.2

6. Urinary tract infection due to candidiasis	112.2

HEMATURIA

Many genitourinary conditions have hematuria as an integral associated symptom. For example, the medical record has a diagnostic statement of hematuria due to renal calculus but only a code of **592.0, Calculus of kidney,** is assigned. The hematuria is integral to this condition and no additional code is assigned. Blood in the urine discovered on laboratory examination is not coded as hematuria but as **791.2, Hemoglobinuria,** an abnormal finding. It is reported only when the physician has indicated its clinical significance. A certain amount of hematuria is expected following a urinary tract procedure or a prostatectomy. It is not considered a postoperative complication, and no code is assigned unless the bleeding is excessive or persistent.

URINARY INCONTINENCE

Stress incontinence causes involuntary urine loss with physical strain such as coughing or sneezing. Although it occurs in both male and female patients, it occurs more frequently in women, typically as a result of physical changes brought on by earlier childbearing. Stress incontinence in female patients is coded as **625.6, Stress incontinence, female;** in male patients it is assigned code **788.32, Stress incontinence, male.** Prostate surgery is the primary cause of incontinence in men.

Other types of incontinence are also classified into subcategory 788, **Symptoms involving urinary system.** When more than one type of incontinence is present, it is classified as mixed incontinence (male) (female), and code 788.33 is assigned. When the underlying cause of incontinence is known, the code for that condition should be sequenced first.

Treatment for incontinence depends, to a large extent, on the particular type of incontinence present. If it is due to an intrinsic sphincter deficiency, collagen injections are sometimes carried out. Code **59.72, Injection of implant into urethra and/or bladder neck,** is assigned for this therapy.

Other treatments for incontinence are surgical in nature. Codes for repair of incontinence depend on the procedure performed. Examples of these procedure codes are:

- 59.3   Plication of urethrovesical junction
- 59.4   Suprapubic sling operation
- 59.5   Retropubic urethral suspension
- 59.6   Paraurethral suspension
- 59.71 Levator muscle operation for urethrovesical suspension
- 59.79 Other repair of urinary stress incontinence

RENAL DISEASE

Renal disease is classified into categories 580 through 593. Glomerulonephritis is a type of nephritis in which there is bilateral inflammatory change without infection. Nephrotic syndrome is a complex clinical state characterized by edema, albuminuria, and increased permeability of the glomerular capillary basement membrane. The syndrome can result from an unknown cause, or it may result from glomerulonephritis or diseases such as diabetes, systemic lupus erythematosus, hypertension, and amyloidosis. Nephropathy is a general term that indicates that renal disease is present. Infection of the kidney is classified to 590.x. Renal disease complicating pregnancy, labor, and the puerperium is reclassified in chapter 11 of *ICD-9-CM.*

Chronic Kidney Disease and End–Stage Renal Disease

Chronic kidney disease (CKD) is considered a more current and precise term than chronic renal failure or chronic renal insufficiency. CKD develops as a complication of other diseases, such as diabetes mellitus, primary hypertension, glomerulonephritis, nephrosis, interstitial nephritis, systemic lupus erythematosus, obstructive uropathy, and polycystic kidney disease. The sequencing of the CKD code in relationship to codes for other contributing conditions is based on the conventions of the Tabular List.

Patients usually live for many years with such chronic kidney disease. When kidney involvement becomes so extensive that kidney function can no longer keep up with the body's needs, dialysis is usually required.

ICD-9-CM classifies CKD on the basis of severity. Based on the glomerular filtration rate (GFR), chronic kidney disease has been categorized into five stages. Category 585, **Chronic kidney disease (CKD),** has been expanded to the fourth-digit subcategory level for further specification of the varying stages of chronic kidney disease. The new fourth-digit subcategory codes are as follows:

- 585.1   Chronic kidney disease, Stage I
- 585.2   Chronic kidney disease, Stage II (mild)
- 585.3   Chronic kidney disease, Stage III (moderate)
- 585.4   Chronic kidney disease, Stage IV (severe)
- 585.5   Chronic kidney disease, Stage V

End-stage renal disease (585.6) is a complex syndrome characterized by a variable and inconsistent group of biochemical and clinical changes that affect volume regulation, acid-base balance, electrolyte balance, excretion of waste products, and several endocrine functions. It is a progression of chronic kidney disease and is defined by clinicians as the point at which regular dialysis sessions or a kidney transplant is required to maintain life. Chronic renal failure not otherwise specified and chronic renal insufficiency are both assigned code

585.9, Chronic kidney disease, unspecified. If both a stage of CKD and end-stage renal disease (ESRD) are documented for the same patient, only code 585.6 would be assigned.

Kidney transplant may be recommended for patients with severe CKD caused by severe, uncontrollable hypertension, infections, diabetes mellitus, or glomerulonephritis. Patients who have undergone kidney transplant may still have some form of CKD because the kidney transplant may not fully restore kidney function. Code V42.0 may be assigned with the appropriate CKD code to indicate that a CKD patient is status post kidney transplant. It is incorrect to assume that mild or moderate CKD following a transplant is a transplant failure unless it is documented as such in the medical record. If transplant failure is documented in patients with severe CKD or ESRD, **code 996.81, Complications of transplanted organ, kidney,** is assigned. If a post kidney transplant patient has CKD, and the documentation is unclear whether there is transplant failure or rejection, it is necessary to query the provider.

Acute Renal Failure

Acute renal failure (584.x) is very different from chronic kidney disease; it is not a phase of the same condition. Chronic kidney disease is a long-term inability of the kidneys to function adequately; acute renal failure is the sudden cessation of renal function following severe insult to normal kidneys. Toxic agents, traumatic or surgical shock, tissue destruction due to injury or surgery, or a variety of other conditions can cause acute renal failure.

Acute renal insufficiency (593.9) is considered an early stage of renal impairment, evidenced by diminished creatinine clearance or mildly elevated serum creatinine or BUN. Clinical symptoms or other abnormal laboratory findings may or may not be present but are usually minimal. Treatment varies, depending on the underlying cause, but serious attention is given to prevent its progression to renal failure. Code **997.5, Urinary complications,** is assigned if renal insufficiency is due to a procedure.

Physicians sometimes use the terms renal insufficiency and renal failure interchangeably. *ICD-9-CM* identifies acute renal insufficiency with code 593.9 and chronic renal insufficiency with code 585.9. Acute renal failure is identified with category 584, chronic kidney disease with category 585, and unspecified renal failure with code 586. It is important for the coder to be guided by the classification. If the physician uses both terms in the medical record, the physician should be queried for clarification as to the correct diagnosis.

Kidney Disease with Hypertension

ICD-9-CM presumes a relationship when a patient has both chronic kidney disease and hypertension, and category **403, Hypertensive kidney disease,** or category **404, Hypertensive heart and kidney disease,** should be assigned. The fifth digit indicates the stage of chronic kidney disease as follows:

- Category 403
  —Fifth digit of 0 is for "chronic kidney disease stage I through stage IV, or unspecified"
  —Fifth digit of 1 is for "chronic kidney disease stage V or end-stage renal disease"
- Category 404
  —Fifth digit of 0 is for "without heart failure and with chronic kidney disease stage I through stage IV, or unspecified"
  —Fifth digit of 1 is for "with heart failure and with chronic kidney disease stage I through stage IV, or unspecified"
  —Fifth digit of 2 is for "without heart failure and with chronic kidney disease stage V or end-stage renal disease"
  —Fifth digit of 3 is for "with heart failure and with chronic kidney disease stage V or end-stage renal disease"

Codes 403.x0, 404.x0, and 404.x1 require an additional code from 585.1–585.4, 585.9 to identify the specific stage of CKD. Codes 403.x1, 404.x2, and 404.x3 require an additional code of 585.5 or 585.6 to identify the specific stage of CKD.

Acute renal failure is not caused by hypertension and is not included in the hypertensive kidney disease codes. When acute renal failure and hypertension are both present, assign a code from category **584, Acute renal failure,** with an additional code for the hypertension.

The use of codes from categories 403 and 404 does not apply in the following situations:

- The renal condition is acute renal failure.
- The hypertension is described as secondary.
- The kidney disease is specifically stated as due to a cause other than hypertension.

Examples of appropriate codes for kidney disease with hypertension include the following:

- Hypertensive kidney disease with chronic kidney disease   403.90 + 585.9
- Hypertensive heart and kidney disease with chronic kidney disease   404.90 + 585.9
- Hypertensive heart and kidney disease with stage V chronic kidney disease and congestive heart failure   404.93 + 585.5 + 428.0
- Acute renal failure; hypertension   584.9 + 401.9

Kidney Disease with Diabetes Mellitus

Diabetic nephropathy is coded as **250.4x, Diabetes with renal manifestations.** A manifestation code is assigned as an additional code to indicate the specific kidney condition, such as glomerulosclerosis, arteriolar nephrosclerosis, chronic interstitial nephritis, papillary necrosis, other tubular lesions, or chronic kidney disease.

Kidney disease sometimes results from both hypertension and diabetes mellitus. In this situation, the combination code from category 403 or category 404 and a code from subcategory 250.4x are assigned. A code from category 585 is assigned to identify the manifestation as chronic kidney disease.

Examples of appropriate codes for kidney disease due to diabetes include the following:

- Diabetic nephrosis   250.40 + 581.81
- Chronic kidney disease due to hypertension and type 1 diabetes mellitus 403.90 + 250.41 + 585.9
- Chronic kidney disease, unspecified due to type 1 diabetic nephropathy 250.41 + 585.9 (+ 583.81 optional)

In the last example, the code for the intervening nephropathy leading to chronic kidney disease can be assigned, but it is not required.

RENAL DIALYSIS

Patients with end-stage renal disease require a regular schedule of dialysis treatments to manage the symptoms arising from kidney disease. They may be admitted to the hospital or seen as outpatients for the sole purpose of dialysis. Code **V56.0, Admission for extracorporeal dialysis (hemodialysis),** or code **V56.8, Admission for other dialysis (peritoneal),** is assigned as the principal diagnosis for such admissions, with an additional code for the kidney disease. If the patient is admitted for other reasons but continues to receive dialysis therapy during the hospital stay, or is known to be maintained on renal dialysis, code **V45.1, Renal dialysis status,** may be assigned as an additional code; the condition responsible for the admission is designated as the principal diagnosis. Code V56.0 may only be used as a principal or first-listed diagnosis code.

The performance of hemodialysis requires the insertion of a venous catheter (38.95) or a totally implantable venous access device (86.07); the associated dialysis is coded **39.95, Hemodialysis.** Peritoneal dialysis is accomplished by instilling a prepared fluid into the peritoneal cavity and removing the uremic toxins along with the prepared fluid. Insertion of a Tenckhoff catheter for this purpose is coded **54.93, Creation of a cutaneoperitoneal fistula;** code **54.98, Peritoneal dialysis,** is assigned for the associated dialysis.

Patients are sometimes admitted for insertion of a catheter or a vascular access device, but no dialysis is performed during the admission. In this case, the condition is coded as the principal diagnosis, and code V56.x is not assigned. When dialysis is performed during the same episode of care, procedure code 39.95 is assigned to specify that the dialysis was actually performed during the encounter. When the admission is for fitting or adjustment of the dialysis catheter, code V56.1 is assigned for an extracorporeal catheter and V56.2 for a peritoneal catheter. If concurrent dialysis is performed, procedure code 39.95 is assigned. Some coding examples follow:

- Patient with end-stage renal disease admitted for insertion of Hickman catheter for renal dialysis (no dialysis performed)   585.6 + 38.95
- Patient with chronic kidney disease, stage V, admitted for hemodialysis   V56.0 + 585.5 + 39.95
- Patient with unspecified chronic kidney disease admitted for creation of AV fistula for renal dialysis; dialysis not performed on this admission   585.9 + 39.27

Patients frequently develop complications as a result of dialysis therapy. Dialysis dementia due to an overload of aluminum from the water used in the procedure is classified as poisoning. Code **985.8, Toxic effect of other metals,** is assigned as the principal diagnosis, with **294.8, Other persistent mental disorders due to conditions classified elsewhere,** or **293.9, Unspecified transient mental disorder in conditions classified elsewhere,** assigned as an additional code.

When dialysis dementia is diagnosed without any reference to aluminum intoxication, code 294.8 is assigned. Dialysis disequilibrium without associated dementia is coded to **276.9, Electrolyte and fluid disorder, not elsewhere classified.** External cause code E879.1 is assigned with any of these codes to indicate that the condition is the result of kidney dialysis. If the complication is the reason for admission, the code for the complication is sequenced first as the principal diagnosis, with an additional code for the chronic kidney disease.

It normally takes two to three months for an arteriovenous fistula to mature. A nonmaturing or nondeveloping fistula is considered a mechanical complication and is coded to **996.1, Mechanical complication of other vascular device, implant, and graft.** Primary causes of a nonmaturing fistula are narrowing of a vein or multiple competing veins. Treatment may consist of performing an arteriovenostomy to create a new arteriovenous fistula (39.27). Other treatment options may be performed by interventional radiologists—such as balloon angioplasty; revision of AV fistula; and/or closing off competing veins, which can be performed using various techniques.

Exercise 17.2

Code the following diagnoses and procedures. Assign E codes as appropriate.

	Code(s)
1. End-stage renal disease	585.6
Peritoneal dialysis	54.98
2. Dialysis disequilibrium with acute delirium	276.9
	293.0
	V45.1
	E879.1

CYSTOSCOPY AS OPERATIVE APPROACH

Cystoscopy is used as the approach for many procedures performed in diagnosing and treating urinary tract conditions; no code is assigned for the cystoscopic approach. A transurethral approach (TUR) is indicated by the title of the procedure and is included in the code.

REMOVAL OF URINARY CALCULUS

Urinary calculi are relatively common and often pass without surgery. Several types of surgical techniques are used when intervention is necessary. Extracorporeal shock wave lithotripsy (ESWL) of the kidney, ureter and/or bladder (98.51) reduces the stones to a slush that can be excreted over a short period of time. This code includes removal of stones from any area in the urinary system, including those in a Koch pouch. Ultrasound destruction of bladder calculi uses two codes, **57.0, Transurethral clearance of the bladder,** and **59.95, Ultrasound fragmentation of urinary stones.** Kidney stones can be removed by percutaneous nephrostomy with fragmentation (55.04) or without fragmentation (55.03). Transurethral ureteroscopic lithotripsy with fragmentation of stones (56.0) removes calculi from the ureter and renal pelvis.

A two-step procedure is sometimes used when it is necessary to manipulate a ureteral stone back into the renal pelvis in order to remove it. This procedure involves the insertion of a ureteral catheter (59.8) for manipulation, followed by either percutaneous nephrostomy with fragmentation of stones (55.04), or by extracorporeal shock wave lithotripsy (98.51).

Exercise 17.3

Code the following diagnoses and procedures. Do not assign E codes.

	Code(s)
1. Right ureteral calculus	592.1
Right calyceal diverticulum	593.89
Left renal cyst, solitary (acquired)	593.2
2. Impacted renal calculus with medullary sponge kidney	592.0 753.17
Extracorporeal shock wave lithotripsy of kidney calculus	98.51
3. Calculus in bladder	594.1
Lithotripsy of urinary bladder with ultrasonic fragmentation	57.0 + 59.95

PROSTATE DISEASE AND THERAPY

Diseases of the male genital organs are classified in categories 600–608, with conditions of the prostate using categories 600–602. Neoplasms of the prostate are classified as follows:

- Malignant neoplasm of the prostate   185
- Benign neoplasm of the prostate   222.2
- In situ neoplasm of the prostate   233.4

Urinary obstruction is a primary symptom of hyperplasia of the prostate. Hyperplasia of the prostate is classified to category 600 with fourth digits providing additional specificity regarding the nature of the hypertrophy. The fifth digits provide a combination code that includes the prostate condition with or without urinary obstruction, as follows:

- Benign hypertrophy of prostate without urinary obstruction and other lower urinary tract symptoms (LUTS)   600.00; with urinary obstruction and other lower urinary tract symptoms (LUTS)   600.01
- Nodular prostate without urinary obstruction (excludes malignant neoplasm)   600.10; with urinary obstruction   600.11
- Benign localized hyperplasia without urinary obstruction and other lower urinary tract symptoms (LUTS)   600.20; with urinary obstruction and other lower urinary tract symptoms (LUTS)   600.21
- Cyst of prostate   600.3
- Hyperplasia of prostate, unspecified, without urinary obstruction and other lower urinary tract symptoms (LUTS)   600.90; with urinary obstruction and other lower urinary tract symptoms (LUTS)   600.91

If a patient with BPH has symptoms of urinary obstruction or retention, such as incomplete bladder emptying, it is allowable to use the fifth digits for "with obstruction" for the BPH code. The fifth digits were created specifically to identify that the prostatic hypertrophy is obstructing urine flow to any degree, not just for complete obstruction. If a patient with BPH has symptoms of urinary incontinence, such as post-void dribbling, the fifth digits for "with obstruction" should **not** be assigned unless the physician has specifically documented a urinary obstruction.

As indicated by the "use additional code" note under codes 600.01, 600.21, and 600.91, an additional code should be assigned in conjunction with the BPH code to identify other lower urinary tract symptoms, such as incomplete bladder emptying (788.21), nocturia (788.43), straining on urination (788.65), urinary frequency (788.41), urinary hesitancy (788.64), urinary incontinence (788.30–788.39), urinary obstruction (599.69), urinary retention (788.20), urinary urgency (788.63), and weak urinary stream (788.62).

Category 601 classifies inflammatory disease of the prostate such as:

- 601.0   Acute prostatitis
- 601.1   Chronic prostatitis

Category 602 classifies other disorders of prostate with such conditions as follows:

- 602.0   Calculus of the prostate
- 602.1   Congestion or hemorrhage of prostate
- 602.3   Dysplasia of prostate

The approach used for prostatectomy usually determines the code assigned, as follows:

- 60.21   Transurethral, (ultrasound) guided laser-induced prostatectomy (TULIP)
- 60.29   Transurethral prostatectomy (TURP), other
- 60.3   Suprapubic prostatectomy
- 60.3   Transvesical prostatectomy
- 60.4   Retropubic prostatectomy
- 60.62   Cryoablation of prostate
- 60.62   Perineal (transperineal) prostatectomy

Code **60.5, Radical prostatectomy,** is assigned for radical prostatectomy regardless of the approach used. In a radical prostatectomy, the seminal vesicles and vas ampullae are excised along with the prostate. A prostatectomy performed with a radical cystectomy is coded **57.71, Radical cystectomy;** this procedure involves removal of the bladder, prostate, and seminal vessels.

In the TULIP procedure, a miniature ultrasound system is combined with a laser, which permits the surgeon to view the prostate on a television monitor. The surgeon then discharges the laser at the blockage caused by the enlarged prostate. The blockage disintegrates over a period of several weeks, passing out of the body without further intervention. The result is the same as that achieved by transurethral prostatic resection (TURP), but the hospital stay is shorter, and there are fewer complications.

A "sweep" of the regional lymph nodes is often carried out in connection with a prostatectomy performed for neoplastic disease. This procedure involves removal of regional lymph nodes and lymphatic drainage of the area, skin, subcutaneous tissue, and fat. Code **40.3, Regional lymph node excision,** is assigned as an additional code when this procedure is also performed. A code for radical lymph node excision is assigned when the excision extends to the muscle and deep fascia.

Other types of therapy utilized for the destruction of prostatic tissue are coded as follows:

- Transurethral destruction of prostate tissue by microwave thermotherapy (TUMT of prostate)   60.96
- Transurethral destruction of prostate tissue by other thermotherapy; this includes radiofrequency thermotherapy and transurethral needle ablation (TUNA)   60.97

ENDOMETRIOSIS

Endometriosis is a condition in which aberrant tissue that almost perfectly resembles the mucous membrane of the uterus is found in various other sites within the pelvic cavity. A code from category **617, Endometriosis,** is assigned for this condition with a fourth digit indicating the site in which the aberrant tissue is found. For example:

- Endometriosis of the ovary   617.1
- Endometriosis of the colon   617.5
- Endometriosis of fallopian tube   617.2

GENITAL PROLAPSE

Prolapse of the vagina and/or the uterus is a relatively common condition. In coding genital prolapse, it is first necessary to determine whether the condition involves the vaginal wall, the uterus, or both; and whether the prolapse is complete or incomplete. For example:

- Uterovaginal prolapse, incomplete (uterus descends into introitus and cervix protrudes slightly beyond)   618.2
- Uterovaginal prolapse, complete (entire cervix and uterus protrude beyond the introitus and vagina is inverted)   618.3

Code 618.5 is assigned for prolapse of vaginal vault occurring after hysterectomy; it is not classified as a surgical complication. This condition may be due to the surgical technique or to the relaxation of supporting structures following surgery. Pelvic or vaginal enterocele, a herniation of the intestine through intact vaginal mucosa, is coded **618.6, Vaginal enterocele, congenital or acquired,** whether it is congenital or acquired. Prolapse of the uterus in an obstetric patient is classified in chapter 11 of *ICD-9-CM.* Examples of appropriate coding for genital prolapse include the following:

- Prolapse of uterus (no vaginal wall involvement)   618.1
- Vaginal enterocele   618.6
- Prolapse of cervical stump   618.84
- Prolapse of gravid uterus (undelivered)   654.43

Subcategory **618.0, Prolapse of vaginal walls without mention of uterine prolapse,** has fifth digits to provide additional specificity regarding the type of vaginal prolapse, such as:

- 618.00   Unspecified prolapse of vaginal walls
- 618.01   Cystocele, midline
- 618.02   Cystocele, lateral
- 618.03   Urethrocele
- 618.04   Rectocele
- 618.05   Perineocele
- 618.09   Other

DYSPLASIA OF CERVIX AND VULVA

Code **622.1x, Dysplasia of cervix (uteri)** is also identified as CIN (cervical intraepithelial neoplasia). CIN I is coded to 622.11, while CIN II is coded to 622.12. Dysplasia of the cervix specified as CIN III, however, is carcinoma in situ of the cervix, and code **233.1, Cervix uteri,** is assigned. Dysplasia of the vulva is coded **624.8, Other specified non-inflammatory disorders of vulva and perineum,** unless it is specified as VIN III, which is classified to **233.3, Carcinoma in situ of other and unspecified female genital organs.** A diagnosis of CIN III or VIN III can be made only on the basis of pathological examination of tissues.

Codes 795.00–795.09 would be assigned for abnormal results from a cervical cytologic examination without histologic confirmation.

ENDOMETRIAL ABLATION

Endometrial ablation is used as an alternative to hysterectomy for women with dysfunctional bleeding that does not respond to hormone therapy. It can also be used to treat women with fibroid tumors or endometrial polyps. A scope equipped with either a roller ball or a u-shaped wire is inserted into the uterus. The lining of the uterus is ablated by laser, radiofrequency electromagnet energy, or electrocoagulation. Code **68.23, Endometrial ablation,** is assigned for this procedure.

DISEASES OF THE BREAST

Neoplasms of the breast are classified in chapter 2 of *ICD-9-CM*. The coder should be aware, however, that terms such as growth, cyst, and lump do not necessarily refer to neoplastic disease. When surgery is performed, the pathology report provides more specific information to assist in code assignment. Examples of appropriate coding include the following:

- Fibrocystic disease of the breast   610.1
- Benign neoplasm of breast   217
- Benign neoplasm of skin of breast   216.5
- Gynecomastia   611.1
- Carcinoma of the male breast   175.9
- Carcinoma of the female breast   174.9

Biopsies of the breast are classified as closed (85.11) or open (85.12). When the procedure is described as an excisional biopsy, it usually refers to excision of the entire lesion rather than a simple biopsy, in which case it is coded to **85.21, Local excision of lesion of breast.** The term lumpectomy also describes a local excision of a breast lesion.

When surgery on the breast is performed for possible neoplasm, it is customary to perform a biopsy before the definitive surgery begins. A rapid-frozen section is reviewed by a pathologist to determine whether malignancy is present. The code for the definitive procedure is sequenced first, followed by the code for the biopsy.

With advances in cancer therapy, radical mastectomy is not performed as often as in the past because a lumpectomy or a modified radical mastectomy appears to be equally effective in most cases. The main distinction between a radical and modified mastectomy is that all or part of the pectoralis major and all of the pectoralis minor are removed in a radical mastectomy, whereas the pectoralis major is preserved in a modified radical mastectomy. Mastectomy codes (85.4x) indicate whether a procedure is performed unilaterally or bilaterally and the extent of the procedure. The coder must review the operative report carefully before assigning these procedure codes.

A **tissue expander (85.95)** is another procedure frequently carried out in conjunction with breast surgery. This tissue insertion permits a flap closure of the site making it not necessary for the patient to undergo a skin graft. Saline is usually injected into the breast expander at regular intervals following its insertion to gradually enlarge the size of the expander. Tissue expanders used in areas other than the breast are coded as **86.93, Insertion of tissue expander.**

BREAST RECONSTRUCTION

Reconstructive breast surgery is performed for a variety of reasons. Prostheses are often implanted for patients who have undergone mastectomies. Breast reconstruction can be performed immediately after the surgery or delayed to a later time. When it is known that patients will undergo postoperative radiation, reconstruction is usually delayed.

If the purpose for reconstruction is to increase breast size for improved appearance, prosthetic implants are usually used. Reduction mammoplasty is sometimes performed for patients whose large breast size interferes with normal daily activities or causes significant discomfort, as well as for cosmetic reasons. When mammoplasty is performed to reduce breast size, code **611.1, Hypertrophy of the breast,** is assigned as the principal diagnosis. When the purpose of the mammoplasty is cosmetic, code **V50.1, Other plastic surgery for unacceptable cosmetic appearance,** is assigned as the principal diagnosis.

Coding examples for reconstruction include the following:

- Total reconstruction of right breast   85.7
- Flaps and microsurgical procedures   85.82–85.85
- Nipple-areola reconstruction   85.75
- Reduction mammoplasty   85.3x

Complications sometime develop in patients who have breast implants, making removal of the implants advisable. In such cases, the code for the principal diagnosis depends on the nature of the complication. For example, if the reason for the surgery is that the implant has ruptured, the principal diagnosis code is **996.54, Mechanical complication due to breast prosthesis.** When the reason for removal is that the patient had a capsular contracture of the right breast, code **996.79, Other complications due to other internal prosthetic device,** is assigned as the principal diagnosis. Code **85.94, Removal of implant of breast,** is assigned for removal of a breast implant.

Patients sometimes request removal of an implant because they are concerned that a complication might occur in the future, although there is no problem at present. In this case, assign **V52.4, Fitting and adjustment of breast prosthesis and implant.** For example:

- A patient experienced a ruptured breast implant on the left side and was admitted for removal of the implant and insertion of a new implant.
  Principal diagnosis: 996.54   Mechanical complications due to breast prosthesis
  Surgery performed: 85.93   Revision of breast implant

- A patient who had undergone a previous right mastectomy with a breast implant inserted at the time of surgery recently suffered from a painful capsule. She was admitted for removal and reinsertion of the implant.
  Principal diagnosis: 996.79   Other complication due to other internal prosthetic device
  Surgery performed: 85.93   Revision of breast implant
- A patient had undergone bilateral breast implantation three years and now admission for elective implant removal. She had no related problems but had become concerned because of newspaper reports describing illnesses associated with breast implants.
  Principal diagnosis: V52.4   Fitting and adjustment of breast prosthesis and implant
  Surgery performed: 85.94   Removal of breast implant (assign code twice to indicate procedure was performed bilaterally)

Review Exercise 17.4

Code the following diagnoses and procedures. Do not assign E codes.

	Code(s)
1. Hydronephrosis with chronic pyelitis	591
Pyelonephritis, focal, chronic, left	590.00
2. Rapidly progressive chronic glomerulonephritis	582.4
3. Syphilitic epididymitis	095.81
	604.91
4. Chronic prostatitis due to Proteus	601.1
	041.6
5. Phimosis and balanoposthitis	605
	607.1
6. Encysted hydrocele, male	603.0
Excision of hydrocele of spermatic cord	63.1

Review Exercise 17.4 *(continued)*

7. Benign prostatic hypertrophy with bladder obstruction

<u>600.01</u>
596.0

Transurethral prostatectomy

60.29

8. Acute and chronic cervicitis

616.0

Vaginal hysterectomy

68.59

9. Chronic pelvic inflammatory disease
Dysmenorrhea

614.4
625.3

10. Menometrorrhagia
Endometrial polyp
Corpus luteum cysts of both ovaries

626.2
621.0
620.1

Total abdominal hysterectomy
Bilateral salpingo-oophorectomy

68.49
65.61

11. Cystocele with incomplete uterine prolapse
and stress incontinence

618.2
625.6

Cystocele repair
Vaginal suspension of uterus

70.51
69.22

12. Pelvic peritoneal endometriosis

617.3

Review Exercise 17.4 *(continued)*

13. Dermoid cyst of ovary   220

    Laparoscopic wedge resection of ovarian cyst   65.24

14. Infertility due to pelvic peritoneal adhesions   614.6
                                                                       628.2

    Hysterosalpingogram, radiopaque dye   87.83

15. Psychogenic dysmenorrhea   306.52

16. Adhesions of ovary and fallopian tubes   614.6

    Laparoscopic lysis of adhesions   65.81

17. Menorrhagia   626.2

    Dilatation and curettage with endometrial ablation   68.23

18. Submucous fibroid of uterus   218.0

    Laparoscopically assisted vaginal hysterectomy   68.51

Coding of Diseases of the Skin and Diseases of the Musculoskeletal System

18 Diseases of the Skin and Subcutaneous Tissue

Chapter 12 of *ICD-9-CM* deals with conditions affecting the skin and subcutaneous tissue. The chapter is organized around the following subdivisions:

- Infections of skin and subcutaneous tissue   680–686
- Other inflammatory conditions of skin and tissue   690–698
- Other diseases of skin and subcutaneous tissue   700–709

Conditions affecting the nails, sweat glands, hair, and hair follicles are included in this chapter. Congenital conditions of skin, hair, and nails are classified in category 757, **Congenital anomalies of the integument.** Neoplasms of skin are classified in chapter 2 of *ICD-9-CM.*

DERMATITIS DUE TO DRUGS

Category 692 is classified for contact dermatitis such as plants other than food and drugs and other medications in contact with skin. Category 693 is assigned for dermatitis such as drugs and medications taken internally. This distinction does not apply to the eyelid and the ear.

In coding dermatitis caused by medicines, the coder must first determine whether the condition represents an adverse effect due to the proper administration of a drug or poisoning due to the incorrect use of the drug. When the dermatitis is due to a medication used correctly as prescribed, the dermatitis code is sequenced first, with an E code from the E930 through E949 series included to indicate the medication responsible. When the dermatitis is due to incorrect use of the drug, it is classified first as a poisoning by drugs, medicinal and biological substances (960–969) with an additional code for the dermatitis, and an E code is assigned to indicate the way in which the poisoning occurred and the type of drug involved. (A more detailed discussion of the distinction between adverse effects and poisoning due to drugs and medications is provided in chapter 28 of this handbook.)

Correct coding examples include the following:

- Dermatitis due to allergic reaction to penicillin tablets, taken as prescribed (adverse reaction)   693.0 + E930.0
- Dermatitis due to accidental ingestion of mother's penicillin tablets (poisoning)   960.0 + 693.0 + E856

In the first example, which indicates an adverse reaction to a prescribed medication taken as directed, the code for dermatitis is sequenced first, followed by an E code to indicate that the drug responsible was penicillin. In the second example, code 960.0, Poisoning due to penicillin, is sequenced first, with an additional code to indicate that the effect of the poisoning is dermatitis and an E code to indicate that the poisoning was accidental.

ULCERS OF THE SKIN

Most chronic ulcers of the skin are classified in category 707, **Chronic ulcer of skin,** with 785.4 assigned as an additional code when gangrene is present. Ulceration associated with arteriosclerosis of the extremities is classified as code **440.23, Atherosclerosis of the**

extremities with ulceration, with an additional code from subcategory of 707.1–707.9 or if gangrene is present, to **440.24, Atherosclerosis of the extremities with gangrene.**

Subcategory **707.0, Decubitus ulcers,** has fifth digits to identify the specific site of the ulcer, such as elbow (707.01), upper back (707.02), lower back (707.03), hip (707.04), buttock (707.05), ankle (707.06), heel (707.07), and other site (707.09). Examples of correct coding for chronic ulcers of the skin include the following:

- Decubitus ulcer, sacral area   707.03
- Decubitus ulcer, sacral area, with gangrene   707.03 + 785.4
- Ulcer of lower limb, except decubitus   707.10–707.19
- Chronic ulcer of other specified sites   707.8
- Chronic ulcer of unspecified site   707.9

Stasis ulcers are ordinarily due to varicose veins of the lower extremities and are coded to category 454.x rather than to the categories for conditions of the skin. When the physician has used the term stasis ulcer but has identified a cause other than varicose veins, code the condition as an ulcer of the skin. A basic rule of coding is that further research must be done when the title of the code suggested by the Alphabetic Index clearly does not identify the condition correctly. In this case, even though the index directs the coder to a code involving varicose veins, the code should not be used when no varicosities are present.

CELLULITIS OF THE SKIN

Cellulitis is an acute, diffuse infection of the skin and soft tissues that commonly results from a break in the skin, such as a puncture wound, laceration, or ulcer. Occasionally, the break is so small that it cannot be identified by either the patient or the examining physician. Clinically, cellulitis usually presents as an abrupt onset of redness, swelling, pain, or heat in the infected area. Coders should not assume, however, that a reference to redness at the edges of a wound or ulcer represents cellulitis. The normal hyperemia associated with a wound usually extends a small distance beyond the edges of the wound rather than extending to the diffuse pattern that characterizes cellulitis.

Coding of cellulitis secondary to superficial injury, burn, or frostbite requires two codes, one for the injury and one for the cellulitis. Sequencing of codes depends on the circumstances of the admission. When the patient is seen primarily for treatment of an open wound, the appropriate code for open wound, complicated, is assigned, with an additional code for the cellulitis. When the wound itself is trivial or when it was treated earlier and the patient is now being seen for treatment of the cellulitis, the code for the cellulitis may be sequenced first, with an additional code for open wound, complicated. For example:

- A patient suffered laceration of the lower leg while on a hiking trip two days ago and came to the hospital on his return. By the time he was seen, cellulitis was beginning to develop. The wound was cleansed, nonexcisional debridement was carried out, and antibiotics were started for the cellulitis.
  Principal diagnosis: 891.1   Open wound, complicated
  Additional diagnosis: 682.6   Cellulitis
  Procedure: 86.28   Nonexcisional debridement of wound, infection or burn
- A patient suffered a minor puncture injury to the finger when removing a staple at the office. Five days later, he was admitted to the hospital because of cellulitis of the finger and was treated with intravenous antibiotics. The wound itself did not require treatment, and therefore no code for injury is assigned.
  Principal diagnosis: 681.00   Cellulitis

Cellulitis of the skin is classified as code **681, Cellulitis and abscess of finger and toe,** and code **682, Other cellulitis and abscess.** Both abscess and lymphangitis are included in the codes for cellulitis of the skin. An additional code should be assigned to indicate the organism responsible, if this information is available. The responsible organism is usually Streptococcus.

Cellulitis may also present as a postoperative wound infection or as a result of the penetration of the skin involved in intravenous therapy. It may develop very early or may not appear until later. Note that code **958.3, Posttraumatic wound infection, NEC,** is not assigned when the infection is identified as cellulitis. For example:

- A patient had an appendectomy six days ago and is now readmitted with evidence of staphylococcal cellulitis of the operative wound.
  Principal diagnosis: 998.59   Postoperative infections
  Additional diagnosis: 682.2   Cellulitis of trunk
  Additional diagnosis: 041.10   Staphylococcus

Cellulitis frequently develops as a complication of chronic skin ulcers, in which case it is assigned to a code from the series 707.00 through 707.9. These codes do not include any associated cellulitis, and so two codes are required to describe these conditions. Designation of the principal diagnosis depends on the circumstances of the admission.

Cellulitis described as gangrenous is classified as code 785.4 rather than in the 681 and 682 categories, when it develops as the result of either injury or ulcer. When gangrene is present, the injury or ulcer is sequenced first, with code **785.4, Gangrene,** assigned as an additional code. This practice is compatible with the usual guidelines concerning the use of chapter 16 codes as principal diagnoses and corresponds to the instructions in the Alphabetic Index.

OTHER CELLULITIS

Although cellulitis most commonly occurs in the skin and subcutaneous tissue, it also occurs in other areas. In such cases, codes from other chapters are assigned as appropriate.

Pelvic cellulitis in women is classified as an inflammatory condition and is assigned to category 614. Occasionally, pelvic cellulitis occurs following abortion, delivery, or molar or ectopic pregnancy, in which case it is classified to chapter 11 of *ICD-9-CM*. In male patients, pelvic cellulitis is coded as **567.21, Peritonitis (acute) generalized.**

DISSEMINATED SUPERFICIAL ACTINIC POROKERATOSIS (DSAP)

Disseminated superficial actinic porokeratosis (692.75) is an autosomal dominantly inherited skin condition that causes multiple, brown, and keratotic lesions on arms and legs and it results from ultraviolet light; the lesions are due to solar radiation. The first average age when this condition is noticed is about 40; its frequency in families increases with age. It is usually not seen on areas covered by clothes or on the scalp, arms, palms, and legs. No ideal treatment has been found to date.

EXCISION OF LESION

Excision or destruction of most skin lesions is classified as code **86.3, Other local excision or destruction of lesion or tissue of skin and subcutaneous tissue,** or as code **86.4, Radical excision of skin lesion.** Simple excisions are coded to 86.3 and involve only the skin. Code 86.3 includes both local excision and destruction carried out by cauterization, cryosurgery, fulguration, or laser beam. A radical or wide excision (86.4) goes beyond the skin and involves underlying and/or adjacent tissue. The surgeon's description should be followed carefully when assigning these codes. Notice that the exclusion notes indicate that skin lesions of several areas (for example, skin of the breast, anus, lip, eyelid, nose, ears, female perineum, scrotum, and penis) are coded elsewhere.

DEBRIDEMENT

Debridement of the skin and subcutaneous tissue is a procedure by which foreign material and devitalized or contaminated tissue are removed from a traumatic or infected lesion until the surrounding healthy tissue is exposed.

Excisional debridement of the skin (86.22) is the surgical removal or cutting away of such tissue, necrosis, or slough. It can be performed either by direct excision or by laser destruction. Depending on the availability of a surgical suite or the extent of the area involved, excisional debridement can be performed in the operating room, in the emergency department, or at the patient's bedside. Excisional debridement may be performed by a physician and/or other health care provider and involves an excisional, as opposed to a mechanical (brushing, scrubbing, washing) debridement. The documentation must reflect actual cutting away of tissue for the procedure to be considered an excisional debridement. Use of a sharp instrument does not always indicate that an excisional debridement was performed. Minor removal of loose fragments with scissors or using a sharp instrument to scrape away tissue is not an excisional debridement. Excisional debridement involves the use of a scalpel to remove devitalized tissue and cutting outside or beyond the wound margin.

Nonexcisional debridement of the skin (86.28) is the nonoperative brushing, irrigating, scrubbing, or washing of devitalized tissue, necrosis, slough, or foreign material. For example, water jet scalpel debridement is coded to **86.28, Nonexcisional debridement of wound, infection, or burn.** This code also includes minor snipping of tissue, such as that loosened by Hubbard tank therapy. Nonexcisional debridement may be performed by a physician or by other health care personnel.

When coding for debridement of areas other than skin, and there is no index entry or guidance provided in the Tabular List, the coder should look for other terms such as excision or destruction of lesion of that site. For example, assign code **83.39, Excision of lesion of other soft tissue,** for debridement of tendon. This code can be located in the index in the following manner:

> Excision, lesion
>   tendon   83.39

When coding multiple-layer debridements of the same site, the coder should assign a code only for the deepest layer of debridement. Debridement carried out in conjunction with another procedure is often included in the code for the procedure, but not always. Index entries and inclusion notes provide guidance for the coder.

DERMAL REGENERATIVE GRAFT

Several new technologies that are able to permanently regenerate or replace skin layers are now being used to treat severe burns. Code **86.67, Dermal regenerative graft,** is assigned for grafts using any of these technologies. Note that this code does not classify heterograft to skin (86.65) or homograft to skin (86.66). The inclusion note for code 86.67 lists biologic skin replacement systems as follows:

- Artificial skin, NOS
- Creation of "neodermis"
- Decellularized allodermis
- Integumentary matrix implants
- Prosthetic implant of dermal layer of skin
- Regenerate dermal layer of skin

Code **996.55, Mechanical complication due to artificial skin graft and decellularized allodermis,** is assigned for failure or rejection of these systems. Code 996.52 is assigned for complication of other skin graft. Status code V43.83 is assigned to indicate that the patient has an artificial skin graft.

Review Exercise 18.1

The following exercise provides examples of conditions classified in chapter 12 of *ICD-9-CM*. Code the following diagnoses and procedures.

	Code(s)
1. Varicose ulcer, lower left leg with severe inflammation	454.2
2. Pilonidal fistula with abscess	685.0
Excision of pilonidal sinus	86.21
3. Large abscess of right flank due to Staphylococcus aureus Infection	682.2 041.11
Incision and drainage of abscess, right flank	54.0
4. Hard corn deformity, right little toe Soft corn deformities, 3rd, 4th, and 5th toes, right	700
5. Keloid scar on left hand from previous burn or Late	701.4 906.6

Review Exercise 18.1 *(continued)*

Radical excision of scar	86.4
6. Chronic purulent inflamed acne rosacea of lower lip	695.3
Wide excision of chronic acne rosacea of lower lip with full-thickness graft over defect, lower lip	27.42 27.55
7. Giant urticaria	995.1
8. Contact dermatitis of eyelid	373.32
9. Seborrheic keratosis underlying the second metatarsal head, right foot	702.19
10. Cellulitis of anus	566
11. Acute lymphangitis, upper arm, due to group A streptococcal infection	682.3 041.01

Review Exercise 18.1 *(continued)*

12. Gangrenous diabetic ulcer of right foot due to peripheral circulatory disorder

250.70
707.14
785.4

13. Surgical (excisional) debridement of skin and fascia of foot   83.39

14. Infected ingrown toenail, right great toe   703.0

15. Cellulitis, buttock   682.5

16. Cellulitis of eyelid   373.13

19 Diseases of the Musculoskeletal System and Connective Tissue

Chapter 13 of *ICD-9-CM* is governed by the general coding guidelines already discussed in this handbook. An understanding of the following terms may be helpful to the coder in assigning codes from chapter 13:

- Arthropathy: disorder of the joint
- Arthritis: inflammation of the joint
- Dorsopathy: disorder of the back
- Myelopathy: disorder of the spinal cord

Most arthropathies are classified in categories 710 through 719 and most dorsopathies in categories 720 through 724 in *ICD-9-CM*.

FIFTH-DIGIT SUBCLASSIFICATION

Many of the categories for diseases of the musculoskeletal system and connective tissue have fifth-digit subclassifications. A note at the beginning of chapter 13 lists fifth digits that apply to categories 711–712, 715–716, 718–719, and 730 to indicate the site involved. This note also indicates the specific bones and joints included in each fifth digit. For example, fifth digit 5 (lower leg) includes the tibia, fibula, patella, and knee joint. The fifth digits are repeated at the beginning of each of the categories and subcategories to which they apply, but the definitions are not repeated. When not all fifth digits apply to a specific subcategory, the appropriate fifth digits are displayed in brackets underneath the code title. Other categories and subcategories use different fifth digits; these are displayed as part of the code title.

BACK DISORDERS

Back pain described as lumbago or low back pain, without further qualification, is coded **724.2, Lumbago.** Back pain not otherwise specified is coded **724.5, Backache, unspecified.** Psychogenic back pain is classified under 724.5 and 307.89, **Other pain disorder related to psychological factors.**

Intervertebral disc disorders are classified in category 722. Careful attention to the terminology is important in coding these conditions. Degeneration and displacement (herniation) of the disc are not the same conditions and require different codes.

The presence or absence of myelopathy is an important distinction to be made in assigning codes for certain back disorders. Myelopathy is a functional disorder and/or pathological change in the spinal cord that often results from compression. Codes for back disorders such as spondylosis and herniation of the intervertebral disc differentiate between conditions with and without myelopathy. Codes for a herniated disc without myelopathy include those with paresthesia but not paralysis. Terms that are included as **Intervertebral disc disorders with myelopathy** are classified into subcategory **722.7,** with a fifth digit used to indicate the site involved. Examples include:

- Herniated intervertebral disc, cervical, without myelopathy 722.0
- Herniated intervertebral disc, lumbosacral, with myelopathy 722.73
- Herniated intervertebral disc, thoracic, without myelopathy 722.11

Back pain associated with herniation of an intervertebral disc is included in the code for the herniated disc; no additional code is assigned.

Surgery for the excision or destruction of a herniated disc is classified in volume 3 of *ICD-9-CM* by the type of surgery performed. For example:

- Excision of herniated intervertebral disc 80.51
- Destruction of displaced intervertebral disc by chemonucleolysis 80.52
- Other destruction (including percutaneous suction diskectomy, automated percutaneous diskectomy, and laser destruction) 80.59
- Diskectomy with corpectomy 80.99

Code 03.09 is assigned for a laminectomy performed for the purpose of exploration or decompression of the spinal canal. Laminectomy performed for the purpose of excision of herniated disc material, however, represents the operative approach and is not coded.

ARTHRITIS

Arthritis is the common term for a wide variety of conditions that primarily affect the joints, muscles, and connective tissue. The associated symptoms are inflammation, swelling, pain, stiffness, and mobility problems. Arthritis may occur independently, but it is also a common manifestation of a variety of other conditions, and dual coding guidelines apply. Examples include:

- Arthritis of the shoulder due to dicalcium phosphate crystals   275.49 + 712.11
- Charcot's arthritis due to diabetes   250.60 + 713.5
- Reiter's arthritis of hand   099.3 + 711.14

Arthritis is also associated with Lyme disease, either as a component of current disease or as a late effect. When the Lyme disease is currently active, code **088.81, Lyme disease,** and *711.8x, Arthropathy associated with other infectious and parasitic diseases,* are assigned. When the arthritis is a late effect of the Lyme disease, the listed codes are **139.8, Late effect of other infectious and parasitic disease,** and 711.8x.

Osteoarthritis is the most common form of arthritis; it is also called polyarthritis, degenerative arthritis, and hypertrophic arthritis. It is a degenerative joint disease, usually occurring in older people, with chronic degeneration of the articular cartilage and hypertrophy of the bone. It is characterized by pain and swelling. Codes from category **715, Osteoarthrosis and allied disorders,** are assigned except when the spine is involved when a code from 720.0–724.9 is assigned.

The primary axis for coding osteoarthritis is whether it is generalized or localized. When localized, it is further subdivided according to whether it is primary (715.1x) or secondary (715.2x). Primary osteoarthritis, also known as polyarticular degenerative arthritis, affects joints in the spine, knee, and hip, as well as certain small joints of the hands and feet. (Note that the codes for localized osteoarthritis include bilateral involvement of the same site.) A code from subcategory 715.3 is assigned for localized arthritis that is not identified as either primary or secondary. Secondary arthritis, also called monarticular arthritis, is confined to the joints of one area and results from some external or internal injury or disease. Osteoarthritis that involves multiple sites but is not specified as generalized is coded as **715.8x, Osteoarthritis involving or with mention of more than one site, but not specified as generalized.**

Rheumatoid arthritis (714.0), another fairly common type of arthritis, is an autoimmune disease that affects the entire body. Pyogenic arthritis (711.0x) is due to infection and is classified with a fifth digit indicating the joints involved. An additional code should be assigned for the responsible organism. Gouty arthritis (274.0) is a recurrent arthritis of the peripheral joints in which excessive uric acid in the blood is deposited in the joints. If the gout is due to lead, code 984.x is assigned.

Exercise 19.1

Code the following diagnoses and procedures. Do not assign E codes.

	Code(s)
1. Acute and chronic gouty <u>arthritis</u>	274.0
2. Chronic nodular rheumatoid <u>arthritis</u> with polyneuropathy	<u>714.0</u> 357.1
3. Traumatic <u>arthritis</u>, left ankle, due to old traumatic dislocation <u>Late</u>	<u>716.17</u> 905.6
Compression <u>arthrodesis</u>, left ankle	81.11
4. <u>Herniated</u> intervertebral disc, L4–5	722.10
Laminectomy with <u>excision</u> of intervertebral disc, L4–5	80.51
5. Chronic lumbosacral <u>sprain</u>	724.6

DERANGEMENT

Derangement of the knee is classified to category 717; derangement of other sites is classified to category 718, with fourth digits indicating the site. Code 718.3x is assigned if the derangement is described as being recurrent. Derangement due to current injury is classified to categories 830–839, Dislocation of joint, with the fourth digit indicating the site and fifth digit indicating whether the dislocation is open or closed. Certain categories also provide fifth digits that indicate the type of dislocation.

Exercise 19.2

Code the following diagnoses. Do not assign E codes.

	Code(s)
1. Recurrent <u>derangement</u> of ankle	718.37
2. Recurrent <u>derangement</u> of knee	718.36
3. <u>Derangement</u> of knee due to a fall from a ladder while working on house	836.2 E881.0 E849.0

PATHOLOGICAL FRACTURES

Pathological fractures occur in bones that are weakened by disease. These fractures are usually spontaneous but sometimes occur in connection with slight trauma that ordinarily would not result in a fracture in healthy bone. There are many different underlying causes for pathological fractures, including osteoporosis, metastatic tumor of the bone, osteomyelitis, Paget's disease, disuse atrophy, hyperparathyroidism, and nutritional or congenital disorders.

Fractures described as spontaneous are always pathological fractures. When the fracture is described as a compression fracture, the record should be reviewed to determine whether any significant trauma has been experienced. A fall from a height, such as a diving board, with compression fracture of the spine would be classified as an injury; but a compression fracture in an older patient resulting from a slight stumble or other minor injury would probably be considered pathological, particularly when the patient also suffers from an underlying condition that frequently causes such fractures. The physician should be asked for clarification.

All pathological fractures are coded as 733.1x, with a fifth digit indicating the bone involved. A pathological fracture is designated as the principal diagnosis only when the patient is admitted solely for treatment of the pathological fracture. Ordinarily the code for the underlying condition responsible for the fracture is listed first with an additional code for the fracture. Never assign a code for both a traumatic fracture and a pathological fracture of the same bone; one or the other would be assigned. (See chapter 26 of this handbook for a discussion of coding traumatic fractures.)

Appropriate coding examples include the following:

- Fracture of tibia and major osseous defects due to senile osteoporosis   <u>733.16 + 733.01 + 731.3</u>
- Pathological fracture due to metastatic carcinoma of bone; ovarian cancer five years ago   <u>733.14 + 198.5 + V10.4</u>

Stress fractures are somewhat different from pathological fractures in that pathological fractures are always due to a physiologic condition such as cancer or osteoporosis that result in damage to the bone. Stress fractures are due to repetitive force applied before the bone and its supporting tissues have had enough time to provide such force. They are usually negative in an X-ray display, and days or weeks may pass before the fracture line is visible on an X-ray. Codes from 733.10–733.19 are assigned for pathological fractures. Stress fractures are coded as follows:

- 733.93   Stress fracture of tibia or fibula
- 733.94   Stress fracture of the metatarsals
- 733.95   Sress fracture of other bone

The term "stress reaction" is included under each code as a synonymous term for stress fracture.

REPLACEMENT OF A JOINT

Replacement of a joint is classified in category 81.5x for joints of the lower extremities and 81.8x for joints of the upper extremities. Code assignment depends on the joint involved and whether the replacement is total or partial. When coding hip replacements, if the type of bearing surface is known, it should be reported using the appropriate codes as follows: 00.74 for metal on polyethylene, 00.75 for metal-on-metal, 00.76 for ceramic-on-ceramic, and 00.77 for ceramic-on-polyethylene. If replacement also involves the placement of a bone-growth stimulator, code 78.9x is assigned as an additional code; the fourth digit indicates the site. Other examples include the following:

- Replacement of acetabulum with prosthesis   81.52
- Total ankle replacement   81.56
- Replacement of femoral head   81.52
- Partial replacement of hip   81.52
- Total elbow replacement   81.84

ICD-9-CM does not provide codes that indicate that a bilateral replacement has been carried out. The procedure code should be assigned twice when the same procedure is performed on bilateral joints.

Occasionally, a prosthesis must be removed because of infection, with a new prosthesis placed after a month or two when the infection has completely cleared. The first admission for such a problem would be coded **996.66, Infection or inflammation due to internal joint prosthesis**, with code **80.0x, Removal of prosthesis**, assigned for the procedure. On the follow-up admission, the principal diagnosis would be acquired deformity of the site (category 736) with a procedure code for revision of the joint.

Anytime a joint replacement is adjusted or removed and replaced, the procedure is coded as a joint revision, which includes any removal of the joint replacement component. However, if there is removal of a joint spacer (e.g., cement), code 84.57 is also assigned. If the type of bearing surface is known, it should be reported using the appropriate code (00.74–00.77).

Codes 00.70–00.73 are assigned for revision of hip replacements to identify the specific joint components revised (acetabular, femoral, and acetabular liner and/or femoral head). The codes are as follows:

- 00.70   Revision of hip replacement, both acetabular and femoral components (this includes total hip revision)
- 00.71   Revision of hip replacement, acetabular component
- 00.72   Revision of hip replacement, femoral component
- 00.73   Revision of hip replacement, acetabular liner and/or femoral head only

When the joint component of the revised hip replacement is not specified, assign code **81.53, Revision of hip replacement, not otherwise specified.**

Codes 00.80–00.84 are assigned for revision of knee replacements. These procedures are classified according to the joint component revised (tibial, femoral, patellar, or tibial insert). The codes are as follows:

- 00.80   Revision of knee replacement, total (all components)
- 00.81   Revision of knee replacement, tibial component
- 00.82   Revision of knee replacement, femoral component
- 00.83   Revision of knee replacement, patellar component
- 00.84   Revision of knee replacement, tibial insert (liner)

When the knee joint component being revised is not specified, assign code **81.54, Revision of knee replacement, not otherwise specified.**

Revision of joint replacements that are not elsewhere classified are assigned to code 81.59 (lower extremity) and code 81.97 (upper extremity). These codes are assigned for both partial or total revision.

New codes have been created for hip resurfacing arthroplasty. These new codes identify the specific joint components resurfaced. Total resurfacing involves both the acetabular and femoral components. Partial resurfacing involves either the femoral head or acetabulum only. These new codes are assigned as follows:

- 00.85 Resurfacing hip, total, acetabulum and femoral
- 00.86 Resurfacing hip, partial, femoral head
- 00.87 Resurfacing hip, partial, acetabulum

Category **V43.6, Joint replacement status,** can be assigned as an additional code when the presence of a joint replacement is significant in terms of patient care.

Exercise 19.3

Code the following diagnoses and procedures. Do not assign E codes.

	Code(s)
1. Primary osteoarthritis of hip	715.15
Replacement, total, of hip with ceramic-on-ceramic bearing surface	81.51, 00.76
2. Bicompartmental total knee replacement	81.54
3. Partial replacement of left shoulder	81.81

SPINAL FUSION

Traditionally, there have been three basic approaches to spinal fusion or spinal refusion: anterior, posterior and lateral transverse. The classic anterior approach (81.02, 81.04, 81.06, 81.32, 81.34, 81.36) requires an incision in the neck or the abdomen and the fusion is carried out from the front of the vertebrae through the anterior annulus. In the classic posterior approach (81.03, 81.05, 81.08, 81.33, 81.35, 81.38) the incision is made in the patient's back directly over the vertebrae. Another approach is the lateral transverse (81.07, 81.37), which involves an incision on the patient's side and the vertebrae is approached through the lamina.

Occasionally, instrumentation called interbody fusion devices are used to stabilize and fuse degenerative disc spaces and to provide an immediately stable segment for fusion and relief of symptoms. These devices are also known as an interbody fusion cage, Bak cage, ray-threaded fusion cage, synthetic cage, spacer or bone dowels. If insertion of an interbody fusion device is performed along with a spinal fusion or refusion, code 84.51 is assigned as an additional procedure code.

A 360-degree spinal fusion is a fusion of both the anterior and posterior portions of the spine performed through a single incision (usually via the lateral transverse approach). When coding this procedure, the coder should carefully review the documentation and first determine whether this is a fusion or refusion. In addition, it should be determined whether the procedure is an anterior lumbar interbody infusion (ALIF), a posterior lumbar interbody fusion (PLIF), or a transforaminal lumbar interbody fusion (TLIF). The PLIF involves an anterior and middle column fusion through a posterior approach. The TLIF involves a transverse lateral interbody fusion through a posterior approach. Codes 81.06 and 81.36 include ALIF. Codes 81.08 and 81.38 include both PLIF and TLIF.

Additional codes are used to capture the number of discs fused when a spinal fusion or refusion is performed. For example:

- 81.62   Fusion or refusion of 2–3 vertebrae
- 81.63   Fusion or refusion of 4–8 vertebrae
- 81.64   Fusion or refusion of 9 or more vertebrae

REFUSION OF SPINE

Pseudarthrosis is a false joint caused by the inadequate immobilization of a fractured bone. The spinal fusion is measured from the time the operation is proposed until the fusion mass is solid. There is a definite relationship between the extent of the fusion and the incidence of pseudarthrosis and progression of the deformity. Findings may include severe pain and tenderness over the fusion of the deformity. Actually only about 50% of patients who have pseudoarthrosis do not have any symptoms.

Codes 81.30–81.39 provide more specific data regarding both the site and the technique utilized. For example:

- 81.34   Refusion of dorsal and dorsolumbar spine, anterior technique
- 81.35   Refusion of dorsal and dorsolumbar spine, posterior technique
- 81.36   Refusion of lumbar and lumbosacral spine, anterior technique
- 81.39   Refusion of spine, not elsewhere classified

An additional code (81.62, 81.63 or 81.64) is used to indicate the number of vertebrae fused.

VERTEBROPLASTY AND KYPHOPLASTY

Vertebroplasty is a technique used to treat vertebral compression fractures. Code 81.65 is assigned for this procedure, which involves the insertion of cement glue-like material (polymethylmethacrylate) into the vertebral body to stabilize and strengthen collapsed or crushed bone.

Kyphoplasty (81.66) is a procedure that utilizes an inflatable balloon that is expanded in order to reestablish vertebral height in compression fractures. After the balloon is removed, the cavity is filled with polymethylmethacrylate, which hardens to further stabilize the bone.

While these procedures are similar, in the vertebroplasty there is no balloon involved, and no attempt is made to restore vertebral height to reduce the compression fractures of the vertebra.

SPINAL DISC PROSTHESES

Minimally invasive arthroplasty procedures are being carried out as an alternative to spinal fusion. These procedures are performed to replace the degenerated disc nucleus and restore or maintain the normal function of the disc by inserting artificial disc prostheses. The prostheses are used to replace the entire spinal disc or replace the disc nucleus.

In order to properly select the procedure code for the insertion of spinal disc prostheses, it is important to determine the type of prosthesis (partial or total), as well as the spinal segment treated, such as cervical (84.61 and 84.62), thoracic (84.63), or lumbosacral (84.64 and 84.65). Note that for the thoracic spine, partial and total prostheses are included in the same code (84.63), unlike for the cervical and lumbosacral spine, where *ICD-9-CM* differentiates between partial and total disc prostheses with unique codes. If information is not available regarding the location of the spine treated, code 84.60 may be used.

Revision/replacement codes (84.66–84.69) are also available to report either the repair or the removal of the artificial disc prosthesis with the synchronous insertion of a new prosthesis. These codes specify the part of the spine treated, but they do not distinguish between partial and total prostheses.

PLICA SYNDROME

Although the plica syndrome can occasionally be found in other areas, it is almost always found in the knee. Plica syndrome occurs when the synovial bands that are present early in fetal development have not combined into one large synovial unit as they develop further. Patients with this syndrome often experience pain and swelling, weakness, and a locking and clicking sensation of the knee. The therapeutic goal is the reduction of the inflammation of the synovium and the thickening of the plica. Usual treatment measures hope to relieve symptoms within three months; if not, arthroscopic or open surgery to remove the plica may be required. Diagnosis code for plica syndrome of the knee is **727.83, Plica Syndrome,** and surgery is **80.76, Synovectomy of knee.**

FASCIITIS

Necrotizing fasciitis is a fulminating infection that begins with severe or extensive cellulitis that spreads to the superficial and deep fascia, producing thrombosis of the subcutaneous vessels and gangrene of the underlying tissue. Group A Streptococcus is the most common organism responsible for this condition, but any bacteria may be the cause. Code 728.86 is assigned for this condition, with an additional code for the organism when this information is known.

Review Exercise 19.4

Code the following diagnoses and procedures. Do not assign E codes.

	Code(s)
1. Acute polymyositis	710.4
Mild thoracogenic scoliosis	737.34
Muscle biopsy	83.21
2. Sclerosing tenosynovitis, left thumb and middle finger	727.05
3. Osteomyelitis of left distal femur due	250.80
to diabetes	731.8
	730.25
Sequestrectomy and excision of sinus tract,	77.05
left femur	77.65

Review Exercise 19.4 *(continued)*

4. Adhesive capsulitis, left shoulder   726.0

5. Nonunion of fracture, left femoral neck   733.82
                                      or Late   905.3

   Inlay type iliac bone graft to nonunion   78.05
   of femoral neck; bone excised for graft   77.79
                                      Excision

6. Second and third hammer toes, left   735.4

   Left second and third hammer toe repair   77.56

7. Recurrent dislocation of patella   718.36

8. Deformity of left ring finger, due to   736.20
   old tendon injury   905.8
                                      Late

   Transfer of flexor tendon from distal   82.56
   phalanx to middle phalanx

Review Exercise 19.4 *(continued)*

9. Cervical spondylosis, C5–6, C6–7   721.0

   Anterior cervical spinal fusion, C5–6, C6–7   81.02
                                                                       81.62

10. Right hallux valgus   735.0

    Resection of hallux valgus with insertion   77.59
    of prosthesis

11. Bunion, left foot   727.1

    Mitchell-type bunionectomy (with osteotomy   77.51
    of first metatarsal)

12. Dupuytren's contracture   728.6

    Incision and division of palmar fascia   82.12

13. Multiple compression fractures of vertebrae   733.13
    and major osseous defects due to senile osteoporosis   733.01
                                                                       731.3

Coding of Pregnancy and Childbirth Complications, Abortion, Congenital Anomalies, and Perinatal Conditions

20 Complications of Pregnancy, Childbirth, and the Puerperium

Conditions that affect the management of pregnancy, childbirth, and the puerperium are classified to categories 630 through 676 in chapter 11 of *ICD-9-CM*. Conditions from other chapters of *ICD-9-CM* are usually reclassified in chapter 11 when they either complicate the obstetrical experience or are themselves aggravated by the pregnancy. Any condition that occurs during pregnancy, childbirth or the puerperium is considered to be a complication unless the attending physician specifically documents that it neither affects the pregnancy nor is affected by the pregnancy.

When the encounter is for a condition totally unrelated to the pregnancy, and the physician so documents, the code for the condition is listed first, with code **V22.2, Pregnant state, incidental,** assigned as an additional code. Chapter 11 codes take precedence over codes from other chapters, but codes from other chapters may be used as additional codes when needed to provide more specificity. Codes from chapter 11 of *ICD-9-CM* refer to the mother only and are assigned only on the mother's record. They are never assigned on the newborn record; other codes are provided for that purpose. (See chapter 23.) Codes from categories 630 through 639 are assigned for ectopic pregnancy, molar pregnancy, and abortion. (Code assignments for these conditions are discussed in chapter 21.)

Codes from categories 640 through 676 apply throughout the entire obstetrical experience, which begins at conception and ends six weeks (42 days) after delivery. *ICD-9-CM* divides this period as follows:

- Complications mainly related to pregnancy   640–649
- Normal delivery and other indications for care in pregnancy, labor and delivery 650–659
- Complications occurring mainly during the course of labor and delivery   660–669
- Complications of the puerperium   670–676

The process of labor and delivery includes three stages. The first stage begins with the onset of regular uterine contractions and ends when the cervical os is completely dilated. The second stage begins with complete dilation and continues until the infant has been completely expelled. The third stage begins with the expulsion of the infant and continues until the placenta and membranes have been expelled and contraction of the uterus is complete. The puerperium begins at the end of the third stage of labor and continues for six weeks.

Occasionally a pregnancy continues for a longer term than usual gestation and is considered to be a long pregnancy. The following two codes are used when this occurs:

- 645.1x   Post term pregnancy (over 40 to 42 weeks of gestation)
- 645.2x   Prolonged pregnancy (advanced beyond 42 weeks of gestation)

FIFTH-DIGIT SUBCLASSIFICATION

Categories 640 through 648 and 651 through 676 use a fourth digit to provide more information regarding the type of complication. A fifth digit provides information regarding the current episode of care, as follows:

- 1   delivered, with or without mention of antepartum condition
- 2   delivered, with mention of postpartum condition
- 3   antepartum condition or complication when delivery has not occurred
- 4   postpartum condition or complication when delivery occurred during a previous episode of care

The episode of care for an obstetrical patient is defined in *ICD-9-CM* as the period between admission and discharge for an inpatient or the conclusion of the current visit to the attending physician, outpatient clinic, or other health care service.

Because certain complications occur only at a given point within the obstetrical experience, only certain fifth digits are appropriate. For example, placenta previa, abruptio placentae, and antepartum hemorrhage occur only during the antepartum period. Postpartum hemorrhage, on the other hand, occurs only after delivery. In some manuals, the fifth digits that can be used with each subcategory code are listed in brackets under the code number in the Tabular List. Because multiple coding is common in this chapter, the coder must be sure that fifth-digit assignments are consistent with each other. Certain fifth-digit combinations are invalid for the same episode of care:

- 0 (for unspecified or not applicable) is inappropriate for acute hospital use, where easily accessible information always permits a more specific assignment. It cannot be used with any other fifth digit in the series.
- 1 and 2 can be used together for the same episode but not with any other fifth digit.
- 3 and 4 cannot be used together or with any other fifth digit.

Figure 20.1 illustrates the decision process for assigning fifth digits for categories 640 through 674.

OUTCOME OF DELIVERY

Because chapter 11 codes do not indicate the outcome of delivery, a code from category V27 is assigned as an additional code to provide this information whenever the patient delivers in the hospital. Fourth digits indicate both whether the outcome was single or multiple and whether liveborn or stillborn. These codes are used only on the mother's record, not the record of the newborn, and are assigned only for the episode of care during which delivery occurred. No code from category V27 is assigned when delivery occurs outside the hospital prior to admission. Examples of appropriate use of codes from category V27 include:

- Term pregnancy, spontaneous delivery, vertex presentation; liveborn male infant <u>650</u> + V27.0
- Term pregnancy with spontaneous delivery; twin pregnancy, with one twin liveborn and one stillborn   <u>651.01</u> + V27.3 + 656.41

To locate the code assignment for outcome of delivery, the coder should refer to the main term **Outcome of delivery** in the Alphabetic Index of Diseases and Injuries. If the mother's record does not state the outcome, the coder should refer to the newborn record for this information.

FIGURE 20.1   Decision Process for Use of Fifth Digits for Categories 640–674

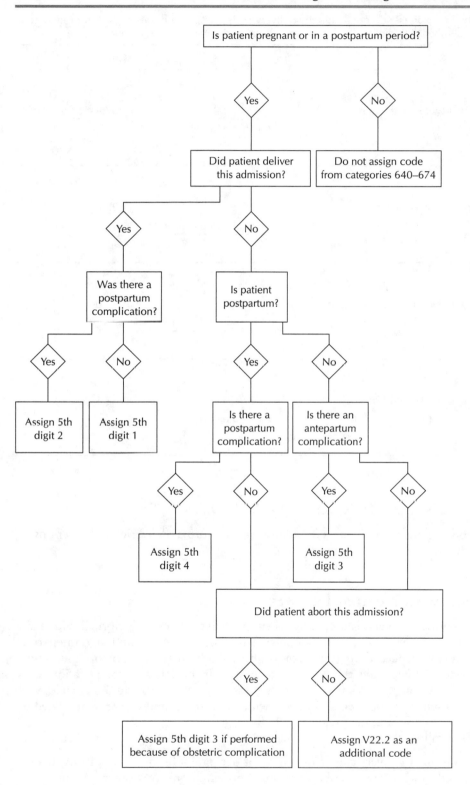

Exercise 20.1

For the following exercise, do not assign the delivery codes; assign only the V codes for outcome of delivery. Remember that in actual practice the delivery code precedes the V code.

	Code(s)
1. Delivery of twins, both stillborn Outcome of delivery	V27.4
2. Delivery of triplets, one stillborn Outcome of delivery	V27.6
3. Delivery of liveborn, female infant Outcome of delivery	V27.0
4. Delivery of single stillborn Outcome of delivery	V27.1

SELECTION OF PRINCIPAL DIAGNOSIS

The selection of principal diagnoses for admissions for normal deliveries and other obstetric care is based on the following guidelines.

Admission with Normal Delivery

Code **650, Normal delivery,** is used only when the delivery is entirely normal with a single liveborn outcome. There can be no postpartum complications, and any antepartum complication experienced during pregnancy must have been resolved before the time of delivery. Code 650 is always the principal diagnosis. If there is any complication, code 650 cannot be assigned. Codes from other chapters may be used as additional codes with code 650 only when the physician has documented that the conditions are not related to, and in no way complicate, the pregnancy.

All of the following criteria must be met in order for code 650 to be used correctly:

- Presentation at delivery can be only head or occipital. (Terms such as ROA, LOA, ROP, LOP, and vertex describe an occipital presentation.) Any other presentation such as breech, face, or brow disallows the use of code 650.

- Any antepartum complication must have been resolved prior to the admission.
- No abnormalities of either labor or delivery can have occurred.
- No postpartum complications can be present.
- No procedures other than the following can have been performed: episiotomy without forceps, episiorrhaphy, amniotomy (artificial rupture of the membranes), manually assisted delivery without forceps, administration of analgesics and/or anesthesia, fetal monitoring, induction of labor (in the absence of medical indications), and sterilization. If any other procedure is performed, code 650 cannot be assigned.
- Outcome of delivery must be single livebirth, V27.0. When there has been a multiple birth or stillbirth, code 650 cannot be assigned.

Examples include the following:

- A patient who had a completely normal delivery suffered a postpartum hemorrhage several hours after delivery. Code **666.12, Other immediate postpartum hemorrhage,** is assigned. Although the delivery itself was normal, complications were present during the episode of care; therefore, code 650 cannot be used.
- The prenatal history for a patient who had a completely normal delivery of a live infant indicates that she had a urinary tract infection at three months' gestation. This was treated with Bactrim on an outpatient basis. There was no recurrence of the infection during the pregnancy, and the patient had no infection at the time of delivery. In this case, code **650, Normal delivery,** is assigned.

Exercise 20.2

Write an "X" in front of each of the following circumstances of delivery that is assigned code **650, Normal delivery**.

_____ 1. Liveborn, full-term, breech presentation

_____ 2. Liveborn, premature, cephalic presentation

_____ 3. Stillborn, full-term, vertex presentation

___X___ 4. Liveborn, full-term, cephalic presentation; episiotomy with repair

_____ 5. Liveborn, full-term, vertex presentation; elective low forceps

_____ 6. Liveborn, full-term, vertex presentation; postpartum breast abscess

_____ 7. Liveborn, full-term, breech presentation changed to vertex presentation by version prior to delivery

---

Admission with Other Delivery

When a delivery does not meet the criteria for assignment of code **650, Normal delivery,** the principal diagnosis should correspond to the main circumstance or complication of the delivery. The principal diagnosis for a cesarean delivery should correspond to the reason for the cesarean unless the reason for admission is unrelated to the condition that resulted in the cesarean delivery. For example:

- A patient who had a previous cesarean delivery was admitted for a second cesarean delivery. She also had type 1 diabetes mellitus. Cesarean delivery was accomplished without complication. Code **654.21, Previous cesarean delivery,** is assigned as the principal diagnosis, with an additional code of **648.01 Diabetes mellitus.** Code 250.01 would also be assigned to provide more specificity.

- A patient was admitted to the hospital in obstructed labor due to a breech presentation. Version was unsuccessful, and the patient was delivered by cesarean section several hours later. The principal diagnosis code is **660.01, Obstruction of labor due to malposition of fetus at onset of labor,** and code **652.21, Breech presentation** is assigned as an additional code to provide more specificity.

Admission for Other Obstetric Care

When the admission or encounter is for obstetric care other than delivery, the principal diagnosis should correspond to the complication that necessitated the admission or encounter. If more than one complication is present, all of which are treated or monitored, any of the complication codes may be sequenced first. If no obstetric complications are present, the following guidelines govern selection of the principal diagnosis:

- If the reason for admission or encounter is not related to an obstetric condition but the patient is pregnant, code **V22.2, Incidental pregnancy,** is assigned as an additional code. This code is never assigned as the principal diagnosis and no codes from chapter 11 can be assigned.
- For routine prenatal visits when no complication is present, one of the following codes is assigned as the reason for encounter:
  V22.0   **Supervision of normal first pregnancy**
  V22.1   **Supervision of other normal pregnancy**
  These codes are assigned only as principal diagnosis and no codes from chapter 11 can be assigned.
- Occasionally, an expectant mother may visit a pediatrician to receive advice on childcare or to evaluate the pediatric office. This is not a visit related to a problem with the pregnancy. Code **V65.11, Pediatric pre-birth visit for expectant mother,** may be assigned for these encounters.
- A code from category **V23.x, Supervision of high risk pregnancy,** can be assigned as the principal diagnosis or as an additional code; codes from chapter 11 can also be assigned. Fourth digits indicate the situation that defines the pregnancy as high risk, such as a poor obstetric history (V23.41 and V23.49) or grand multiparity (V23.3). An exception is that code **V23.2, Pregnancy with history of abortion,** is not assigned for a pregnant patient; code **646.3x, Habitual aborter,** is assigned.
- *ICD-9-CM* also defines a high risk pregnancy as those who will be 35 years of age or over or 16 years of age or less at the expected time of delivery. Codes for supervision of such patients include the following:
  V23.81   **Elderly primigravida**
  V23.82   **Elderly multigravida**
  V23.83   **Young primigravida**
  V23.84   **Young multigravida**
  If the patient's age has become a complication, code 659.5x is assigned for an elderly primigravida, or code 659.6x for an elderly multigravida. Code 659.8x is assigned for a young patient whether this is the first or a later pregnancy.
- When a patient delivers outside the hospital and is then admitted for routine postpartum care with no complications present, code **V24.0, Postpartum care and examination immediately after delivery,** is assigned as the principal diagnosis. When a postpartum complication is present, the code for that condition is designated as the principal diagnosis and code V24.0 is not assigned.

  For example: A woman was admitted following delivery in the parking lot of the hospital. On admission, it was noted that she had sustained a first-degree perineal laceration. Code **664.04, First-degree laceration,** postpartum, is assigned rather than code V24.0.

Exercise 20.3

Code the following diagnoses.

	Code(s)
1. Antepartum supervision of <u>pregnancy</u> in patient with history of three previous stillbirths	V23.5
2. Office visit for routine prenatal <u>care</u>, for primigravida patient with no complications	V22.0
3. Office visit for care of elderly patient who is in the fourth month of her third pregnancy	V23.82
4. Hospital admission of patient in good condition after delivering a single liveborn infant in taxi on the way to the hospital <u>Admission</u> for	V24.0
5. Admission for intravenous antibiotic therapy of patient who delivered a single liveborn at home three days ago; patient now suffering an abscess of the breast <u>Postpartum</u>	675.14

FETAL CONDITIONS AFFECTING MANAGEMENT OF PREGNANCY

Codes from categories **655, Known or suspected fetal abnormality affecting management of the mother,** and **656, Other fetal and placental problems affecting management of the mother,** are assigned only when the fetal condition is actually responsible for modifying the mother's care. Such an effect may be documented by additional diagnostic studies based on the fetal problem, additional observation, special care, or termination of the pregnancy. The fact that the fetal condition exists does not in itself justify assigning a code from these categories; this applies only when the condition affects the management of the mother's care.

For example, when fetal distress results in a decision to perform a cesarean delivery or early induction of labor in the mother, code **656.8x, Other specified fetal and placental problems,** is assigned. On the other hand, fetal distress may be noted during delivery with no change made in the mother's care. In this case, code 656.8x is not assigned because the fetal distress is not considered to have affected the management of the mother significantly, given that the only procedures performed were the administration of fluids and/or oxygen and the repositioning of the mother. This guideline also applies to code **659.7x, Abnormality in fetal heart rate or rhythm.**

Code **656.3x, Fetal distress,** is assigned when fetal metabolic acidosis is documented as affecting the management of the mother's care.

In Utero Surgery

Surgery performed in utero on a fetus is considered an obstetric encounter. Codes from chapter 15, perinatal codes, should not be used on the mother's record to identify fetal conditions. Instead, when surgery is performed on the fetus in utero, a diagnosis code from category **655, Known or suspected fetal abnormalities affecting management of the mother,** should be assigned for the fetal condition. Procedure code **75.36, Correction of fetal defect,** is assigned.

OTHER CONDITIONS COMPLICATING PREGNANCY, CHILDBIRTH, OR THE PUERPERIUM

Some conditions inevitably complicate the obstetrical experience or are themselves aggravated by pregnancy. Hypertension, for example, is classified in category 642 during pregnancy, delivery, and the puerperium. Other designated conditions, such as urinary tract infection and liver disorders, are classified in category 646 when they complicate the obstetrical experience. Certain infectious diseases such as rubella, malaria, tuberculosis, and venereal disease are classified in category 647, and conditions such as diabetes mellitus, anemia, and thyroid dysfunction are reclassified in category 648. Conditions classifiable in categories 642 and 646 through 648 should be assumed to complicate the obstetrical experience unless the physician specifically indicates otherwise. These codes are also used when such conditions are present during childbirth or the puerperium.

Some codes for such complications are very specific, and others are rather broad. When a code from chapter 11 describes the condition adequately, only that code is assigned. It is appropriate, however, to assign an additional code when it provides needed specificity. For example, a diagnosis of diabetes mellitus, insulin-dependent, with ketoacidosis, complicating pregnancy, is coded 648.0x, but this code indicates only that the patient has diabetes mellitus. It provides no information about the type of diabetes or any complication associated with it, making an additional code from category 250 useful in fully describing the patient's condition. Code **V58.67, Long-term (current) use of insulin,** may also be assigned if the diabetes mellitus is being treated with insulin. Gestational diabetes can occur during pregnancy in women who were not diabetic before the pregnancy. Gestational diabetes can complicate the pregnancy, and there is an increased risk in women with gestational diabetes to develop diabetes mellitus following delivery. Gestational diabetes is coded to 648.8x. Code V58.67 should also be assigned if the gestational diabetes is being treated with insulin. On the other hand, the code for varicose veins of the legs complicating pregnancy or the puerperium (671.0x) provides complete information, and assignment of an additional code would be redundant. Other examples of the appropriate use of these codes follow:

- Term pregnancy, delivered, spontaneous; patient has a chronic cystitis and has had recurrent bouts of acute cystitis during her pregnancy with an acute episode at time of admission   646.61 + 595.0
- Asymptomatic bacteriuria; pregnancy, near-term, undelivered   646.53
- Diabetes mellitus, type 1, out of control and in coma; intrauterine pregnancy, 28 weeks, undelivered   648.03 + 250.33

Category 649 has been created to describe certain conditions or status of the mother that affect the pregnancy, childbirth, or the puerperium. For example:

- 649.0x   Tobacco use disorder complicating pregnancy, childbirth, or the puerperium
- 649.1x   Obesity complicating pregnancy, childbirth, or the puerperium
- 649.2x   Bariatric surgery status complicating pregnancy, childbirth, or the puerperium
- 649.3x   Coagulation defects complicating pregnancy, childbirth, or the puerperium
- 649.4x   Epilepsy complicating pregnancy, childbirth, or the puerperium
- 649.5x   Spotting complicating pregnancy
- 649.6x   Uterine size date discrepancy

Hypertension

Other examples show the use of codes for a patient who has both pregnancy and hypertension. Pre-existing hypertension is always considered to be a complicating factor in pregnancy, childbirth, or the puerperium and is classified in category 642 as follows:

- Benign essential hypertension 642.00–642.04
- Hypertension secondary to chronic kidney disease 642.10–642.14
- Other preexisting hypertension 642.20–642.24

Patients who do not have pre-existing hypertension frequently develop transient or gestational hypertension during pregnancy. This condition is essentially an elevated blood pressure and clears relatively quickly once the pregnancy is over. This condition is coded to the 642.30 through 642.34 series.

Hypertension in pregnancy sometimes leads to a pathological condition described as eclampsia or pre-eclampsia. When these conditions are superimposed on a pre-existing hypertension, a code from subcategory 642.7x is assigned. When they arise without any pre-existing hypertension, they are classified in subcategories 642.4 through 642.6.

Gestational hypertension associated with albuminuria (albumin in urine) or edema (abnormal accumulation of fluid in body tissues) or both is generally considered to be pre-eclampsia or eclampsia. Codes for eclampsia or pre-eclampsia are never assigned solely on the basis of an elevated blood pressure, an abnormal albumin level, or the presence of edema. The physician must specify the condition as eclampsia or pre-eclampsia before any of these codes may be assigned.

CERCLAGE OF CERVIX

Cerclage of the cervix is a surgical technique to reinforce the cervical muscle by placing sutures above the opening of the cervix to narrow the cervical canal. This procedure is used in the treatment of incompetent cervix. Cervical incompetence, a cause of miscarriage and preterm birth in the second and third trimesters, is a condition in which the cervix begins to open and thin before pregnancy has reached term. Dilation and effacement of the cervix occurs without pain or uterine contraction in a woman with cervical incompetence. Instead of developing uterine contractions as it happens in normal pregnancy, these events occur because of the weakness of the cervix, which opens under the growing pressure of the uterus as the pregnancy progresses. If the changes are not delayed, rupture of the membranes and birth of a premature baby can result. These cerclage procedures usually close the cervix through the vagina using a speculum. The transabdominal cerclage makes it possible to place the stitch exactly at the level needed. Another approach involves performing the cerclage through an abdominal incision. It can be carried if the cervix is very short, effaced or totally distorted.

The codes for repair of the cervical os are as follows:

- 67.51 Transabdominal cerclage of cervix
- 67.59 Other cerclage of cervix

The Shirodkar operation, transvaginal cerclage, McDonald operation, and cerclage of isthmus uteri are included in code 67.59.

POSTPARTUM COMPLICATIONS

The postpartum period, clinically termed the puerperium, begins immediately after delivery and includes the subsequent six weeks. A postpartum complication is defined as any complication that occurs during that six-week period. Postpartum complications that occur during the same admission as the delivery are identified by a fifth digit 2. Fifth digit 4 is used for a postpartum complication that occurs after discharge. For example:

- A patient is admitted three weeks postpartum and treated for acute pyelonephritis due to E. coli infection. Code **646.64, Infections of genitourinary tract, postpartum complication,** is assigned as the principal diagnosis. Code **590.10, Acute pyelonephritis,** and code **041.4, Escherichia coli (E. coli),** are assigned as additional codes to provide specificity regarding the infection.
- A patient is admitted five weeks postpartum with acute cholecystitis and cholelithiasis. Code **646.84, Other specified complication of pregnancy,** and code **574.00, Calculus of gallbladder with acute cholecystitis without mention of obstruction,** are assigned.

The narrative for code 669.8x, Other complications of labor and delivery, has been revised to include uterine atony without hemorrhage. This change is intended to differentiate uterine atony with and without hemorrhage. Code 666.1x, Other immediate postpartum hemorrhage, describes uterine atony with hemorrhage. Uterine atony can lead to postpartum hemorrhage when the uterus is unable to contract and compress the blood vessels that previously supplied blood to the placenta. As previously discussed, postpartum complications that occur during the same admission as the delivery are identified by fifth digit 2. Fifth digit 4 is used for a postpartum complication that occurs after discharge. For example:

- A patient developed uterine atony with hemorrhage immediately following delivery of the placenta. Code **666.12, Other immediate postpartum hemorrhage, delivered with mention of postpartum complication,** is assigned.

LATE EFFECT OF COMPLICATION OF PREGNANCY, CHILDBIRTH, OR THE PUERPERIUM

Code **677, Late effect of complication of pregnancy, childbirth, or the puerperium,** is assigned when an initial complication of the obstetrical experience develops a sequela that requires care or treatment at a later date. This code can be used at any time after the initial postpartum period. Like all late effect codes, code 677 is sequenced after the code describing the residual condition. Examples include the following:

- A patient was admitted for repair of uterine prolapse secondary to trauma sustained during childbirth two years earlier. Code **618.1, Uterine prolapse,** is assigned first with code **677, Late effect of complication of pregnancy, childbirth, or the puerperium,** assigned as an additional code.
- A patient presented with fatigue and cold intolerance. Her history indicated that she had experienced a severe hemorrhage during delivery of a normal liveborn seven months earlier. She was diagnosed with Sheehan's syndrome and treated with replacement hormones. Code **253.2, Panhypopituitarism,** is assigned for Sheehan's syndrome, followed by code **677, Late effect of complication of pregnancy, childbirth, or the puerperium.**

Exercise 20.4

Code the following diagnoses and procedures. Assign V codes where applicable.

	Code(s)
1. Intrauterine pregnancy, spontaneous delivery, single liveborn	650 V27.0
Induction of labor by cervical dilation	73.1

Exercise 20.4 *(continued)*

2. Intrauterine pregnancy, 12 weeks gestation,   643.03
   undelivered, with mild hyperemesis
   Gravidarium

3. Intrauterine pregnancy, 39 weeks,   661.01
   delivered, left occipitoanterior, single liveborn   V27.0
   Primary uterine inertia

4. Cesarean delivery of stillborn at 38 weeks   656.71
   gestation owing to placental infarction   V27.1
        656.41

5. Intrauterine pregnancy, with pernicious   648.23
   anemia, not delivered   281.0

6. Intrauterine pregnancy, term   650
   Spontaneous delivery, left occipitoanterior   V27.0
   Single liveborn

   Assisted spontaneous delivery   73.59

7. Intrauterine pregnancy, twins, 33 weeks   644.21
   Premature rupture of membranes   658.11
   Spontaneous delivery of premature twins,   651.01
   vertex presentation, both liveborn   673.22
   Postpartum pulmonary embolism   V27.2

8. Premature delivery, frank breech   644.21
   presentation, single female liveborn   652.21
   First-degree tear, vaginal wall   664.01
        V27.0

9. Term pregnancy, delivered, single stillborn,   641.21
   left occipitoanterior   663.11
   Terminal abruptio placentae   656.41
   Cord tightly around neck with compression   V27.1

10. Intrauterine pregnancy, 12 weeks;   642.03
    long-standing essential hypertension
    being monitored closely

PROCEDURES ASSISTING DELIVERY

Delivery can be assisted in a number of ways. Labor may be induced by artificial rupture of membranes (73.01) or by other surgical induction such as cervical dilatation (73.1). Artificial rupture of membranes may also be performed after labor has begun (73.09). Amnioinfusion (75.37) may also be performed. If rotation is carried out, code **72.4, Forceps rotation of fetal head,** or code **73.51, Manual rotation of fetal head,** is assigned. For a routine delivery, code **73.59, Other manually assisted delivery,** may be assigned.

Forceps Delivery and Vacuum Extraction

Forceps, vacuum extraction, or internal and combined version may also assist delivery. Codes are provided for low-forceps, mid-forceps, or high-forceps delivery. In a low-forceps or outlet-forceps delivery (72.0–72.1), forceps are applied to a visible fetal head after it has entered the pelvic floor. Mid-forceps (72.2x) are applied to the head during its entry into the pelvic floor, and high-forceps (72.3x) are applied to the head before it enters the pelvic brim. Breech presentations may require partial or total breech extraction (72.5x), with or without forceps to the aftercoming head. Vacuum extraction (72.7) uses a traction device rather than forceps applied to the fetal head for extraction of the fetus.

Episiotomy

Episiotomy is ordinarily performed to assist delivery; code 73.6 is assigned for a routine episiotomy. When an episiotomy is performed in connection with a forceps delivery, a combination code is provided for the type of forceps and episiotomy (72.1, 72.21, 72.31). Repair of the episiotomy is included in the episiotomy code.

Perineal Lacerations

Perineal lacerations are classified as first, second, or third degree in subcategories 664.0x through 664.3x. Inclusion notes for these codes indicate what is involved in each degree. When more than one degree is mentioned, only the code for the highest degree is assigned. Code **75.69, Repair of other current obstetric laceration,** is assigned for repair of an obstetrical perineal laceration. Occasionally, an episiotomy extends spontaneously to become a perineal laceration or tear; in this case, the laceration is coded as a diagnosis, and no code is assigned for the episiotomy. Repair of the laceration is included in code 75.69.

Fetal Pulse Oximetry

Fetal oxygen monitoring technology provides the physician with a direct measure of fetal oxygen status when an irregular fetal heart rate is present. The intrapartum fetal oxygen monitor uses a single-use, disposable sensor that is inserted through the birth canal when one of the amniotic membranes has ruptured and the cervix is dilated over 2 centimeters. The oxygen saturation is displayed on a monitor screen as a percentage. The Food and Drug Administration has indicated that this monitor should be used only after maternal membranes have ruptured and on a singleton fetus in vertex presentation with a gestational age greater than or equal to 36 weeks. The code for this fetal pulse oximetry is 75.38 and the title for **75.34** is changed to **Other fetal monitoring.**

Cesarean Delivery

Cesarean delivery is an operative delivery that is carried out when, for some reason, spontaneous delivery is not possible or does not seem advisable. A **Classical cesarean section,**

74.0, removes the fetus through an incision into the upper part of the uterus using an abdominal peritoneal approach. A **Low cervical cesarean, 74.1,** uses an incision into the lower portion of the uterus, with a pelvic cavity or abdominal peritoneal incision. Other fourth digits with category 74 indicate other types of cesarean delivery.

SERVICES RELATED TO CONTRACEPTIVE MANAGEMENT

Category **V25, Encounter for contraceptive management,** is assigned as the principal diagnosis for admissions or outpatient encounters for the purpose of contraceptive management. This category covers services such as initiation of contraceptive measures (V25.0x), insertion of intrauterine contraceptive device (V25.1), sterilization (V25.2), surveillance of previously implemented contraceptive measures (V25.4x), and insertion of implantable subdermal contraceptive device (V25.5). Procedure codes must also be assigned when appropriate.

Exercise 20.5

Code the following procedures.

	Code(s)
1. Family planning counseling	V25.09
2. Encounter for insertion of intrauterine contraceptive device	V25.1
Insertion of intrauterine contraceptive device	69.7
3. Encounter for removal of intrauterine contraceptive device	V25.42
Removal of intrauterine contraceptive device	97.71

STERILIZATION

When a patient seeks health care for the purpose of contraceptive sterilization, code **V25.2, Sterilization,** is assigned as the principal diagnosis. If there are underlying medical or psychological conditions that led to the decision to undergo sterilization, codes for these conditions may be assigned as additional diagnoses. Because sterilization may be performed as an elective procedure without any predisposing medical or psychological reasons, code V25.2 can be used as a solo diagnosis code.

When an elective sterilization procedure is performed during a hospital episode in which an obstetrical delivery has occurred, V25.2 is assigned as a secondary code, with a code from chapter 11 of *ICD-9-CM* assigned as the principal diagnosis.

Note that code V25.2 is assigned for both female and male patients for whom a contraceptive sterilization procedure is performed. Sterilization procedures for females are classified in subcategories 66.2x and 66.3x; sterilization procedures for males are classified in subcategory 63.7x.

Code V25.2 is not assigned as either a principal or a secondary diagnosis when sterilization results from other treatment or when a sterilization procedure is performed as part of the treatment for another condition. In such cases, the original condition, any complications or comorbidities, and the procedures performed are coded. For example, when a hysterectomy is performed because of injury or damage to the uterus during delivery, only the obstetrical diagnoses and procedures are coded, even though the procedure results in sterility. Code V25.2 is used only for a sterilization performed specifically for contraception; assigning it when a sterilization is incidental to other treatment is inappropriate.

Other examples of appropriate coding of situations involving sterilization follow:

- A patient with multiparity (five children) with reactive depression is admitted for elective sterilization; bilateral endoscopic ligation and division of the fallopian tubes is carried out for sterilization   V25.2 + 300.4 + V61.5 + 66.22
- Term pregnancy, delivered; breech presentation; delivery by partial breech extraction; endoscopic bilateral partial salpingectomy for sterilization   652.21 + V25.2 + 72.52 + 66.29

Exercise 20.6

Code the following diagnostic statements and procedures.

	Code(s)
1. Malignant hypertension	V25.2
Admitted for sterilization	401.0
Endoscopy with bilateral tubal ligation and division	66.22

Exercise 20.6 *(continued)*

2. Endometriosis of uterus | V25.2
   Admitted for sterilization | 617.0

Bilateral partial salpingectomy for sterilization | 66.39

3. Term pregnancy, with breech delivery, | 652.21
   female infant, followed by sterilization | V25.2
   | V27.0

Breech extraction | 72.52
Bilateral partial salpingectomy | 66.39

4. Elective sterilization, patient request | V25.2

Vasectomy, bilateral | 63.73

PROCREATIVE MANAGEMENT

A code from category **V26, Procreative management,** is assigned when a patient who is having difficulty in becoming pregnant is seen for help in correcting this problem.

Admission for a tuboplasty or vasoplasty to reverse a previous sterilization procedure is coded **V26.0, Tuboplasty or vasoplasty after previous sterilization.** This is performed to reverse a previous sterilization. Encounters for investigations such as sperm counts or fallopian tube insufflation are coded to **V26.21, Fertility testing.**

There are codes to describe testing and counseling of male counterparts for genetic disease. The following codes distinguish between genetic testing for a female and male:

- V26.31   Testing of female for genetic disease carrier status
- V26.32   Other genetic testing of female
- V26.33   Genetic counseling
- V26.34   Testing of male for genetic disease carrier status
- V26.35   Encounter for testing of male partner of habitual aborter
- V26.39   Other genetic testing of male

Review Exercise 20.7

Code the following diagnostic statements and procedures. Assign V codes where applicable.

	Code(s)
1. Elderly primigravida (37 years old); term delivery, spontaneous, of living female infant	659.51
	V27.0
Outcome of delivery	
Episiotomy and repair	73.6
2. Term pregnancy, living twins, cesarean delivery performed because fetal distress noted prior to labor	656.81
	651.01
	V27.2
Outcome of delivery	
Low cervical cesarean delivery	74.1
3. Delivery, term birth, living child, ROA presentation	650
	V27.0
Outcome of delivery	
Fetal monitoring during labor	75.34
Episiotomy and episiorrhaphy	73.6
4. Uterine pregnancy, term, delivered with obstructed labor due to transverse presentation Preexisting hypertension with mild pre-eclampsia, single liveborn	660.01
	652.31
	642.71
Outcome of delivery	V27.0

Review Exercise 20.7 *(continued)*

5. Intrauterine pregnancy, near-term, <u>delivered</u>,   <u>651.01</u>
   spontaneous   666.02
   Third-stage hemorrhage with <u>anemia</u>   648.22
   secondary to acute blood loss   285.1
   Twins, both liveborn   V27.2
   <u>Outcome of delivery</u>

6. Pregnancy, <u>delivered</u>, frank breech   <u>652.21</u>
   presentation with liveborn male infant   V27.0
   <u>Outcome of delivery</u>

   Partial breech <u>extraction</u> with forceps   72.51
   to aftercoming head

7. Term pregnancy, <u>delivered</u>, spontaneous   <u>650</u>
   Liveborn, male infant   V27.0
   <u>Outcome of delivery</u>

   Assisted spontaneous <u>delivery</u>   73.59

   Elective <u>sterilization</u> following delivery   V25.2

   Bilateral endoscopic <u>ligation</u> and crushing of   66.21
   fallopian tubes

8. Intrauterine <u>pregnancy</u>, with complicating   654.53
   incompetent cervix, undelivered

   Modified <u>Shirodkar</u> operation   67.59

Review Exercise 20.7 *(continued)*

9. Gestational hypertension   642.33
   <u>Pregnancy</u>, third trimester, undelivered

10. Intrauterine pregnancy, term, <u>delivered</u>,   664.11
    right occipitoanterior, liveborn male infant   V27.0
    Second-degree <u>lacerations</u>, perineum

         <u>Outcome of delivery</u>

    <u>Amniotomy for induction of labor</u>   73.01
    Low-forceps <u>delivery</u>   72.0
    Repair of perineal laceration   75.69

11. <u>Delivery</u>, stillborn, male infant,   660.01
    brow presentation; obstructed labor   652.41
         <u>Outcome of delivery</u>   656.41
                                                              V27.1

    <u>Version</u> and <u>extraction</u>   73.22
    <u>Episiotomy</u> and repair   73.6

12. Twin pregnancy with <u>malposition</u> of one fetus   652.61
    One liveborn twin, one stillborn   651.01
                                                              656.41
                                                              V27.3

    Classical <u>cesarean</u> section   74.0

13. <u>Outpatient evaluation of fetal bradycardia</u>   659.73

21 | Abortion and Ectopic Pregnancy

Abortion is defined as the expulsion or extraction of all or part of the placenta or membrane with or without an identifiable fetus weighing less than 500 grams. When the fetus's weight cannot be determined, an estimated gestation of less than 22 completed weeks is considered an abortive outcome (abortion). Although requirements for fetal death reporting vary from state to state, these requirements should not be confused with *ICD-9-CM* rules for classifying abortions; they are entirely separate. If an expelled fetus weighs more than 500 grams or if the period of gestation is more than 22 weeks but less than 37 weeks, it is considered an early delivery and code **644.21, Early onset of delivery,** is assigned.

Pregnancy with abortive outcome is classified in categories 634 through 639. Note that the term abortion in the disease classification of *ICD-9-CM* refers to a fetal death; the codes for the abortion procedure used to terminate a pregnancy are located in volume 3. The abortion code is assigned as the principal diagnosis when the admission or encounter is for the purpose of dealing with a spontaneous abortion or performing an elective abortion. If a procedure to terminate the pregnancy is performed in the hospital, the procedure code is also required.

TYPES OF ABORTION

The primary axis for coding abortion is the type of abortion. Abortive outcome is classified by type in *ICD-9-CM* as follows:

- **Spontaneous abortion (634):** one that occurs without any instrumentation or chemical intervention
- **Legally induced abortion (635):** one performed for either therapeutic or elective termination of pregnancy (terms such as elective abortion, induced or artificial abortion, and termination of pregnancy are used when this type of abortion is performed)
- **Illegally induced abortion (636):** one not performed in accordance with provisions of state law or not meeting regulatory requirements in regard to the qualifications of the individual performing the abortion or to the location in which it is performed. This category is used for inpatient coding only when a patient who had an abortion performed outside the hospital is admitted to ensure that the abortion is complete or to treat a complication.
- **Failed abortion (638):** one in which an elective abortion procedure has failed to evacuate or expel the fetus and the patient is still pregnant

ICD-9-CM provides default category 637 for coding an abortion of unspecified type; the use of this code in an acute care facility is not appropriate.

FIFTH-DIGIT SUBCLASSIFICATION

A fifth-digit subclassification is used with categories 634 through 637 to indicate whether the abortion is complete or incomplete. When the patient is admitted because of spontaneous abortion, the fifth digit is based on whether it was complete or incomplete at the time of admission. Abortions performed in the hospital are not ordinarily discharged as incomplete. The fifth digits are assigned as follows:

- 0   unspecified (not stated as either complete or incomplete)
- 1   incomplete; all products of conception have not been expelled from the uterus
- 2   complete; all products of conception have been expelled from the uterus

The coder should not assume that an abortion is complete or incomplete without a specific statement by the physician or other concrete information in the medical record. The fact that a follow-up dilatation and curettage (D & C) is performed is not evidence in itself that an abortion is incomplete; the physician on the basis of the pathology report makes this determination.

COMPLICATIONS ASSOCIATED WITH ABORTION

Fourth digits are used with categories 634–639 to indicate whether a complication is present and the general type of complication, such as a metabolic disorder or genital infection. The abortion code is assigned as the principal diagnosis and an additional code is assigned to provide more specificity for the complication.

- A patient was admitted with spontaneous abortion, and a D & C was performed to remove any retained products of conception. None were found but there was evidence of pelvic infection. The patient was discharged on the fourth hospital day with the infection cleared. The principal diagnosis is **634.02, Spontaneous abortion complicated by genital tract and pelvic infection.** An additional code should be assigned for the infection.

When a patient is readmitted because a complication has developed following discharge, a code from category 639 is assigned as the principal diagnosis. The same fourth digits used with the abortion codes are used and an additional code is assigned to provide more specificity regarding the complication. For example:

- A patient was readmitted one week following discharge after an abortion because she had developed endometritis. Code **639.0, Complication of genital tract and pelvic infection following abortion,** was assigned as the principal diagnosis with an additional code for the endometritis.
- A patient is admitted in renal failure one week after discharge following an abortion. Code **639.3, Complications following abortion and ectopic and molar pregnancies, Renal failure,** is assigned as the principal diagnosis.

Note that category codes 634 through 638 cannot be assigned with a code from category 639.

If the readmission is for the purpose of dealing with retained products of conception, however, a code from the 634 through 637 series is assigned along with fifth digit 1 to indicate that it was incomplete. This advice should be followed even though the patient was discharged previously with a diagnosis of complete abortion. For example:

- A patient who underwent an elective abortion one week earlier was admitted because of continued bleeding. A dilation and curettage (D & C) was performed, and the pathology report showed retained products of conception. Code **635.11, Legally induced abortion complicated by delayed or excessive hemorrhage,** is assigned. Code 639 is not assigned because the abortion was incomplete.

- Five days following discharge for spontaneous abortion, a patient is admitted with a diagnosis of infection due to retained fetal tissue. The retention of fetal tissue indicates that the abortion was not complete, and so code **634.01, Spontaneous abortion complicated by genital tract and pelvic infection, incomplete,** is assigned even though the patient was hospitalized for the abortion previously.

Exercise 21.1

Code the following diagnoses, assigning fifth-digit codes. Consider the diagnostic statements given below as the only information available in the medical record. Do not assign procedure codes.

	Code(s)
1. Failed attempted abortion complicated by hemorrhage	638.1
2. Incomplete early abortion (spontaneous)	634.91
3. Therapeutic abortion, complete, with electrolyte imbalance	635.42
4. Electively induced abortion, complete, with amniotic fluid embolism	635.62
5. Patient readmitted with bleeding due to retained placenta one week following previous hospital admission for spontaneous abortion	634.11
6. Discharge #1: Electively induced abortion, complete	635.92
Discharge #2 (same patient): Sepsis following induced abortion during previous admission	639.0

MATERNAL CONDITION AS REASON FOR ABORTION

Codes from categories 640 through 648 and 651 through 657 can be assigned as an additional code to indicate a maternal condition that assisted in the decision to proceed with an elective abortion. Pregnancy can be terminated on a purely elective basis, however, and it is not necessary to assign a code to indicate a reason for the abortion. For example:

- A patient is admitted for elective abortion, based on her physician's advice that her severe congenital heart disease indicates that an abortion might be advisable to prevent cardiac complications. In this case, the principal diagnosis code is **635.92, Legal abortion, and 648.53, Congenital cardiovascular disorders,** is also assigned, along with an additional code to identify the particular heart disease.
- A patient who had rubella at six weeks gestation requests abortion because of the possibility of fetal abnormality. Code **635.92, Legally induced abortion without mention of complication,** is designated as the principal diagnosis, with an additional code of **655.33, Suspected damage to fetus from viral disease in the mother.**
- A patient is admitted with placenta previa. She does not request abortion, but after evaluating various treatment possibilities, her physician concludes that an abortion is necessary. The patient consents, and the abortion is carried out. In this case, the code for placenta previa (641.0x) is sequenced first, followed by the abortion code.

INADVERTENT ABORTION

An inadvertent abortion sometimes occurs when a pregnant patient suffers major trauma or undergoes surgery for another condition. In this situation, the code for the condition that occasioned the admission is designated as the principal diagnosis, with an additional code for the abortion.

When abortion occurs because of surgery performed on the uterus for a condition unrelated to the pregnancy, the code for the condition that required surgery is sequenced first, with an additional code from category **637, Unspecified abortion,** used to indicate that an abortion occurred. For example:

- Hysterectomy was performed after a diagnosis of uterine carcinoma. When the excised uterus was examined, a six-week-old fetus was found.
  Principal diagnosis: Carcinoma of uterus   182.8
  Additional diagnosis: Unspecified abortion, complete   637.92

When abortion occurs as a result of major trauma or surgery other than on the uterus, a code for the traumatic injury or the condition that required the surgery is sequenced as the principal diagnosis. A code from category **634, Spontaneous abortion,** is assigned as an additional code. For example:

- Appendectomy was performed because of acute appendicitis with peritonitis. On second postoperative day, patient experienced an inadvertent abortion (complete).
  Principal diagnosis: Appendicitis with peritonitis   540.0
  Additional diagnosis: Spontaneous abortion   634.92

Exercise 21.2

Code the following diagnoses. Do not assign procedure codes.

	Code(s)
1. Therapeutic abortion, complete, performed because of severe reactive psychosis	635.92 648.43 298.8
2. Inadvertent abortion (complete) prompted by radiation treatment damage to fetus, necessitating termination of pregnancy	635.92 655.63 E926.9
3. Elective abortion (complete) performed because of chromosomal abnormality of fetus	635.92 655.13

ABORTION PROCEDURE RESULTING IN LIVEBORN INFANT

Occasionally, an attempt to terminate a pregnancy results in a liveborn infant. Note that a fetus that has any heartbeat, respiration, or involuntary muscle movement after expulsion is considered to be a live birth, no matter how short a time it survives. In this situation, code **644.21, Early onset of delivery,** is assigned rather than an abortion code because, by definition, an abortion cannot result in a livebirth. A code for the procedure used in the attempt to terminate the pregnancy should also be assigned. For example:

- A patient delivered a liveborn infant with extreme immaturity following attempted abortion by insertion of laminaria. Code **644.21, Early onset of delivery, delivered,** is assigned, along with code **V27.0** (for the **single liveborn**) and code **69.93** (for the **insertion of the laminaria**).

LOSS OF FETUS WITH REMAINING FETUS

Occasionally, a patient with multiple gestation is admitted for what appears to be a spontaneous abortion during which one or more fetuses are expelled but one or more live fetuses remain in utero. In such cases, no code from 634 through 639 is assigned, and one of the following complication of pregnancy codes is assigned instead:

- 651.33 twin pregnancy with fetal loss and retention of one fetus
- 651.43 triplet pregnancy with fetal loss and retention of one or more fetuses
- 651.53 quadruplet pregnancy with fetal loss and retention of one or more fetuses
- 651.63 other multiple pregnancy with fetal loss and retention of one or more fetuses

MULTIPLE GESTATION FOLLOWING FETAL REDUCTION

Subcategory code 651.7 identifies multiple gestation following fetal reduction during the current pregnancy. These pregnancies are considered high-risk, and there is a need to identify them, even if the pregnancy is reduced to a single fetus. For example, when the woman delivers the single newborn, these codes make it possible to identify that this was originally a multiple gestation that underwent fetal reduction. Note that subcategory 651.7 refers to fetal reduction, while subcategories 651.3, 651.4, 651.5, and 651.6 described in the preceding section are for spontaneous abortion or involuntary fetal loss. For example:

- A patient with an initial twin pregnancy had previously undergone fetal reduction of one fetus because of suspected chromosomal anomalies. The patient is now admitted and delivers a normal single liveborn infant. Code **651.71, Multiple gestation following (elective) fetal reduction, delivered, with or without mention of antepartum condition,** is assigned as the principal diagnosis. Code **V27.0, Single liveborn,** is assigned to indicate the outcome of the delivery.

The codes for multiple gestation following fetal reduction are as follows:

- 651.70   Multiple gestation following (elective) fetal reduction, unspecified as to episode of care or not applicable
- 651.71   Multiple gestation following (elective) fetal reduction, delivered, with or without mention of antepartum condition
- 651.73   Multiple gestation following (elective) fetal reduction, antepartum condition or complication

PROCEDURES FOR TERMINATION OF PREGNANCY

Abortion may be induced by dilatation and curettage (69.01), aspiration curettage (69.51), injection of prostaglandin or saline (75.0), insertion of laminaria (69.93), or insertion of prostaglandin suppository (96.49). *ICD-9-CM* also provides a code for hysterotomy to terminate pregnancy (74.91), but this procedure is seldom performed.

ECTOPIC AND MOLAR PREGNANCIES

Ectopic and molar pregnancies and other abnormal products of conception are classified as follows, with an additional code from category 639 when any complication occurs:

- 630   Hydatidiform mole
- 631   Other abnormal product of conception
- 632   Missed abortion
- 633   Ectopic pregnancy

A molar pregnancy occurs when a blighted ovum within the uterus develops into a mole or benign tumor. The hydatidiform mole is a particular type of molar pregnancy and is classified separately (630) in *ICD-9-CM*. All other molar pregnancies are included in code 631.

Utilization of assisted technologies has resulted in an increase in multiple gestational pregnancies in which an intrauterine pregnancy may coexist with an ectopic pregnancy. An ectopic pregnancy (633) occurs when a fertilized ovum is implanted and develops anywhere outside the uterus. The fourth digit indicates the extrauterine location of the ectopic pregnancy. Fifth digits are assigned to indicate whether there is an intrauterine pregnancy in addition to the extrauterine pregnancy. The codes are as follows:

- 633.00 and 633.01   Abdominal pregnancy
- 633.10 and 633.11   Tubal pregnancy

- 633.20 and 633.21   Ovarian pregnancy
- 633.80 and 633.81   Other ectopic pregnancy

Tubal pregnancy is the most common type of ectopic pregnancy. Surgical procedures for removing a tubal ectopic pregnancy include **66.01, Salpingotomy,** or **66.02, Salpingostomy;** in both procedures, the ectopic pregnancy is removed from the tube by means of an incision into the fallopian tube. It can also be removed by salpingectomy (excision of the fallopian tube) with the ectopic pregnancy intact (66.62). Code **74.3, Removal of extratubal ectopic pregnancy,** is assigned for removal of any other type of ectopic pregnancy. For example:

- Tubal pregnancy   633.1x
  Removal of ectopic fetus from fallopian tube by salpingotomy   66.01
- Tubal pregnancy   633.1x
  Salpingectomy with removal of tubal pregnancy   66.62
- Abdominal pregnancy   633.0x
  Removal of abdominal pregnancy   74.3
- Cornual pregnancy   633.8x
  Removal of cornual pregnancy   74.3

Complications of Molar and Ectopic Pregnancy

Unlike complications of abortions, complications of ectopic and molar pregnancies are classified in category 639, whether they occur during the initial episode of care or during a later episode. When the complication occurs during an episode of care for the purpose of treating the ectopic or molar pregnancy, a code from the 630 through 633 series is sequenced first, followed by a code from category 639. When the patient is readmitted after a code from this series, the code from category 639 is assigned as the principal diagnosis. An additional code that describes the complication more specifically can be assigned as needed. Sample codes include the following:

- Pelvic peritonitis following ectopic tubal pregnancy (this admission)
  633.1x + 639.0
- Hemorrhage following ruptured ectopic tubal pregnancy removed on previous admission   639.1

MISSED ABORTION

The term missed abortion refers to fetal death that occurs prior to the completion of 22 weeks of gestation, with the dead fetus retained for a period of time in the uterus. This condition may be indicated by a cessation of growth, hardening of the uterus, or by actual diminution in size of the uterus. Absence of fetal heart tones after they had been previously heard is also indicative of a missed abortion. The retained fetus may be expelled spontaneously, or surgical or chemical intervention may be required. For example:

- A patient in the 20th week of gestation reports that she is no longer feeling any fetal movement. The physician cannot hear any fetal heart tones, although they were present one month ago. On examination, the uterus is hard and possibly smaller than on the last visit. Code **632, Missed abortion,** is assigned.

When the period of gestation is longer than 22 weeks, retention of a dead fetus is considered a missed intrauterine death (656.4x).

Review Exercise 21.3

Code the following diagnoses. Do not assign procedure codes.

	Code(s)
1. Therapeutic <u>abortion</u>, complete, with embolism	635.62
2. Failed attempted induction of <u>abortion</u>	638.9
3. Ruptured right tubal <u>pregnancy</u> with <u>peritonitis</u> due to group A streptococcus	633.10 639.0 041.01
4. Incomplete early <u>abortion</u> (spontaneous)	634.91
5. Spontaneous <u>abortion</u>, complete, with excessive hemorrhage	634.12
6. Electively induced <u>abortion</u> with liveborn	644.21 V27.0
7. Electively induced <u>abortion</u>, complete, complicated by shock	635.52
8. Ectopic <u>pregnancy</u>, right fallopian tube	633.10

Review Exercise 21.3 *(continued)*

9. Carneous <u>mole</u>   631

10. Hydatidiform <u>mole</u>   630

11. <u>Missed abortion</u>, 19 weeks gestation   632

12. Electively induced <u>abortion</u>, complete   <u>635.92</u>
    Family <u>problems</u> due to multiparity   V61.5

22 Congenital Anomalies

Congenital anomalies are classified in categories 740–759 in chapter 14 of *ICD-9-CM*. Congenital anomalies are abnormal conditions that are present at birth, although they may be recognized later. Codes from chapter 14 may be used throughout the life of the patient. If a congenital anomaly has been corrected, a personal history code should be used to identify the history of the anomaly.

LOCATION OF TERMS IN THE ALPHABETIC INDEX

A distinction between acquired and congenital conditions is often noted in the Alphabetic Index by a nonessential modifier associated with the main term or a subterm. When either term appears in parentheses with the main term, the alternative term can ordinarily be located as a subterm.

Note that some conditions are congenital by definition and have no acquired version; others are always considered to be acquired. For many conditions, of course, no distinction is made. When the diagnostic statement does not describe a condition as being either acquired or congenital, however, *ICD-9-CM* often makes a presumption that it is one or the other.

The following example from the Alphabetic Index demonstrates this usage:

Deformity. . .
   breast (acquired) 611.8
     congenital 757.9
   bronchus (congenital) 748.3
     acquired 519.1

In this example, the Alphabetic Index assumes that deformity of the breast without other qualification is classified as acquired, whereas deformity of the bronchus is classified as congenital if not otherwise specified. The Tabular List may offer additional guidance by means of an exclusion note. For example, the entry under category **562, Diverticula of intestine,** refers the coder elsewhere for congenital diverticulum of colon, coded **751.5, Other anomalies of intestine.** For code **751.5,** the inclusion note indicates that congenital diverticulum of the colon is appropriately classified here.

Congenital anomalies are classified first by the body system involved. Many congenital anomalies have specific codes in *ICD-9-CM*; others are located under such general terms as anomaly and deformity rather than under the name of the specific condition. For example:

- Congenital malposition of gastrointestinal tract 751.8
- Prader-Willi syndrome 759.81
- Congenital hiatus hernia 750.6
- Strawberry nevus 757.32
- Congenital hydrocephalus 742.3

Because approximately 4,000 congenital anomalies have been identified, it is impossible for the classification to provide a specific code for each. When the type of anomaly is specified, but no specific code is provided, the code for other specified anomaly of that type and site should be assigned. Often, only the code for unspecified anomaly of that general type or site can be assigned. When a specific code is not available, additional codes for manifestations of the anomaly should be assigned to the extent possible. Use additional secondary codes from other chapters to specify conditions associated with the anomaly.

RELATIONSHIP OF AGE TO CODES

Codes from chapter 14 can be reported for a patient of any age. Many congenital anomalies, although actually present at birth, do not manifest themselves until later in life. In addition, many cannot be corrected and persist throughout life and these conditions may be reported for an adult patient. Patient age is not the determining factor in assigning these codes. Here are some examples:

- A patient, 30 years of age, with Marfan syndrome was admitted for a heart valve replacement and repair of an abdominal aortic aneurysm. In this case, the code for **Marfan syndrome, 759.82,** is assigned in spite of the patient's age because the condition is an inherited disorder of the connective tissue that is transmitted as an autosomal dominant trait.
- A patient, age 25, was admitted for brain surgery, which revealed a colloid cyst of the right third ventricle. In this case, code **742.4, Other specified anomaly of the brain,** is assigned because a colloid cyst of the third ventricle is always congenital and the patient's age does not influence code assignment.

NEWBORN WITH CONGENITAL CONDITIONS

When a diagnosis of a congenital condition is made during the hospital episode in which an infant is born, the appropriate code from chapter 14 of *ICD-9-CM* should be assigned as an additional code, with the appropriate code from the V30 through V39 series used as the principal diagnosis. (See chapter 23 of this handbook.) For example:

- Term birth, male; incomplete cleft lip on right side   V30.00 + 749.12
- Term birth, male; hypospadias   V30.00 + 752.61

Note that this is an exception to the guidelines for reporting other conditions. Congenital conditions that may have future health care implications are reported for newborns even though they are not further evaluated or treated during the current episode of care.

CONGENITAL DEFORMITIES
VS. PERINATAL DEFORMITIES

Certain musculoskeletal deformities that result from a mechanical factor during gestation, such as intrauterine malposition or pressure, are classified in category **754, Certain congenital musculoskeletal deformities,** with a fourth-digit axis indicating the site or type of deformity. Conditions due to birth injury are classified as perinatal conditions in category 767 in chapter 15 of *ICD-9-CM*, with an additional code assigned to identify the specific condition whenever possible. Examples include the following:

- Bilateral congenital dislocation of hip   754.31
- Congenital dislocation of knee   754.41
- Fracture of clavicle due to birth trauma   767.2

CYSTIC KIDNEY DISEASE

There are major differences in the clinical characteristics, pathophysiology, and prognosis of the various types of congenital cystic kidney disease. This fact augments the importance of being as specific as possible about the type when assigning a code. For example, medullary sponge kidney (753.17) is relatively common and has a good prognosis, but medullary cystic kidney (753.16) can lead to chronic renal failure. When the diagnostic statement does not indicate whether a renal cyst is congenital or acquired, *ICD-9-CM* presumes that the cyst is congenital.

Review Exercise 22.1

Code the following diagnoses and procedures. Do not assign E codes.

	Code(s)
1. Polycystic kidneys, adult type	753.13
2. Hypospadias with congenital chordee	752.61
	752.63
Repair of hypospadias and release of chordee	58.45
	64.42
3. Congenital pyloric stenosis	750.5
Ramstedt procedure	43.3
4. Congenital dislocation of left hip with subluxation of right hip	754.35
Closed reduction of dislocation of both hips with immobilization in plaster casts	79.75

Review Exercise 22.1 *(continued)*

5. Congestive heart failure in patient with congenital   428.0
   interatrial septal defect   745.5

6. Posterior subcapsular cataract, OS, congenital   743.31

   Intracapsular cataract extraction with peripheral   13.19
   iridectomy and insertion of intraocular lens prosthesis   13.71

7. Accessory fifth-digit, right foot   755.02

8. Esophageal web with esophageal spasm and reflux   750.3
   esophagitis   530.5
                                          530.11

9. Left trigger thumb, congenital   756.89

   Tenolysis of flexor sheath of left thumb   82.91

10. Urachal cyst and patent urachus   753.7

Review Exercise 22.1 *(continued)*

11. Thoracoabdominal coarctation of aorta   747.10

12. Hallux rigidus, left   735.2

13. Down's syndrome   758.0

14. Bilateral talipes equinovarus, congenital   754.51

    Heel cord lengthening   83.85

15. Unilateral cleft lip and cleft palate, complete   749.21

    Rotation-advancement repair of cleft lip   27.54
    Repair cleft palate   27.62

16. Cystic lung, congenital   748.4

23 | Perinatal Conditions

Conditions other than anomalies that originate in the perinatal period are classified in chapter 15 of *ICD-9-CM* and categories 760–779. The perinatal period is defined as before birth through the 28th day following birth.

LOCATING CODES FOR PERINATAL CONDITIONS IN THE ALPHABETIC INDEX

Codes for perinatal conditions are located in the Alphabetic Index (volume 2) by referring to the main term **Birth** or to the main term for the condition and then to such subterms as neonatal, fetal, and infantile. If the Alphabetic Index does not provide a specific code for a perinatal condition, assign code **779.89, Other specified conditions originating in the perinatal period,** followed by the code from another chapter that specifies the condition.

GENERAL PERINATAL GUIDELINES

Codes from chapter 15 are never used on maternal records. By the same token, codes from chapter 11, Complications of pregnancy, childbirth and the puerperium, should never be reported on the newborn record.

Generally, chapter 15 codes are sequenced as the principal or first-listed diagnosis on the newborn record, except for the appropriate code from the V30 through V39 series for the birth episode. Codes from other chapters may be assigned as secondary diagnoses to provide additional detail.

The perinatal guidelines for secondary diagnoses are the same as the general coding guidelines for "additional diagnoses" (refer to chapter 3). In addition, assign codes for any conditions that have been specified by the provider as having implications for future health care needs. Assign codes from chapter 15 only for definitive diagnoses established by the provider. If a definitive diagnosis has not been established, codes for signs and symptoms may be assigned.

Sometimes a newborn may have a condition that may be either due to the birth process or community-acquired. If the documentation does not specify which it is, the default code selected should be due to the birth process, and a chapter 15 code should be selected. When the condition is community-acquired, do not report a chapter 15 code.

RELATIONSHIP OF AGE TO CODES

Most conditions originating during the perinatal period are transitory in nature. Other conditions that originate during the perinatal period, however, persist, and some do not manifest themselves until later in life. Such conditions are classified in chapter 15, no matter how old the patient is, and may be reported throughout the life of the patient if the condition is still present. For example:

- A 33-year-old woman was admitted for treatment of vaginal carcinoma due to intrauterine exposure to DES (diethylstilbestrol) taken by her mother during pregnancy. Code **184.0, Malignant neoplasm of vagina,** and code **760.76, Diethylstilbestrol,** are assigned because the intrauterine exposure was still an important element in the patient's condition even though the problem did not present itself until later in the patient's life.

- An 18-year-old man was admitted for workup because he had begun experiencing respiratory problems. A diagnosis of bronchopulmonary dysplasia was made, and the patient was discharged to be seen in the physician's office in two weeks. Code **770.7, Chronic respiratory disease arising in the perinatal period,** is assigned because bronchopulmonary dysplasia is a congenital condition even though it may not become a problem until later in the patient's life.

CLASSIFICATION OF BIRTHS

A code from categories V30 through V39 is assigned as the principal diagnosis for any newborn. The first axis for coding is whether the birth is single or multiple; codes for multiple births indicate whether mates are liveborn or stillborn. The fourth-digit axis indicates that the birth occurred in the hospital (0) or immediately before admission to the hospital (1). Fourth digit 2 indicates that the birth took place outside the hospital and that the newborn was not admitted; therefore, it is not assigned except for an outpatient encounter. For live births in the hospital, a fifth digit indicates whether there was a cesarean delivery. Note that categories V33, V37, and V39 should not be used in the acute care hospital; the medical record will provide sufficient information to permit assignment of a more specific code.

A code from this series is assigned only on the newborn record and is assigned only for the episode in which the birth occurred. If a newborn is discharged and readmitted or transferred to another facility, the code for the condition responsible for the transfer or readmission is designated as the principal diagnosis. For example:

- A single liveborn in the hospital with an associated diagnosis of subdural hemorrhage due to birth trauma would be coded as **V30.00, Single liveborn, + 767.0, Subdural and cerebral hemorrhage,** with the V code sequenced first.
- If the infant is discharged and readmitted or transferred to another facility for treatment of the hemorrhage, the principal diagnosis for that admission would be 767.0; no code from the V30 through V39 series would be assigned.
- If the admission of an infant born outside the hospital is delayed and the newborn is admitted later because of complication, the complication code would be assigned as the principal diagnosis; no code from the V30 through V39 series would be assigned.

OTHER DIAGNOSES FOR NEWBORNS

A code from the V30 through V39 series indicates only that a birth occurred. Additional codes are assigned for all clinically significant conditions noted on the examination of the newborn. A newborn condition is clinically significant when it has implication for the newborn's future health care. This is an exception to the UHDDS guidelines.

Insignificant or transient conditions that resolve without treatment are not coded. Medical records of newborns sometimes mention conditions such as fine rashes, molding of the scalp, and minor jaundice. Because these conditions usually resolve without treatment and require no additional workup, they would not be coded. For example:

- The physician documented diagnoses of syndactyly and hydrocele on the newborn's diagnostic statement. Even though no treatment was given and no further evaluation was done during the infant's hospital stay, both of these conditions will require treatment at some time in the future, and so they are reported.
- The physician mentioned on the newborn delivery record that the infant had slight jaundice. No further evaluation was done, and the jaundice cleared by the following day. No code for jaundice is assigned.

PREMATURITY, LOW BIRTH WEIGHT, AND POSTMATURITY

Newborns delivered before full term are defined as either immature or premature and are classified in category 765 as follows:

- Immaturity (765.0x) implies a birth weight of less than 1000 grams.
- Prematurity (765.1x) implies a birth weight of 1000–2499 grams.

Even when a newborn is not premature, it may be appropriate to assign a code from category **764, Slow fetal growth and fetal malnutrition.** This code does not imply prematurity but indicates that the newborn is smaller than expected for the length of gestation. A code to specify the number of completed weeks of gestation (765.20–765.29) should only be used with category 764 and codes 765.0x and 765.1x to report: (1) the number of weeks of gestation for preterm infants, (2) infants with extreme immaturity, and/or (3) infants with slow fetal growth and malnutrition.

To indicate the birth weight, fifth digits are assigned to codes for immaturity (765.0), prematurity (765.1), and slow fetal growth and fetal malnutrition (764.0–764.9). Care should be taken to ensure that the weight expressed by the fifth digit is reasonably consistent with the four-digit code to which it is applied. For example, a diagnosis of immaturity would appear to be inconsistent with fifth digit 9 because a birth weight of 2500 grams falls far outside the criteria for immaturity even though there is no indication in the manual that the heavier weight is excluded. The physician should be queried when there is a significant discrepancy.

Codes from category 764 and subcategories 765.0 and 765.1 are never assigned on the basis of birth weight or estimated gestation alone, but only on the physician's clinical evaluation of the maturity of the newborn, as indicated in the diagnostic statement.

Post-term is defined as a gestational period over 40 completed weeks to 42 completed weeks. Prolonged gestation or postmaturity is defined as a gestational period of more than 42 completed weeks. Category 766 classifies a long gestation and/or a high birth weight as follows:

- 766.0   Exceptionally large baby (usually implies weight of 4500 grams or more)
- 766.1   Other "heavy for dates" infants, regardless of gestation period
- 766.21   Post-term infant
- 766.22   Prolonged gestation of infant

There is no time frame that limits the use of these codes; a code can be assigned as long as the physician considers the birth weight an important element of the infant's condition. For example, an infant born at Hospital A at 34 weeks gestation and transferred to Hospital B after 14 days for further evaluation of a congenital anomaly could still have a code for prematurity assigned as an additional diagnosis. The fifth digit for these codes is always based on birth weight, not the infant's weight at the time of transfer or readmission.

FETAL DISTRESS AND ASPHYXIA

Fetal distress may be defined as signs that indicate a critical response to stress. It implies metabolic abnormalities such as hypoxia and acidosis that affect the functions of vital organs to the point of temporary or permanent injury or even death. Code 768.x is assigned for fetal distress in a liveborn, with the fourth digit indicating when it was first noted as follows:

- 768.2   First noted before onset of labor
- 768.3   First noted during labor and delivery
- 768.4   Unspecified as to time of onset

A new code has been created to identify hypoxic ischemic encephalopathy (HIE). HIE is a life-threatening condition that usually results from damage to the cells of the brain and spinal cord secondary to inadequate oxygen during the birth process. HIE can cause brain damage resulting in neurological problems such as developmental delay, mental retardation, epilepsy, and/or cerebral palsy. The incidence of HIE is infrequent, occurring in roughly two in 1,000 births. The new code for HIE is as follows:

- 768.7   Hypoxic-ischemic encephalopathy (HIE)

Subcategory 763.8 distinguishes abnormalities of heart rate or rhythm from the more serious fetal stress indicators classified in category 768:

- 763.81   Abnormality in fetal heart rate or rhythm before onset of labor
- 763.82   Abnormality in fetal heart rate or rhythm during labor
- 763.83   Abnormality in fetal heart rate or rhythm, unspecified as to time of onset

Codes for fetal distress or abnormality of heart rate and rhythm are assigned to the newborn record only when the condition is specifically identified by the physician. These codes are never assigned on the basis of other information in the newborn record.

Subcategory 770.8, **Other respiratory problems after birth,** classifies respiratory problems, including apnea, cyanotic attacks, respiratory failure, hypoxia and asphyxia, noted after birth. New codes have been created to describe other respiratory problems occurring after birth such as respiratory arrest of newborn and hypoxemia of newborn. The new codes are as follows:

- 770.87   Respiratory arrest of newborn
- 770.88   Hypoxemia of newborn

FETAL AND NEWBORN ASPIRATION

Subcategory code 770.1, **Fetal and newborn aspiration,** further specifies aspiration conditions as follows:

- 770.10   Fetal and newborn aspiration, unspecified
- 770.11   Meconium aspiration without respiratory symptoms
- 770.12   Meconium aspiration with respiratory symptoms
- 770.13   Aspiration of clear amniotic fluid without respiratory symptoms
- 770.14   Aspiration of clear amniotic fluid with respiratory symptoms
- 770.15   Aspiration of blood without respiratory symptoms
- 770.16   Aspiration of blood with respiratory symptoms
- 770.17   Other fetal and newborn aspiration without respiratory symptoms
- 770.18   Other fetal and newborn aspiration with respiratory symptoms

If applicable, an additional code, 416.8, should be assigned to identify any secondary pulmonary hypertension.

Meconium aspiration in newborns occurs when the fetus gasps while still in the birth canal and inhales meconium-stained amniotic, vaginal, or oropharyngeal fluids. Massive aspiration syndrome is synonymous with massive fetal aspiration. Although meconium aspiration syndrome and massive meconium aspiration are somewhat different conditions with similar clinical presentation and course, code **770.12, Meconium aspiration with respiratory symptoms,** is assigned for both. Code 779.84 would be assigned for meconium staining.

A diagnosis of meconium in liquor is considered an abnormal finding, and code **792.3, Abnormal findings in other body substances, Amniotic fluid,** is assigned. Code 763.84 is assigned for meconium passage during delivery.

Tachypnea, wheezing, and apnea are sometimes present in meconium aspiration; these conditions may resolve over a short period or may take a more prolonged course. In the milder forms of this condition, dyspnea occurs soon after birth, lasts two or three days, and is followed by rapid recovery. Therapy includes bronchoscopic suction of meconium, oxygen administration, humidity control, and prophylactic antibiotics.

HEMOLYTIC DISEASE OF THE NEWBORN

Infants born to Rh-negative mothers often develop hemolytic disease owing to fetal-maternal blood group incompatibility. These conditions are classified in category **773, Hemolytic disease of fetus or newborn, due to isoimmunization.** Note that an indication of incompatibility on a routine cord blood test is not conclusive. Do not assign a code from category 773 on the basis of this finding alone; a diagnosis of isoimmunization or hemolytic disease requires confirmation by a positive Coomb's (direct antibody or direct antiglobulin) test.

PERIVENTRICULAR LEUKOMALACIA (PVL)

Periventricular leukomalacia occurs with increasing frequency in births with very low birth weight infants. It refers to necrosis of white matter adjacent to lateral ventricles with formation of cyst and is a major risk factor for cerebral palsy and other neurological disorders. While the cause of this condition is still obscure, recent studies have associated it with intrauterine growth retardation, intrauterine infections, and pregnancies involving monozygotic twins. PVL is frequently associated with severe intraventricular hemorrhage but it is not necessarily the cause of the problem. Severity of the grade of bleeding is important in the outcome of the newborn. The codes assigned for PVL and associated intraventricular hemorrhage, if it is present, are as follows:

    779.7 Periventricular leukomalacia
          Use additional code for any associated intraventricular hemorrhage (772.1)
    772.1 Intraventricular hemorrhage
        772.10 Unspecified grade
        772.11 Grade I
             Bleeding into germinal matrix
        772.12 Grade II
             Bleeding into ventricle
        772.13 Grade III
             Bleeding with enlargement of ventricle
        772.14 Grade IV
             Bleeding into cerebral cortex

OBSERVATION AND EVALUATION OF NEWBORNS AND INFANTS

A code from category **V29, Observation and evaluation of newborns for suspected condition not found,** is assigned when a healthy newborn or infant is evaluated for a suspected condition that is found not to be present when study is complete. These codes may be assigned as an additional code along with a code from categories V30 through V39 when the newborn is further evaluated during the hospital episode in which birth occurred.

A code from category V29 may also be assigned as the principal diagnosis for a later readmission or encounter when a code from V30 through V37 no longer applies. It is used only for healthy newborns and infants for whom no reportable condition is identified after study, and is assigned only during the perinatal period of 28 days. When the newborn presents signs or symptoms of a suspected problem, or when a definite condition is identified, a code for the symptom or condition is assigned; a code from V29 is not assigned. For example:

- The physician was concerned that a newborn with a drug-dependent mother may have been adversely affected. Drug screens were carried out on the newborn, and the newborn was placed in the intensive care nursery temporarily for closer observation of potential withdrawal symptoms. Drug screens were negative. Codes **V30.00, Single liveborn,** without mention of cesarean delivery, and **V29.8, Observation for other specified suspected condition,** are assigned.

- A newborn infant was readmitted two days after discharge because of slight cyanosis and the possibility of a perinatal respiratory problem. Complete workup disclosed no problem, and the newborn was discharged without any diagnosis having been established. Code **V29.2, Observation for suspected respiratory condition,** is assigned as the principal diagnosis.
- A newborn infant was readmitted two days after discharge because of cyanosis and the possibility of a perinatal respiratory problem. The infant was diagnosed as having type I respiratory distress syndrome. Code **769, Respiratory distress syndrome,** is assigned. No code from category V29 should be assigned.

Although ordinarily no additional code is assigned when V29 is the principal diagnosis, codes can be assigned for a perinatal or congenital condition that requires continuing therapy or monitoring during the stay. Codes for congenital conditions that do not receive further evaluation or therapeutic treatment are not assigned when a newborn is admitted for observation.

INFECTIONS ORIGINATING DURING THE PERINATAL PERIOD

Many infections specific to the perinatal period are considered to be congenital and may be classified in chapter 15 of *ICD-9-CM* when they are acquired before birth via the umbilicus (for example, rubella) or during birth (for example, herpes simplex). Codes are located by referring to the main term for the infection and then identifying subterms such as neonatal, newborn, congenital, or maternal, affecting fetus or newborn. Certain perinatal infections (for example, congenital syphilis), however, may appear in chapter 1 of *ICD-9-CM*, Infections and Parasitic Diseases.

Infections that occur after birth but appear during the 28-day perinatal period may or may not be classified in chapter 15. When none of the subterms mentioned above are listed, the usual infection code is assigned. If an infection does not appear for a week or more after birth, the record should be reviewed to see whether there is any indication that it may be due to exposure to the infection rather than being congenital. Clarification should be sought from the physician when the record is not completely clear.

If a newborn has sepsis, assign code **771.81, Septicemia [sepsis] of newborn.** In addition, identify the organism with a secondary code from category **041, Bacterial infections in conditions classified elsewhere and of unspecified site.** A code from category **038, Septicemia,** should not be used on a newborn record. Code 771.81 describes the sepsis. It is not necessary to assign a code from subcategory **995.9, Systemic inflammatory response syndrome (SIRS),** on a newborn record.

As mentioned in chapter 10 of this handbook, ELISA or Western blot tests of newborns with HIV-positive mothers are often positive. This result usually indicates the antibody status of the mother rather than that of the newborn. Code **795.71, Nonspecific serologic evidence of human immunodeficiency virus (HIV),** is assigned to the newborn chart because the HIV antibodies can cross the placenta into the newborn and may persist for as long as 18 months, producing a false positive test result in the newborn. The newborn may later lose these antibodies, which means that there was never any actual HIV infection.

MATERNAL CONDITIONS AFFECTING THE FETUS OR NEWBORN

Codes from categories 760 through 763 are assigned only on the newborn's record and only when the maternal condition is the cause of morbidity or mortality in the newborn. Unless there is an adverse effect, no code from this series is assigned. The fact that the mother has a related medical condition or has experienced a complication of pregnancy, labor, or delivery does not warrant assignment of a code from these categories on the newborn's record. For example:

- Term birth, living child, mother diabetic, delivered by cesarean section, is coded as V30.01. No code from the series 760 through 763 is assigned because the medical record does not document a problem affecting the newborn.
- Newborn delivered of mother addicted to cocaine showed no sign of dependence, but a drug screen was positive. In this case, code **760.75, Noxious influence affecting fetus or newborn, via placenta or breast milk, cocaine,** is assigned as an additional code on the newborn's record.

When a specific condition in the infant that resulted from the mother's condition is identified, a code for that condition is assigned rather than a code from categories 760 through 763. For example, infants born to diabetic mothers sometimes experience a transient abnormally low blood glucose level (hypoglycemia), classified as **775.0, Syndrome of infant of a diabetic mother.** Others may have a transient diabetic state (hyperglycemia), sometimes referred to as pseudodiabetes, which is coded as **775.1, Neonatal diabetes mellitus.**

When these fetal or newborn conditions affect the management of the mother, codes 655.x and 656.x are assigned on the maternal record.

ENDOCRINE AND METABOLIC DISTURBANCES SPECIFIC TO THE FETUS AND NEWBORN

ICD-9-CM provides codes to describe acidosis of newborn and other neonatal endocrine and metabolic disturbances. Causes of respiratory acidosis include, but are not limited to, asphyxia, obstruction to the respiratory tract, respiratory distress syndrome, pneumonia, pulmonary edema, and/or apnea. Metabolic acidosis may be caused by renal failure, septicemia, hypoxia, hypothermia, hypotension, cardiac failure, dehydration, electrolyte disturbances, hyperglycemia, anemia, intraventricular hemorrhage, and/or metabolic disorders. The underlying cause of acidosis must be treated in order to correct the problem. The following codes are used for acidosis of newborn and other neonatal endocrine and metabolic disturbances:

- 775.81   Other acidosis of newborn
- 775.89   Other neonatal endocrine and metabolic disturbances

ROUTINE VACCINATION OF NEWBORNS

Newborns are vaccinated shortly after birth against hepatitis B and varicella. When the need for vaccination is indicated during the newborn stay, codes V05.3 for hepatitis B and V05.4 for varicella may be assigned. Code **99.55, Prophylactic administration of vaccine against other diseases,** would be assigned for the vaccination performed.

HEALTH SUPERVISION OF INFANT OR CHILD

Category **V20, Health supervision of infant or child,** is assigned for routine encounters of infants when no problem has been identified. V20.2 is assigned when an infant is seen for routine examination of a newborn or child (for example, at a well-baby clinic) but would not be assigned for a hospital admission. Code V20.2 has been modified to include initial and subsequent routine newborn check.

Review Exercise 23.1

Code the following diagnoses and procedures as they would be assigned to a newborn's record. Presume that all births occurred in the hospital unless stated otherwise.

	Code(s)

1. Term birth, living male, cesarean delivery,
    with hemolytic disease due to ABO isoimmunization
                         Newborn
	V30.01
	773.1

2. Term birth, living child
    Physiological neonatal jaundice
                         Newborn
	V30.00
	774.6

3. Normal, full-term female, spontaneous delivery
    Congenital left hip subluxation
                         Newborn
	V30.00
	754.32

4. Newborn, male, premature (1400 grams) Hyaline membrane disease	V30.00 765.15 765.20 769

5. Term birth, living male
    Ophthalmitis of the newborn due to
    maternal gonococcal infection
                         Newborn
	V30.00
	098.40

6. Near-term birth, living male, delivered by
    cesarean section with neonatal hypoglycemia
                         Newborn
	V30.01
	775.6

7. Term birth, living child
    Intrauterine growth retardation
                         Newborn
	V30.00
	764.90

Review Exercise 23.1 *(continued)*

8.	Premature birth, living female infant (1850 grams) Withdrawal syndrome in infant due to maternal heroin addiction	V30.00 765.17 765.20 779.5
	Newborn	

9.	Term birth, twin, with fracture of right clavicle during birth (mate stillborn)	V32.00 767.2
	Newborn	

10.	Five-year-old child with Erb's palsy secondary to birth trauma	767.6

11.	Infant with hemolytic disease due to Rh isoimmunization (patient received by transfer from other facility)	773.0

	Phototherapy	99.83

12.	Patient born in Community Hospital, with erythroblastosis fetalis due to ABO incompatibility; transferred immediately after birth to intensive care nursery at University Hospital for exchange transfusion and further care	
	Newborn	
	a. Codes for Community Hospital stay	V30.00 773.1
	b. Codes for University Hospital stay	773.1 99.01

13.	Normal, male infant, delivered by cesarean when fetal distress was noted early in labor Fetal distress due to cord compression	V30.01 768.3 762.5
	Newborn	

Review Exercise 23.1 *(continued)*

14. Newborn born on the way to the hospital and admitted directly to newborn nursery		V30.1
		776.5
Anemia due to acute blood loss from umbilical stump		772.3

15. Term birth with fetal sepsis due to amnionitis		V30.00
		771.81
	Newborn	762.7

16. Term birth, delivered with meconium aspiration syndrome due to prolonged labor, first stage		V30.00
		770.12
		763.89
Cord around neck of infant two times		762.5
	Newborn	

17. Term birth, living male, with partial facial paralysis		V30.00
	Newborn	767.5

18. Premature infant (1300 grams) transferred from Community Hospital to intensive care nursery at University Hospital for supervision of weight gain		765.15
		765.20
	Newborn	

19. Newborn twins, #1 delivered in parking lot of hospital, #2 delivered after admission of mother		#1: V31.1
		#2: V31.00
	Newborn	

20. Term birth, living child; mother known to be a chronic alcoholic; newborn placed in intensive care nursing for observation for possible alcohol-related problems; none found		V30.00
		V29.8
	Observation	
	Newborn	

21. Routine visit to well-baby clinic for checkup; healthy infant		V20.2

Coding of Circulatory System Diseases and Neoplastic Diseases

24 Diseases of the Circulatory System

Chapter 7 of *ICD-9-CM* classifies circulatory disorders except for those that have been reclassified to chapter 11 (obstetrical conditions) or to chapter 14 (congenital anomalies). This chapter covers a broad range of conditions, many of which are commonly seen for patients admitted to acute-care hospitals. Because these are complex disorders, and many of them are interrelated, it is particularly important for the coder to be alert to all instructional terms.

RHEUMATIC HEART DISEASE

Rheumatic heart disease occurs as the result of an infection with group A hemolytic Streptococcus. *ICD-9-CM* classifies rheumatic fever with and without rheumatic heart disease. The first axis distinguishes whether the fever is acute (390–392) or quiescent (393–398), and the second axis determines whether there is heart involvement.

Chronic rheumatic heart disease (393–398) includes heart disease that has resulted from a previously active rheumatic infection. The heart valves are most often involved. *ICD-9-CM* presumes that certain mitral valve disorders of unspecified etiology are rheumatic in origin. When the diagnostic statement includes more than one condition affecting the mitral valves, one of which is presumed to be rheumatic, all are classified as rheumatic. For example:

- Mitral valve stenosis 394.0
- Mitral valve insufficiency 424.0
- Mitral valve stenosis and insufficiency 394.2

In these examples the mitral valve stenosis is presumed to be of rheumatic origin, but the mitral valve insufficiency is not. In the third example, the combination code presumes both to be rheumatic because the stenosis is presumed to be rheumatic.

ICD-9-CM presumes that a disorder affecting both the mitral and aortic valves is rheumatic in origin. Otherwise, the aortic condition is classified as rheumatic only when specifically stated as such. Examples follow:

- Aortic valve insufficiency 424.1
- Mitral valve insufficiency with aortic valve insufficiency 396.3
- Aortic valve stenosis 424.1
- Rheumatic aortic stenosis 395.0
- Mitral stenosis and aortic stenosis 396.0

A diagnosis of heart failure in a patient who has rheumatic heart disease, whether specified or presumed, is classified as **398.91, Rheumatic heart failure,** unless the physician specifies a different cause. For example:

- End-stage congestive heart failure due to rheumatic heart disease and dilated cardiomyopathy with mitral valve insufficiency 398.91 + 425.4 + 394.1

Exercise 24.1

Code the following diagnoses.

	Code(s)
1. Mitral regurgitation	424.0
2. Mitral valve stenosis with congestive heart failure	394.0 398.91
3. Severe mitral stenosis and mild aortic insufficiency	396.1
4. Aortic and mitral insufficiency Atrial fibrillation	396.3 427.31
5. Mitral insufficiency, congenital	746.6
6. Mitral valve insufficiency with aortic regurgitation	396.3
7. Chronic aortic and mitral valve insufficiency, rheumatic, with acute congestive heart failure	398.91 396.3

ISCHEMIC HEART DISEASE

Ischemic heart disease is the general term for a number of disorders affecting the myocardium caused by a decrease in the blood supply to the heart due to coronary insufficiency.

The insufficiency is usually caused by deposits of atheromatous material in the epicardial portions of the coronary artery that progressively obstruct its branches so that the lumen of the arteries become either partially or completely occluded. Other common terms for ischemic heart disease are arteriosclerotic heart disease (ASHD), coronary ischemia, coronary artery disease, and coronary arteriosclerosis (atherosclerosis).

Ischemic heart disease is classified in categories 410 through 414 as follows:

- Acute myocardial infarction   410
- Other acute and subacute forms of ischemic heart disease   411
- Old (healed) myocardial infarction   412
- Angina pectoris   413
- Other forms of chronic ischemic heart disease   414

Myocardial Infarction

Acute myocardial infarction is an acute ischemic condition that ordinarily appears following prolonged myocardial ischemia. It is usually precipitated by an occlusive coronary thrombosis at the site of an existing arteriosclerotic stenosis. Although ischemic heart disease is a progressive disorder, it is often silent for long periods with no clinical manifestations, then appears suddenly in an acute form without any intervening symptoms having been experienced.

A myocardial infarction described as acute or with a duration of eight weeks or less is classified in category **410, Acute myocardial infarction,** with a fourth digit indicating the wall involved. Codes 410.0x through 410.6x identify transmural infarctions; code 410.7x identifies subendocardial infarctions that do not extend through the full thickness of the myocardial wall. Diagnostic statements do not always mention the affected wall, but this information can almost always be found in the electrocardiographic report. A code from subcategory **410.9, Myocardial infarction, unspecified site,** should not be assigned unless no information regarding the site is documented in the medical record. Myocardial infarctions can also be classified according to whether there is ST-segment elevation (codes 410.0–410.6 and 410.8) or non-ST-segment elevation (code 410.7). If there is no information regarding whether there is ST elevation or non-ST elevation, or information regarding the site of the myocardial infarction, coders should assign code 410.9. If a myocardial infarction is documented as nontransmural or subendocardial, but the site is provided, it is still coded as a subendocardial MI. If a non-ST elevation myocardial infarction (NSTEMI) evolves to ST-elevation myocardial infarction (STEMI), assign the code for the STEMI. If STEMI converts to NSTEMI due to thrombolytic therapy, assign the code for STEMI. Be careful to note that these codes are used for documented acute myocardial infarctions and should not be confused with abnormal findings on electrocardiograms of ST-segment elevation.

A fifth-digit subclassification is provided for category 410 to indicate whether the current admission is the initial episode of care or a subsequent one for the same infarction. Note that the significant terms are initial and subsequent, not acute and chronic. Fifth digit 0, episode of care unspecified, is assigned only when the medical record does not contain sufficient information for a more specific assignment. Although physicians do not ordinarily use the terms initial or subsequent in the diagnostic statement, it is safe to consider an admission for infarction as the initial episode of care when the history makes no mention of a previous infarction.

Fifth digit 1 indicates the initial (first) episode of care for an infarction. It is used in both the first hospital to which a patient is admitted as well as to any other acute-care facility to which the patient is transferred without an intervening discharge. For example, if a patient is admitted to Hospital A for an initial episode of care for an acute anteroseptal myocardial infarction, transferred to Hospital B for further diagnostic workup or therapy, and then transferred back to Hospital A without being discharged from acute care, code **410.11, Acute myocardial infarction, of other anterior wall, initial episode of care,** would be assigned for all three admissions.

Fifth digit 2, subsequent episode of care, is assigned when the patient is admitted for further care of the cardiac condition any time during the first eight weeks after the infarction occurred. Myocardial infarction described as chronic or with a duration of more than eight weeks is classified as **414.8, Other specified forms of chronic ischemic heart disease.**

Patients sometimes experience a second infarction involving another wall during a hospital admission for an acute myocardial infarction. In this case, both infarctions are coded according to the sites involved.

An associated postinfarction hypotension is sometimes experienced by patients with acute myocardial infarction. In this situation, the code for the infarction is sequenced first, with an additional code of **458.8, Other specified hypotension.**

Evolving Infarction

An evolving myocardial infarction sometimes precipitates right ventricular failure that progresses to congestive heart failure. The patient may then be admitted because of this precursor condition, which then progresses to an acute myocardial infarction. After study, the principal diagnosis in this situation is the infarction, with an additional code assigned for the heart failure. Additional codes should also be assigned for any mention of cardiogenic shock, ventricular arrhythmia, and fibrillation. For example:

- Congestive heart failure with acute myocardial infarction of anterolateral wall with ventricular fibrillation   410.01 + 428.0 + 427.41

Exercise 24.2

Code the following diagnoses; do not code procedures.

	Code(s)
1. A patient felt well until around 10 p.m., when he began having severe chest pain, which continued to increase in severity. He was brought to the emergency department by ambulance. There was no previous history of cardiac disease, but the EKG showed an acute anterolateral myocardial infarction, and the patient was admitted immediately for further care.	410.01
2. A patient with compensated congestive heart failure on Lasix began to have extreme difficulty in breathing and was brought to the emergency department, where he was found to be in congestive failure. Because it was felt that an impending infarction was possible, a PTCA was carried out, but the patient went on to have an acute inferolateral infarction.	410.21 428.0

Exercise 24.2 *(continued)*

3. A patient was admitted with acute anterior myocardial infarction with no history of previous infarction or previous care for this episode. During the hospital stay, he also experienced an acute anterolateral infarction.

   410.11
   410.01

4. A patient was admitted to Community Hospital on 3/3 with severe chest pain, which was identified as an acute anterolateral wall infarction (no history of earlier care). Patient was transferred to University Hospital later on 3/3 for angioplasty and returned to Community Hospital on 3/6 to continue recovery. Patient was discharged on 3/8.

First admission to Community Hospital	410.01
Transfer to University Hospital	410.01
Transfer back to Community Hospital	410.01

5. The patient in the previous situation was readmitted to Community Hospital on 3/12 because he was having severe chest pains. Extension of the infarction was suspected but ruled out.

   410.02

If the infarction is described as old or healed, the coder should review the medical record to determine whether the infarction is actually old and/or healed or whether the diagnosis refers to a more recent infarction still under care. A diagnosis of old myocardial infarction is usually made on the basis of electrocardiographic findings or some other investigation in a patient who is not experiencing symptoms. Code **412, Old myocardial infarction,** is essentially a history code, even though it is not included in the V-code chapter of *ICD-9-CM*. It should not be assigned when current ischemic heart disease is present and should be assigned as an additional code only when it has some significance for the current episode of care.

Other Acute and Subacute Ischemic Heart Disease

Code **411.1, Intermediate coronary syndrome,** includes conditions described as unstable angina, crescendo angina, preinfarction angina, accelerated angina, and impending myocardial infarction. These conditions occur after less exertion than angina pectoris; the pain is more severe and is less easily relieved by nitroglycerin. Without treatment, unstable angina often progresses to acute myocardial infarction.

Code 411.1 is designated as the principal diagnosis only when the underlying condition is not identified and there is no surgical intervention. Patients with severe coronary arteriosclerosis and unstable angina may be admitted for cardiac bypass surgery or a percutaneous coronary angioplasty to prevent further progression to infarction. In such cases, the code for coronary arteriosclerosis (414.0x) is assigned as the principal diagnosis, with an additional code for the unstable angina. Examples of appropriate coding follow:

- A patient was admitted with unstable angina and underwent right and left heart catheterization, which showed coronary arteriosclerosis. A coronary bypass procedure was recommended, but the patient felt he needed some time to think it over and to discuss it with his family. For this admission, the coronary arteriosclerosis (414.0x) is the principal diagnosis, with an additional code for the unstable angina.
- A patient was admitted with unstable angina and a history of myocardial infarction five years ago. She was treated with IV nitroglycerin, and the angina subsided by the end of the first hospital day. No other complications were noted and no additional diagnostic studies were carried out. In this case, the unstable angina is the principal diagnosis.

A diagnosis of acute ischemic heart disease or acute myocardial ischemia does not always indicate an infarction. It is often possible to prevent infarction by means of surgery and/or the use of thrombolytic agents if the patient is treated promptly. If there is occlusion or thrombosis of the artery without infarction, code **411.81, Acute coronary occlusion without myocardial infarction,** is assigned. Code **411.89, Other acute and subacute forms of ischemic heart disease,** includes coronary insufficiency and subendocardial ischemia.

Postmyocardial Infarction Syndrome

Patients with acute myocardial infarction sometimes experience postmyocardial infarction syndrome (411.0) or angina described as postinfarction angina. Postmyocardial infarction, also called Dressler's syndrome, is a pericarditis characterized by fever, leukocytosis, pleurisy, pleural effusion, joint pains, and occasionally pneumonia. Except for these two conditions, no code from category 411 is assigned with a code from category 410.

Exercise 24.3

Code the following diagnoses.

	Code(s)
1. Acute myocardial infarction, inferolateral wall (initial care) Third-degree atrioventricular block	410.21 426.0
2. Acute myocardial infarction of inferoposterior wall (initial) Congestive heart failure Hypertension	410.31 428.0 401.9
3. Impending myocardial infarction (crescendo angina) resulting in occlusion of coronary artery	411.81
4. Acute coronary insufficiency	411.89

Chronic Ischemic Heart Disease

Category **414, Other forms of chronic heart disease,** includes such conditions as coronary atherosclerosis, chronic coronary insufficiency, myocardial ischemia, and aneurysm. Diagnoses of coronary artery disease or coronary heart disease without any further qualification are too vague to be coded accurately; the physician should be asked to provide a more specific diagnosis. Code **414.9, Unspecified chronic ischemic heart disease,** should rarely be assigned in an acute-care hospital setting.

Code **414.0x, Coronary atherosclerosis,** includes conditions described as arteriosclerotic heart disease, coronary arteriosclerosis, coronary stricture, and coronary sclerosis or atheroma. A fifth-digit subclassification indicates the nature of the coronary artery involved. For example:

- Native coronary artery   414.01
- Autologous vein bypass graft   414.02
- Nonautologous biological bypass graft   414.03
- Artery bypass graft, including internal mammary artery   414.04
- Native coronary artery of transplanted heart   414.06
- Bypass graft (artery) (vein) of transplanted heart 414.07
- Unspecified type of bypass graft   414.05
- Unspecified type of vessel, native or graft   414.00

Physicians rarely include information regarding the type of graft in the diagnostic statement, but it is almost always available in the medical record. If the medical record makes it clear that there has been no previous bypass surgery, code **414.01, Coronary atherosclerosis of native coronary arteries,** can be assigned. If there is a history of previous bypass, code 414.02, 414.03, or 414.04 should be assigned when information indicating the material used in the bypass is available. Note that arteriosclerosis of a bypass vessel is not classified as a postoperative complication.

When atherosclerosis of a native coronary artery in a transplanted heart is identified in the diagnostic statement, code 414.06 would be assigned. Code **414.07, Coronary atherosclerosis of bypass graft (artery) (vein) of transplanted heart,** is assigned to identify atherosclerosis of a bypass graft in a transplanted heart.

ANGINA PECTORIS

Angina pectoris (413.9) is an early manifestation of ischemic heart disease, although in rare instances it occurs as a result of congenital abnormalities of the coronary arteries or such conditions as aortic stenosis, valvular insufficiency, aortic syphilis, and Raynaud's phenomenon. It is characterized by chest pain, usually perceived by the patient as a sensation of tightness, squeezing, pressing, choking, burning, heartburn or gas, or an ill-defined discomfort. This type of angina can be produced by anything that increases the oxygen requirements of the myocardium, such as exercise, walking into the wind, cold weather, consumption of a large meal, emotional stress, and elevation of blood pressure. This type of pain is similar to that of unstable angina, but it is less severe, more easily controlled, and usually relieved in a predictable manner, either by rest or the administration of nitroglycerin.

Angina pectoris sometimes occurs even when the patient is at rest, apparently without any stimulation, such as during the night. This condition is referred to as nocturnal or decubitus angina and is classified as 413.0. A variant type that also occurs at rest is known as Prinzmetal angina. Angina described as angiospastic or with coronary spasm at rest is coded to **413.1, Prinzmetal angina.**

In today's health care environment, it is unlikely that a patient would be admitted to the hospital for treatment of stable angina except for the purpose of undergoing diagnostic studies to determine its underlying cause. In this case, the underlying cause, not the stable angina, is sequenced as the principal diagnosis.

Exercise 24.4

Code the following diagnoses and procedures.

	Code(s)
1. Crescendo angina due to coronary arteriosclerosis	414.00 411.1
Right and left cardiac catheterization	37.23
2. Angina pectoris with essential hypertension	413.9 401.9

HEART FAILURE

Heart failure occurs when an abnormality of cardiac function results in the inability of the heart to pump blood at a rate commensurate with the body's needs, or the ability to do so only from an abnormal filling pressure. This decrease in blood supply to body tissue results in unmet needs for oxygen, as well as a failure to meet other metabolic requirements. This in turn results in pulmonary and/or systemic circulatory congestion and reduced cardiac output. Precipitating causes of heart failure include cardiac arrhythmias, pulmonary embolism, infections, anemia, thyrotoxicosis, myocarditis, endocarditis, hypertension, and myocardial infarction. All codes for heart failure include any associated pulmonary edema; therefore, no additional code is assigned. A diagnosis of acute pulmonary edema in the absence of underlying heart disease is classified with conditions affecting the respiratory system. (See chapter 15 of this handbook for more information on the respiratory system.)

There are two main categories of heart failure: systolic and diastolic. Systolic heart failure (428.2x) occurs when the ability of the heart to contract decreases. Diastolic heart failure (428.3x) occurs when the heart has a problem relaxing between contractions (diastole) to allow enough blood to enter the ventricles. Fifth digits further specify whether the heart failure is unspecified, acute, chronic, or acute on chronic.

Heart failure is differentiated clinically by whether the right or left ventricle is primarily affected. Left-sided heart failure (left ventricular failure) is due to the accumulation of excess fluid behind the left ventricle. Code **428.1, Left heart failure,** includes associated conditions such as dyspnea, orthopnea, bronchospasm, and acute pulmonary edema; no additional codes are assigned. Heart failure, unspecified, is coded to 428.9. This is a vague code, however, and an effort should be made to determine whether a code from the series 428.0 through 428.4 would be more appropriate.

Right-sided failure ordinarily follows left-sided failure and is classified in *ICD-9-CM* as congestive heart failure (428.0). This code includes any left-sided failure that is present; therefore, codes 428.0 and 428.1 are not assigned for the same episode of care; code 428.0 takes precedence.

The term "congestive heart failure" is often mistakenly used interchangeably with " heart failure." Congestion, pulmonary or systemic fluid build-up, is one feature of heart failure, but it does not occur in all patients.

Hypertensive heart failure with congestive failure is classified in category 402, with code 428.0 assigned as an additional diagnosis. If chronic kidney disease is present, a code from category 403 is assigned, and the appropriate code from 585.1–585.6, 585.9 to identify the stage of chronic kidney disease is assigned as an additional diagnosis. If both congestive failure and chronic kidney disease are present, a code from category 404 is used, with code 428.0 and a code from 585.1–585.9 assigned as additional diagnoses. Fifth digits indicate with or without heart failure and/or the stage of the chronic kidney disease. Further information in classifying hypertension and other associated conditions is provided later in this chapter.

Compensated and Decompensated Heart Failure

When heart failure occurs, the heart muscle commonly develops compensatory mechanisms such as cardiac hypertrophy, raised arterial pressure, ventricular dilation, or increased force of contraction. When this occurs, the heart failure may be described as compensated, permitting near-normal function. When these compensatory mechanisms can no longer meet the increased workload, decompensation of the heart function results; this situation is often described as decompensated heart failure. Code assignment is not affected by the use of these terms; the code for the type of heart failure is assigned.

CARDIOMYOPATHY

Cardiomyopathy (425.x) presents a clinical picture of a dilated heart, flabby heart muscles, and normal coronary arteries. Common types of cardiomyopathy are those due to the long-term consumption of alcohol (425.5) and those described as congestive, constrictive, hypertrophic, and obstructive, which are classified as code **425.4, Other primary cardiomyopathies.**

The symptoms of congestive cardiomyopathy (425.4) are essentially the same as those of congestive heart failure, and the condition is often associated with congestive heart failure. Treatment ordinarily revolves around management of the congestive heart failure, and so the heart failure (428.0–428.43) is designated as the principal diagnosis, with an additional code assigned for the cardiomyopathy.

Two codes may be required for cardiomyopathy due to other underlying conditions; for example, cardiomyopathy due to amyloidosis is coded **277.30, Amyloidosis, unspecified,** and **425.7, Nutritional and metabolic cardiomyopathy.** The underlying disease, amyloidosis, is sequenced first. Hypertensive cardiomyopathy should be coded to category 402, **Hypertensive heart disease,** with an additional code of **425.8, Cardiomyopathy in other diseases classified elsewhere.**

The term ischemic cardiomyopathy is sometimes used to designate a condition in which ischemic heart disease causes diffuse fibrosis or multiple infarction, leading to heart failure with left ventricular dilation. This is not a true cardiomyopathy and is coded to **414.8, Other specified forms of chronic ischemic heart disease,** when no further clarification is provided by the attending physician.

TAKOTSUBO SYNDROME

Takotsubo syndrome is a newly recognized reversible form of left ventricular dysfunction, seen in patients without coronary disease. Code **429.83, Takotsubo syndrome,** is assigned for Takotsubo syndrome, broken heart syndrome, reversible left ventricular dysfunction following sudden emotional stress, stress induced cardiomyopathy, and transient left ventricular apical ballooning syndrome. This syndrome is usually precipitated by emotional or physiological stress with sudden onset of chest symptoms, electrocardiographic changes characteristic of myocardial ischemia, transient left ventricular dysfunction, low-grade troponin elevation, and insignificant coronary stenosis by ventriculography. Patients presenting with Takotsubo syndrome are usually monitored and treated for left heart failure, intraventricular obstruction, and/or cardiac arrhythmias, if they develop. Apical ballooning syndrome previously indexed to code **429.89, Other ill-defined heart disease,** is now assigned to code 429.83.

CARDIAC ARREST

Code **427.5, Cardiac arrest,** may be assigned as a principal diagnosis only when a patient arrives at the hospital in a state of cardiac arrest and cannot be resuscitated, or is resuscitated briefly and pronounced dead before the underlying cause of the arrest is identified. It may be assigned as a secondary code when cardiac arrest occurs during the hospital episode and the patient is resuscitated (or resuscitation is attempted). In this case, the code for the underlying cause is designated the principal diagnosis, with code 427.5 assigned as an additional code. Note that codes are not assigned for symptoms integral to the condition, such as bradycardia and hypotension. Cardiac arrest that occurs as a complication of surgery is coded as **997.1, Cardiac complications.** Code 669.4x is assigned for cardiac arrest complicating abortion, ectopic pregnancy, or labor and delivery. None of these codes are assigned to indicate that a patient has died. Do not code cardiac arrest to indicate the patient's death.

ANEURYSM

An aneurysm is a localized abnormal dilation of blood vessels. A dissecting aneurysm is one in which blood enters the wall of the artery and separates the layers of the vessel wall. As the aneurysm progresses, tension increases and the aneurysm is likely to rupture, which usually results in death.

Aneurysms are diagnosed primarily according to their location, such as the following:

- Aneurysm of coronary vessels   414.11
- Dissecting aneurysm of abdominal aorta   441.02
- Aneurysm of abdominal aorta with rupture   441.3
- Aneurysm of thoracic artery   441.2
- Ruptured aneurysm of thoracic artery   441.1
- Thoracoabdominal aneurysm   441.7

Occasionally, a term describing the aneurysm's appearance is used, such as berry aneurysm (430), or a term may describe its etiology, such as syphilitic aneurysm of aorta (093.0) or traumatic aneurysm (901.0, 901.2).

An aneurysm of a vessel may be treated by resection with anastomosis (38.3x) or replacement (38.4x) with the fourth digit indicating the vessel involved. Repair is achieved by clipping (39.51) or a variety of other procedures such as electrocoagulation, suture, or wiring (39.52). Several new procedures are now being used for aneurysm repair. Endoluminal endovascular prosthesis is a new technique for transfemoral graft placement and aneurysm exclusion in patients with abdominal aortic aneurysm. This is an alternative to open surgery, is minimally invasive, and avoids laparotomy. Hospital stays are shorter and there is less intensive postoperative management. Another new technique is the use of the Corvita endovascular graft for abdominal aortic aneurysm and common iliac aneurysm. Placement of a Vanguard endograft is used for treatment of aortoiliac aneurysmal disease. The following codes are used for endovascular repair of aneurysms:

- 39.71   Endovascular implantation of graft in abdominal aorta
- 39.72   Endovascular repair or occlusion of head and neck vessels
- 39.73   Endovascular implantation of graft in thoracic aorta
- 39.74   Endovascular removal of obstruction from head and neck vessels
- 39.79   Other endovascular repair (of aneurysm) of other vessels

Code 36.91 is assigned for repair of an aneurysm of a coronary vessel, and code 37.32 is assigned for excision or repair of an aneurysm of the heart.

CEREBROVASCULAR DISORDERS

Acute organic (nontraumatic) conditions affecting the cerebral arteries include hemorrhage, occlusion, and thrombosis and are coded in the 430 through 437 series. Category

433, Occlusion and stenosis of precerebral arteries, and category **434, Occlusion of cerebral arteries,** use a fifth-digit subclassification to indicate whether there is mention of associated cerebral infarction. Fifth digit 1, indicating the presence of cerebral infarction, is not assigned unless cerebral infarction is clearly documented in the medical record and the physician has indicated a relationship between cerebral artery stenosis or occlusion and the infarction. The coder should never assume that infarction has occurred. Note that these fifth digits apply for the current episode of care only; they do not indicate that the patient has had a cerebral infarction in the past. Code **433.10, Occlusion and stenosis of precerebral arteries, carotid artery, without mention of cerebral infarction,** is used to describe carotid artery stenosis without cerebral infarction. If the documentation describes bilateral carotid artery stenosis, code **433.30, Occlusion and stenosis of precerebral arteries, multiple and bilateral, without mention of cerebral infarction,** is assigned along with code 433.10 to further describe the laterality. Assigning both codes will allow information on both the specific artery involved and the laterality to be captured.

Diagnostic statements often are not specific regarding the site or type of the cerebrovascular condition. When the diagnosis is stated as cerebrovascular accident, CVA, or stroke without any further qualification, it is important for the coder to review the medical record for more definitive information or to consult with the physician. When no further information is available, code **434.91, Cerebral artery occlusion, unspecified, with cerebral infarction,** is assigned for the diagnosis of stroke or CVA to allow for improved uniformity in coding and statistical data. The use of code 436 with a code from categories 430 through 435 or 437 is redundant; the more specific code always takes precedence.

Each component of a diagnostic statement identifying cerebrovascular disease should be coded unless the Alphabetic Index or the Tabular List instructs otherwise. For example:

- Cerebrovascular arteriosclerosis with subarachnoid hemorrhage due to ruptured berry aneurysm   430 + 437.0

A new therapy (99.75) is now being used in which a neuroprotective agent is administered directly on nerve cells to minimize ischemic injury, particularly for acute subarachnoid hemorrhage.

In the event of a postoperative stroke, assign code **997.02, Iatrogenic cerebrovascular infarction or hemorrhage.** Assign an additional code to identify the specific type of stroke/cerebrovascular accident. The general coding rule for postoperative complications is that when the complication code does not specifically identify the condition, an additional code should be assigned to more fully explain it.

Conditions classifiable in categories 430 through 437 are reclassified in subcategory **674.0x, Cerebrovascular disorders in the puerperium,** when they occur during pregnancy, childbirth, or the puerperium. Although the code title mentions puerperium, the inclusion note indicates that these conditions are included when they occur any time during the obstetrical experience. Because code 674.0x does not indicate the nature of the cerebrovascular condition, it is appropriate to assign an additional code from chapter 7 of *ICD-9-CM* for greater specificity.

Late Effects of Cerebrovascular Disease

Codes from category **438, Late effect of cerebrovascular disease,** have been expanded by fourth and fifth digits to provide greater specificity regarding the residual effects as follows:

- 438.0   Cognitive deficits
- 438.1x   Speech and language deficits
- 438.2x   Hemiplegia/hemiparesis
- 438.3x   Monoplegia of upper limb
- 438.4x   Monoplegia of lower limb
- 438.5x   Other paralytic syndrome
- 438.6   Alternations of sensations
- 438.7   Disturbances of vision
- 438.8x   Other late effects of cerebrovascular disease
- 438.9   Unspecified late effects of cerebrovascular disease

Instructions to use an additional code have been added to 438.5, 438.6, and 438.7 to indicate the specific residual condition. An additional code should also be added to 438.89 to indicate the specific late effect.

Codes from this category are assigned for any remaining deficits when the patient is admitted at a later date. Like other history codes, however, a code from category 438 is assigned only when it is significant for the current episode of care. Code **V12.5x, Personal history of disease of circulatory system,** may be used when the patient has had a prior CVA with no residual conditions, but this code would rarely meet the criteria for a reportable diagnosis. Codes from category 438 differ from other late effect codes in two ways:

- These codes can be assigned as the principal diagnosis when the purpose of the admission is to deal with the late effect. If the admission is for the purpose of rehabilitation, however, a code from category V57 is assigned as the principal diagnosis with an additional code from category 438.
- These codes can be assigned as additional codes when a new CVA is present and deficits from an earlier episode remain. This distinction permits the identification of those deficits due to the current CVA and those remaining from an earlier episode.

Unlike other late effects, neurological deficits such as hemiplegia and aphasia due to cerebrovascular accidents are often present from the onset of the disease rather than arising after the original condition itself has cleared. Such deficits are frequently transient and are no longer present at discharge; if they have cleared by the time of discharge, codes for the deficits are not assigned. Residual effects still present at discharge are coded as additional diagnoses, but not as late effects. For example, a patient admitted because of subarachnoid hemorrhage with associated aphasia and hemiplegia would have only the arachnoid hemorrhage code assigned if the other conditions had cleared by the time of discharge. If these deficits are still present at discharge, the following codes are assigned:

- 430   Subarachnoid hemorrhage
- 784.3   Aphasia
- 342.90   Hemiplegia

Exercise 24.5

Code the following diagnoses.

	Code(s)
1. Occlusion of right internal carotid artery with cerebral infarction with mild hemiplegia resolved before discharge	433.11
2. Hemiplegia on right (dominant) side due to old cerebral thrombosis	438.21

Exercise 24.5 *(continued)*

3. Admission for treatment of new <u>cerebral</u> <u>embolism</u> with cerebral infarction and with <u>aphasia</u> remaining at discharge (patient suffered cerebral embolism one year ago, with residual apraxia and dysphagia)	434.11 784.3 438.81 438.82

<u>Late</u>

4. Cerebral <u>thrombosis</u> with right <u>hemiparesis</u> and <u>aphasia</u> still present at discharge	434.00 342.90 784.3

5. Cerebrovascular <u>accident</u> due to cerebral <u>embolism</u>, with infarction	434.11

6. <u>Insufficiency</u> of vertebrobasilar arteries	435.3

7. <u>Admission</u> for rehabilitation because of monoplegia of the right arm and left leg, each affecting dominant side (patient suffered a nontraumatic extradural hemorrhage one month ago)	V57.89 438.31 438.41

<u>Late</u>

8. <u>Quadriplegia</u> due to ruptured berry aneurysm five years ago	438.53 344.00

HYPERTENSION

ICD-9-CM classifies hypertension by type (primary or secondary) and nature (benign, malignant, or unspecified). Categories 401 through 404 classify primary hypertension according to a hierarchy of the disease from its vascular origin (401) to the end-organ involvement of heart (402), chronic kidney disease (403), or heart and chronic kidney disease combined (404). Primary hypertension is also described as essential hypertension, hypertensive vascular disease, or systolic hypertension.

Benign and Malignant Hypertension

Malignant hypertension is an accelerated, severe hypertensive disorder, with progressive vascular damage and a poor prognosis. It is characterized by rapidly rising blood pressure, usually in excess of 140 millimeters of mercury diastolic. Without effective treatment, malignant hypertension can lead to congestive heart failure, hypertensive encephalopathy, intracerebral hemorrhage, uremia, and even death. *ICD-9-CM* includes hypertension described as accelerated or necrotizing in the code for malignant hypertension.

The term "benign hypertension" refers to a relatively mild degree of hypertension of prolonged or chronic duration. Although malignant hypertension is almost always identified in the diagnostic statement, benign hypertension is rarely specified as a diagnosis, perhaps because the term benign has a different significance for the physician than it does in the classification system. Hypertension not classified as malignant would rarely be designated as the principal diagnosis, although occasionally a patient may be admitted for careful monitoring while a new medication regimen is being implemented.

Secondary hypertension (405) is the result of some other primary disease. When the condition causing the hypertension can be cured or brought under reasonable control, the secondary hypertension may stabilize or disappear entirely. The underlying cause is sequenced first, followed by the code for the hypertension. For example:

- Hypertension due to systemic lupus erythematosus   710.0 + 405.99
- Acromegaly with secondary hypertension   253.0 + 405.99

Location of Hypertensive Disease Codes

The Alphabetic Index includes a table under the main term **Hypertension** with subterms indexed in the usual manner. Three columns to the right provide codes for the malignant, benign, and unspecified versions of that type of hypertension. For example, a reference to cardiorenal hypertension provides codes for all three types of hypertension, but a reference to accelerated hypertension shows only a code for malignant hypertension because accelerated hypertension is only malignant. Codes should always be verified with the Tabular List and any instructional terms should be noted. There are also subentries for hypertensive and due to hypertension under the main term for certain other conditions.

Diagnostic statements of hypertension frequently include the terms "uncontrolled" or "controlled" or "history of." Hypertension described as "uncontrolled" is coded by its type and nature; *ICD-9-CM* does not have a code to indicate this uncontrolled status. Hypertension described as "controlled" or "history of" hypertension usually refers to an existing hypertension that is under control by means of continuing therapy. The coder should review the medical record to determine whether the hypertension is still under treatment; if so, the appropriate code from categories 401 through 405 should be assigned.

HYPERTENSIVE HEART DISEASE

Certain heart conditions are assigned to category **402, Hypertensive heart disease,** when a causal relationship is stated (due to hypertension) or implied (hypertensive). Hypertensive heart disease includes cardiomegaly, cardiovascular disease, myocarditis, and degeneration of the myocardium. Category 402 includes a fifth-digit subclassification that indicates whether heart failure is present. However, an additional code is still required to specify the type of heart failure (428.0–428.43), if known.

A cause-and-effect relationship between hypertension and heart disease cannot be assumed, however, and careful attention must be given to the exact wording of the diagnostic statement. When the diagnostic statement mentions both conditions but does not indicate a causal relationship between them, separate codes are assigned. For example:

- Congestive heart failure due to hypertension   402.91 + 428.0
- Hypertensive heart disease with congestive heart failure   402.91 + 428.0
- Congestive heart failure with hypertension   428.0 + 401.9

A causal relationship is presumed to exist for a cardiac condition when it is associated with another condition classified as hypertensive heart disease. For example:

- Hypertensive myocarditis with congestive heart failure   402.91 + 428.0
- Hypertensive cardiovascular disease with congestive heart failure   402.91 + 428.0

The coder should review the medical record for any reference to the presence of conditions such as coronary arteriosclerosis or chronic coronary insufficiency that could merit additional code assignments.

HYPERTENSION AND CHRONIC KIDNEY DISEASE

When the diagnostic statement includes both hypertension and chronic kidney disease, *ICD-9-CM* usually assumes that there is a cause-and-effect relationship. A code from category **403, Hypertensive chronic kidney disease,** is provided in the Alphabetic Index; a causal relationship need not be indicated in the diagnostic statement. A fifth digit is used with category 403 to indicate the stage of the chronic kidney disease. Note that category 403 does not include acute renal failure, which is an entirely different condition from chronic kidney disease and is not caused by hypertension. Kidney conditions that are not indexed to hypertensive chronic kidney disease may or may not be hypertensive; if the physician indicates a causal relationship, only the code for hypertensive chronic kidney disease is assigned. Sample codes for cases of hypertensive chronic kidney disease include the following:

- Hypertensive nephropathy, benign   403.10
- Hypertensive nephrosclerosis   403.90
- Accelerated hypertension with chronic kidney disease   403.00 + 585.9
- Acute renal failure with renal papillary necrosis and hypertension   584.7 + 401.9

HYPERTENSIVE HEART AND CHRONIC KIDNEY DISEASE

When a heart condition ordinarily coded to category 402 and a kidney condition coded to category 403 both exist, a combination code from category **404, Hypertensive heart and chronic kidney disease,** is assigned. Fifth digits are provided to indicate with or without heart failure, as well as the stage of the chronic kidney disease, as follows:

- 0   without heart failure and with chronic kidney disease stage I through stage IV, or unspecified
- 1   with heart failure and with chronic kidney disease stage IV, or unspecified
- 2   without heart failure and with chronic kidney disease stage V or end-stage renal disease
- 3   with heart failure and chronic kidney disease stage V or end-stage renal disease

An additional code (585.1–585.6, 585.9) should be used with categories 403 and 404 to identify the specific stage of chronic kidney disease.

When the diagnostic statement indicates that both hypertension and diabetes mellitus are responsible for chronic kidney disease, both the appropriate code from category 403 or 404 and code 250.4x, from the subcategory for diabetes with renal manifestations, are assigned, with sequencing optional. An additional code is assigned for the stage of chronic kidney disease (585.1–585.6, 585.9), if known.

HYPERTENSION WITH OTHER CONDITIONS

Although hypertension is often associated with other conditions and may accelerate their development, *ICD-9-CM* does not provide combination codes. Codes for each condition must be assigned to fully describe the condition. For example:

- Atherosclerosis of aorta with benign essential hypertension   440.0 + 401.1
- Coronary atherosclerosis and systemic benign hypertension   414.00 + 401.1
- Arteriosclerotic heart disease   414.00
- Arteriosclerotic heart disease with essential hypertension   414.00 + 401.9

Exercise 24.6

Code the following diagnoses.

	Code(s)
1. Left heart failure with benign hypertension	428.1 401.1
2. Hypertensive cardiomegaly	402.90
3. Congestive heart failure Cardiomegaly Hypertension	428.0 429.3 401.9
4. Acute congestive heart failure due to hypertension	402.91 428.0
5. Hypertensive heart disease Myocardial degeneration	402.90
6. Acute cerebrovascular insufficiency	437.1

Exercise 24.6 *(continued)*

7. Cerebral thrombosis   434.00
   Moderate arterial hypertension   401.9

8. Arteriosclerotic cerebrovascular disease   437.0
   Hypertension, benign   401.1

9. Chronic coronary insufficiency   414.8
   Essential hypertension   401.9

10. Acute coronary insufficiency   411.89
    Hypertensive heart disease   402.90

HYPERTENSION COMPLICATING PREGNANCY, CHILDBIRTH, AND THE PUERPERIUM

Hypertension associated with pregnancy, childbirth, or the puerperium is considered to be a complication unless the physician specifically indicates that it is not. This condition includes both preexisting hypertension as well as transient hypertension of pregnancy or hypertension arising during pregnancy. Hypertension complicating pregnancy, childbirth, and the puerperium is reclassified in category 642. (See chapter 20 of this handbook.)

ELEVATED BLOOD PRESSURE VS. HYPERTENSION

Blood pressure readings vary from time to time and tend to increase with age. Because of these variables, a diagnosis of hypertension must be made on the basis of a series of blood pressure readings rather than a single reading. A diagnosis of elevated blood pressure reading, without diagnosis of hypertension, is assigned code 796.2. This code is never assigned on the basis of a blood pressure reading documented in the medical record; the physician must have specifically documented a diagnosis of elevated blood pressure.

True postoperative hypertension is classified as a complication of surgery, and code **997.91, Complications affecting other specified body systems, hypertension,** is assigned along with an additional code to identify the type of hypertension. However, a diagnosis of postoperative hypertension often refers only to an elevated blood pressure that reflects the patient's agitation or inadequate pain control, and would be coded to 796.2. When the patient has a preexisting hypertension, only a code from categories 401 through 405 is assigned; neither preexisting hypertension nor simple elevated blood pressure is classified as a postoperative complication. Any other diagnosis of transient hypertension, except that occurring in pregnancy, or a diagnosis of postoperative hypertension not clearly documented in the medical record should be discussed with the physician to determine whether it represents an elevated blood pressure reading or a true hypertension.

ATHEROSCLEROSIS OF EXTREMITIES

Atherosclerosis of the native arteries of the extremities is classified into subcategory 440.2. Fifth digits used with subcategory **440.2, Atherosclerosis of the extremities,** indicate the progression of the disease as follows:

- Code 440.21 indicates atherosclerosis of the extremities with intermittent claudication.
- Code 440.22 indicates the presence of rest pain; it includes any intermittent claudication.
- Code 440.23 indicates a condition that has progressed to ulceration; it includes any rest pain and/or intermittent claudication.
- Code 440.24 indicates the presence of gangrene; it includes any or all of the preceding conditions. An additional code is assigned for any associated ulceration (707.10–707.9).

Atherosclerosis of extremities involving a graft is coded to 440.3x as follows:

- 440.30   unspecified graft
- 440.32   autologous vein bypass graft
- 440.33   nonautologous biological bypass graft

THROMBOSIS AND THROMBOPHLEBITIS OF VEINS OF EXTREMITIES

A diagnosis of thrombosis of a vein indicates only that a clot has formed; a diagnosis of thrombophlebitis indicates that the clot has become inflamed. A code from category 451, Thrombophlebitis, is assigned when the diagnosis is stated as thrombosis and thrombophlebitis. An additional code for thrombosis is not assigned. When the diagnosis is stated only as thrombosis or deep vein thrombosis (DVT) without further qualification, the coder should review the medical record for evidence of thrombophlebitis. Evidence includes swelling, redness, or pain. When such evidence is documented, the coder should query the physician to determine whether a code for thrombophlebitis should be assigned. Thrombophlebitis of the extremities is classified according to the veins involved, as follows:

- 451.0   superficial veins of lower extremities
- 451.1x   deep veins of lower extremities
- 451.2   unspecified veins of lower extremities
- 451.82   superficial veins of upper extremities
- 451.83   deep veins of upper extremities
- 451.84   unspecified veins of upper extremities

Atheroembolism is separate and distinct from atherosclerosis, thrombosis or embolism. Thrombosis and embolism involve true clots, while atheroembolism involves cholesterol crystals from atheromatous plaques from vessels like the aorta or the renal artery. Atheroembolism is most commonly associated with the extremities. Category 445 is used to report atheroembolism.

OTHER CIRCULATORY CONDITIONS

In general, the coding principles applicable throughout *ICD-9-CM* apply to other sections of the *ICD-9-CM* chapter on circulatory diseases, such as categories 415 through 417 and 451 through 459, which are not discussed specifically in this handbook.

Exercise 24.7

Code the following diagnoses and procedures.

	Code(s)
1. Bleeding internal and external hemorrhoids	455.2
Stasis ulcer, left lower extremity	455.5
	454.0
Hemorrhoidectomy	49.46
2. Thrombophlebitis, femoral vein, left leg	451.11
Chronic iatrogenic hypotension	458.29
3. Arteriosclerosis of legs with intermittent claudication	440.21
4. Postoperative infarction of pulmonary artery	415.11
Saphenous phlebitis, right leg	451.0
5. Pulmonary hypertension	416.0
6. Raynaud's syndrome with gangrene	443.0
	785.4

Exercise 24.7 *(continued)*

7. Esophageal <u>varices</u>, hemorrhagic	456.0
8. Bleeding esophageal <u>varices</u> due to portal <u>hypertension</u>	572.3 456.20
<u>Ligation</u> of esophageal varices	42.91
9. <u>Arteriosclerotic</u> ulcer and gangrene of lower leg	440.24 707.10
10. Patient was admitted with acute headache and problems with vision; condition deteriorated rapidly, and patient died within four hours of admission; final diagnosis: ruptured berry <u>aneurysm</u>	430
11. Dissecting <u>aneurysm</u> of thoracic aorta	441.01
<u>Excision</u> of the aneurysm with anastomosis	38.34

STATUS V CODES

ICD-9-CM provides several V codes to indicate that the patient has a health status related to the circulatory system, such as the following:

- Heart valve transplant   V42.2
- Cardiac pacemaker in situ   V45.01
- Aortocoronary bypass status   V45.81

These codes are assigned only as additional codes and are reportable only when the status affects the patient's care for a given episode.

PROCEDURES INVOLVING THE CIRCULATORY SYSTEM

Several complex diagnostic tests have been developed for evaluating a patient's circulatory status, and several intensive procedures are currently in use for treating diseases of the circulatory system. The coronary artery bypass, used for patients with severe blockage in the coronary arteries, has been augmented by less invasive procedures, such as angioplasty. Some of these tests and procedures are described briefly in this section.

Intravascular Imaging Procedures

A new imaging technique for diagnosing intravascular vessels is known as Intravascular Vessel Imaging. This procedure utilizes a catheter-based ultrasound imaging method that allows viewing of the vessels from within. The codes for the intravascular imaging procedures are as follows:

- 00.21 Intravascular imaging of extracranial cerebral vessels
- 00.22 Intravascular imaging of intrathoracic vessels
- 00.23 Intravascular imaging of peripheral vessels
- 00.24 Intravascular imaging of coronary vessels
- 00.25 Intravascular imaging of renal vessels
- 00.28 Intravascular imaging, other specified vessel(s)
- 00.29 Intravascular imaging, unspecified vessel(s)

Diagnostic Cardiac Catheterization

Cardiac catheterization is an invasive diagnostic procedure performed for diagnosing and assessing the severity of cardiovascular disease. Codes 37.21–37.23 are assigned for this procedure and include recording intracardiac and intravascular pressures, recording tracings, obtaining blood for blood-gas testing, and measuring cardiac output. A number of other tests involve the insertion of cardiac catheters, but they are not classified as diagnostic catheterization unless a separate procedure with a report including the measurements listed in the preceding sentence has been documented.

Angiocardiography

Cardiac angiography (88.5x) is a diagnostic test ordinarily performed in conjunction with diagnostic cardiac catheterization. Ergovine provocation testing is often performed in association with coronary arteriograms to diagnose coronary spasm and is included in the code for the coronary arteriogram. Arteriography involving other arteries is classified into subcategory **88.4x, Arteriography,** with the fourth digit indicating the artery. The same codes are assigned for digital subtraction angiography, which is the same procedure as standard angiography except for the manner in which the image is detected and stored.

Bundle of His Study

The His bundle is part of the heart's conduction system, and a bundle of His study (37.29) records the heart's electrical activity. The technique involves introducing a transvenous electrode catheter through the femoral vein and then positioning it in the right ventricle near the tricuspid valve. Characteristic atrial, His bundle, and ventricular depolarizations are recorded and the intervals are timed. This study is frequently performed in conjunction with cardiac catheterization, in which case codes for both procedures are assigned, with the code for the cardiac catheterization sequenced first.

Electrophysiologic Stimulation and Recording Studies

Electrophysiologic stimulation and recording studies, commonly referred to as EP studies (EPS), are performed as part of the diagnosis and therapeutic management of patients with ventricular tachycardia or ventricular fibrillation, both forms of cardiac arrhythmia that carry a high risk of sudden death. The studies are also performed for patients who have unexplained syncope and palpitation or supraventricular tachycardia. After cardiac access is obtained either percutaneously or via cutdown, specialized electrophysiologic catheter electrodes are inserted and guided into position under fluoroscopy. Code **37.26, Catheter based invasive electrophysiologic testing,** is assigned for these studies. Code **37.20, Noninvasive programmed electrical stimulation (NIPS),** is assigned for noninvasive electrical stimulation.

Implant of Automatic Defibrillator/Cardioverter

The automatic implantable cardioverter defibrillator (AICD) is an electronic device designed to detect and treat life-threatening tachyarrhythmias by means of countershocks. Patients receiving this therapy have usually had one or more episodes of life-threatening arrhythmias that cannot be controlled by other therapy.

A total cardioverter defibrillator system implant (37.94) is usually performed as a single procedure. It includes the formation of a subcutaneous tissue pocket or abdominal fascia pocket, implantation or replacement of the defibrillator with epicardial patches and any transvenous leads, intraoperative procedures for evaluation of the lead signal, defibrillator threshold measurements, and tests of the implanted device with induction of arrhythmia. The implant is sometimes performed in two stages, however, with the leads implanted first (37.95) and the generator implanted on a subsequent day during the same hospital admission (37.96). Any extracorporeal circulation (39.61) or any other concomitant surgical procedure should also be coded. Code 37.26 is not assigned for an intraoperative EP study performed for device testing during implantation of an AICD. Code **37.79, Revision or relocation of cardiac device pocket,** includes creation of a loop recorder pocket and also creation of a pocket for an implantable, patient-activated cardiac event recorder. Insertion and relocation of both devices are included in this code.

When a patient is admitted for replacement or adjustment of an automatic cardioverter/defibrillator, code **V53.32, Automatic implantable cardiac defibrillator,** is assigned as the principal diagnosis unless the procedure is being performed because of a mechanical complication, in which case code **996.04, Mechanical complication of cardiac device, implant, and graft, due to automatic implantable cardiac defibrillator,** is assigned. Replacement of the entire system is included in the code for the initial insertion, and code **37.94, Implantation or replacement of cardioverter/defibrillator, total system (AICD),** is assigned. When only the leads are replaced, code **37.97, Replacement of automatic cardioverter/defibrillator lead(s) only,** is assigned; when only the pulse generator is replaced, code **37.98, Replacement of cardioverter/defibrillator pulse generator only,** is assigned. Removal without replacement or simple repositioning is coded to **37.99, Other.**

Automatic implantable cardioverter/defibrillators (AICDs) sometimes require checking of the pacing thresholds or interrogation without arrythmia induction. This procedure is coded to **89.49, Automatic implantable cardioverter/defibrillator (AICD) check.** For example, a bedside check or interrogation of an AICD device is assigned to code 89.49.

Cardiac Pacemaker Therapy

Cardiac pacemaker therapy involves electrical control of the heart rate. *ICD-9-CM* codes differentiate between the insertion of temporary pacemakers and the insertion of permanent pacemakers. In a temporary pacemaker insertion (37.78), leads are inserted via a catheter and attached to an external pulse generator. This type of pacemaker is generally used for an acutely ill patient until a permanent one can be inserted. Another type of temporary pacemaker is used intraoperatively or immediately following surgery, with the leads inserted into the myocardium in an already-opened chest (39.64). No codes are assigned for insertion of the leads or for removal of a temporary or intraoperative pacemaker.

A temporary transmyocardial pacemaker in which a needle is inserted into the chest and into the myocardium with leads fed through the needle directly into the heart muscle and attached to an external pacing device is sometimes used in an effort at cardiopulmonary resuscitation. This procedure is considered an integral part of cardiopulmonary resuscitation (99.60), and no additional code is assigned. Two codes are required for the initial insertion of a permanent pacemaker. One code indicates the type of device, commonly called a pulse generator (37.81–37.83); the other indicates the insertion of the leads (37.71–37.74).

Pacemaker leads (electrodes) can be placed either transvenously into the inside of the heart or epicardially onto the outside of the heart. In order to insert a transvenous lead into the ventricle, an incision is made in the skin and the lead is passed into the subclavian vein, down the superior vena cava, across the right atrium, and into the right ventricle. When transvenous leads are used, the pacemaker device is ordinarily placed in a subcutaneous pocket in the upper chest wall. Code 37.79 is assigned for the revision or relocation of a pocket for a pacemaker, defibrillator, or other implanted cardiac device.

No incision into the chest cavity is needed for the insertion of an epicardial lead. The most common site for the pacemaker pocket when epicardial leads are used is the abdominal wall.

There are three types of pacemaker devices on the market, each of which has a unique *ICD-9-CM* code for its insertion:

- Single chamber   37.81
- Single chamber, rate responsive   37.82
- Dual chamber   37.83

A single-chamber device uses a single lead; a dual-chamber device requires two leads, one in the atrium and one in the ventricle (37.72). It is important to be sure that the code for the lead insertion and the code for the pacemaker device are compatible because errors in this area have serious implications for reimbursement. A rate-responsive device is one in which the pacing rate is determined by physiological variables other than the atrial rate. This type of pacemaker permits patients to lead a more normal life and is strongly preferred for a potentially active patient. Physicians use various terms for this ability to respond and in many cases mention only the device number in documenting an insertion. The coding department should work with the hospital operating room staff and/or physicians to identify the devices commonly used in the facility and how they might be consistently identified in the operative report.

Total replacement of a permanent pacemaker system also requires two codes, one that identifies the replacement of leads (37.74 or 37.76) and one that identifies the replacement of the pacemaker device (37.85–37.87). When an existing pacemaker device is replaced with a new device, the type of device removed does not affect the code; only the type of new device inserted should be coded (37.85–37.87). Removal of the old device is included in the replacement code. Removal of lead(s) (electrode) without replacement is coded as 37.77 for leads and 37.89 for revision or removal of the pacemaker device.

When a patient is admitted for removal, replacement, or reprogramming of a cardiac pacemaker, code **V53.31, Fitting and adjustment of a cardiac pacemaker,** is assigned as the principal diagnosis. Reprogramming is a simple nonoperative procedure that does not require a procedure code. Physicians sometimes indicate that a patient is being admitted for battery replacement. This is something of a misnomer because pacemakers no longer use batteries and the whole device is actually replaced. When the pacemaker device is being replaced only because it is nearing the end of its expected life, code V53.31 is assigned as the principal diagnosis. When it is being replaced because of a mechanical complication of the device, diagnosis code **996.01, Mechanical complication due to cardiac pacemaker (electrode),** is assigned.

Cardiac Resynchronization Therapy

Cardiac resynchronization therapy (CRT) is a new technology similar to conventional pacemaker therapy and implantable cardioverter-defibrillators (ICDs). CRT is different because it requires the implantation of a special electrode within the coronary vein to attach the device to the exterior wall of the left ventricle. CRT treats heart failure by providing strategic electrical stimulation to the right atrium, right ventricle and left ventricle of the heart to recoordinate ventricular contractions and improve cardiac output. CRT is also sometimes referred to as biventricular pacing. ICD-9-CM codes distinguish between the insertion of cardiac resynchronization pacemaker without internal cardiac defibrillator (CRT-P) and the insertion of cardiac resynchronization defibrillator, total system (CRT-D). CRT-P implantations are coded to 00.50 and CRT-D implantations are coded to 00.51. No additional codes are assigned for the creation of the pocket to hold the device, implantation of the device, insertion of transvenous leads as well as the lead into the coronary venous system and intraoperative procedures to evaluate lead signals.

Over time, there may be a need to replace the lead into the left ventricular coronary venous system (00.52), replace the pacemaker pulse generator on a CRT-P (00.53), or replace the defibrillator pulse generator on a CRT-D (00.54). Code **37.75, Revision of lead [electrode],** is assigned for repositioning of the CRT-D or CRT-P lead only.

Percutaneous Balloon Valvuloplasty

Percutaneous balloon valvuloplasty (PBPV) (35.96) is a noninvasive treatment for pulmonary valve stenosis. It involves a balloon wedge catheter that is advanced via the femoral vein into the heart and across the stenotic valve. The balloon is then inflated by hand pressure. There is no need for general anesthesia, the hospital stay is short, and no scarring results from the procedure. The code includes any nondiagnostic cardiac catheterization done as a part of the procedure.

Percutaneous Transluminal Coronary Angioplasty

Code 00.66 is assigned for percutaneous transluminal coronary angioplasty (PTCA) and includes arteriectomy (atherectomy). Codes 00.40–00.43 identify the number of vessels on which the PTCA was performed. An additional code is assigned for the thrombolytic agent administered (99.10). These codes are as follows:

- 00.40   Procedure on single vessel
- 00.41   Procedure on two vessels
- 00.42   Procedure on three vessels
- 00.43   Procedure on four or more vessels

Code **00.44, Procedure on vessel bifurcation,** is used to describe the presence of a vessel bifurcation and is provided to capture data regarding the procedural differences between interventional procedures on a straight vessel and a vessel bifurcation. Bifurcation lesions usually involve blockages of a main coronary vessel and an adjacent side vessel, resulting in a lesion that is more complex to treat. Code 00.44 does not identify a specific bifurcation stent. This code is only used once per operative episode, irrespective of the number of bifurcations present in vessels.

Because reclosure often occurs following angioplasty, a stent is frequently inserted to prevent reclosure. In this procedure, a small stainless steel mesh stent is inserted during angioplasty to prop open the blocked coronary arteries. After the balloon has been threaded into the coronary artery and inflated to squash plaque deposits against the vessel wall, the process is repeated with a second balloon carrying the stent. Expansion of the balloon pushes the stent against the artery wall, where it remains to maintain patency. To report the insertion of stents, it is necessary to assign two codes. One code is used to identify the number of vascular stents inserted (00.45–00.48), and another code to identify the type of coronary stent (non-drug-eluting, 36.06, or drug-eluting, 36.07). These codes cannot be used alone since an angioplasty is needed to insert the stent. The codes are as follows:

- 00.45 Insertion of one vascular stent
- 00.46 Insertion of two vascular stents
- 00.47 Insertion of three vascular stents
- 00.48 Insertion of four or more vascular stents

Minor intimal tears often occur during angioplasty or the newer rotational atherectomy procedures; these are considered to be an unavoidable part of the procedure and are not classified as complications.

Angioplasty of Non-coronary Vessels

Code **39.50, Angioplasty or atherectomy of other non-coronary vessel(s),** is assigned for percutaneous angioplasty of vessels other than coronary vessels. Code **39.90, Insertion of non-drug-eluting, peripheral vessel stent or stents,** or code **00.55, Insertion of drug-eluting peripheral vessel stent(s),** is assigned for any associated stent insertion. If a thrombolytic agent is used, code **99.10, Injection or infusion of thrombolytic agent,** should be assigned as an additional code. The number of vascular stents inserted is identified with codes 00.45–00.48.

Assign code 00.61 for a percutaneous angioplasty or atherectomy of precerebral vessels, and code 00.62 for intracranial vessels. Assign code 00.63 for the percutaneous insertion of carotid artery stents, code 00.64 for other precerebral artery stents, and code 00.65 for intracranial vascular stents. Use codes 00.45–00.48 to report the number of stents inserted, codes 00.40–00.43 to report the number of vessels treated, and code 00.44 to report vessel bifurcation.

Coronary Artery Bypass Graft

Coronary artery bypass grafts (CABGs) are performed to revascularize the myocardium when a blockage in a coronary artery limits the blood supply to the heart. The grafts bypass the obstructions in the coronary arteries.

Coronary circulation consists of two main arteries, right and left, each with several branches, which are counted as arteries in coding aortocoronary bypass grafts:

- Right coronary artery (RCA)
  —Right marginal
  —Right posterior descending (PDA)
- Left main coronary artery (LMCA)
  —Left anterior descending branch (LAD)
  —Diagonal
  —Septal
  —Circumflex (LCX)
  —Obtuse marginal (OM)
  —Posterior descending
  —Posterolateral

The abbreviation CABG is commonly used to indicate a coronary artery bypass graft; separate codes are provided to indicate the type of bypass carried out.

The aortocoronary artery bypass is the one most commonly used. It brings blood from the aorta into the obstructed coronary artery, bypassing the obstruction by means of a segment of the patient's own saphenous vein, nonautologous biological material, or occasionally a segment of the internal mammary artery. The graft material used in an aortocoronary bypass does not affect code assignment. The axis for coding aortocoronary bypass grafts is the number of coronary arteries involved in the bypass (see figure 24.1):

- (Aorto)coronary bypass of one coronary artery   36.11
- (Aorto)coronary bypass of two coronary arteries   36.12
- (Aorto)coronary bypass of three coronary arteries   36.13
- (Aorto)coronary bypass of four or more coronary arteries   36.14

All coronary bypass procedures do not involve the aorta. The internal mammary-coronary artery bypass graft is accomplished by loosening the internal mammary artery from its normal position and using it as a conduit to bring blood from the subclavian artery to the occluded coronary artery. The axis for coding internal mammary-coronary artery bypass grafts is whether one or both internal mammary arteries are used, regardless of the number of coronary arteries involved:

- Single internal mammary-coronary artery bypass   36.15
- Double internal mammary-coronary artery bypass   36.16

It is rare for only one coronary artery to be bypassed, and it is also fairly common to perform both an internal mammary-coronary artery bypass and an aortocoronary bypass at the same operative episode (see figure 24.2). The surgeon's brief statement of the operation performed does not always distinguish the types of bypasses involved, which makes it necessary for the coder to refer to the body of the operative report when the statement is not clear.

FIGURE 24.1   Direct Myocardial Revascularization by Triple Aortocoronary Artery Bypass Using Autogenous Vein Grafts

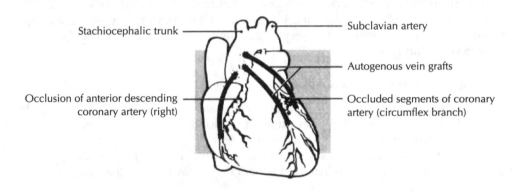

Reprinted, with permission, from *Coding Clinic for ICD-9-CM,* 4th quarter 1989. ©1989 American Hospital Association.

FIGURE 24.2   A Combination of Aortocoronary and Internal Mammary Artery Bypass Grafts for Myocardial Revascularization

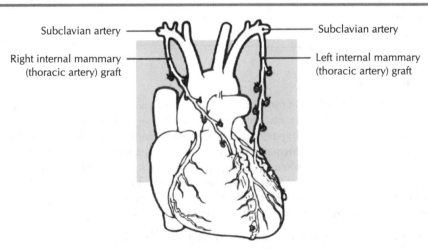

Reprinted, with permission, from *Coding Clinic for ICD-9-CM,* 4th quarter 1989. ©1989 American Hospital Association.

Other arteries are also used to bypass an obstruction in the coronary artery. Code **36.17, Abdominal-coronary artery bypass,** is used when an abdominal artery such as the gastric or gastroepiploic artery is used for the graft. Code **36.19, Other bypass anastomosis for heart revascularization,** is assigned when any other bypass anastomosis is performed.

An additional code should also be assigned for any use of extracorporeal circulation (39.61), or pressurized treatment of venous bypass graft with pharmaceutical substance (00.16). However, procedures such as hypothermia, cardioplegia, intraoperative pacing, and chest tube insertions are considered to be integral to bypass surgery; no separate codes are assigned.

In coding coronary artery bypass procedures, it is important to keep the following points in mind:

- The fact that a detached segment of the internal mammary artery is used as graft material instead of saphenous vein in performing an aortocoronary bypass does not make it an internal mammary-coronary artery bypass. The internal mammary-coronary artery bypass involves the use of the internal mammary itself as a still vascularized conduit for the blood supply and does not involve the aorta.
- When more than one coronary artery is involved in either type of graft, the anastomosis is sometimes carried out in a sequential manner, bypassing more than one artery. The mention of sequential anastomoses does not affect the code in any way.

The following examples may provide further assistance in coding coronary bypass grafts:

1. Coronary artery vascularization was carried out with four grafts: the aorta to the diagonal branch of the left coronary and in sequential fashion to the obtuse marginal branch of the circumflex, the right coronary artery, and the left anterior descending coronary artery. This procedure involved only the aorta and the coronary arteries. Because four coronary arteries were bypassed, **36.14, (Aorto)coronary bypass of four or more coronary arteries,** is assigned.

2. Grafts from the aorta to the coronary arteries were carried out by grafting the bifurcated left anterior descending system with a 1.5-millimeter section of the left internal mammary artery. The first diagonal was then grafted side-to-side with a 4-millimeter section of the saphenous vein. The obtuse marginal was then grafted with a 4-millimeter section of the saphenous vein. The posterior descending was diffusely diseased and was grafted with a 4-millimeter section of the saphenous vein. All four grafts brought blood from the aorta to the coronary arteries. Sections of both the saphenous vein and the internal mammary artery were used for this purpose, but the materials used for the graft do not affect the code. Because four arteries (LAD, diagonal, obtuse marginal, and posterior descending) were bypassed, code **36.14, (Aorto)coronary bypass of four or more coronary arteries,** is assigned.

3. Bypass grafts were performed by bringing the left internal mammary artery to the left anterior ascending; a saphenous vein graft was then used to bring blood from the aorta to the obtuse marginal branch of the circumflex artery, to the diagonal artery, and to the proximal PDA. In this case, a single internal mammary-coronary artery bypass and three aortocoronary bypass grafts were placed (OM, diagonal, PDA). The codes assigned are **36.15, Single internal mammary-coronary artery bypass,** and **36.13, (Aorto)coronary artery bypass of three coronary arteries.** The sequence of the codes is optional.

4. The left internal mammary artery was loosened and used to bypass the left anterior descending artery; grafts of the saphenous vein were bypassed to the posterior descending artery and to the obtuse marginal branch of the circumflex. In this case, three coronary arteries were bypassed, one by an internal mammary-coronary artery bypass and two by aortocoronary bypasses. The codes assigned are **36.15, Single internal mammary-coronary artery bypass,** and **36.12, (Aorto)coronary artery bypass.**

As mentioned earlier, coronary artery bypass grafts often become occluded, sometimes because of a continuation of the arteriosclerotic disease process. Arteriosclerosis of an artery involved in a bypass graft is coded **414.02, Coronary atherosclerosis of autologous vein bypass graft** or **414.03, Coronary atherosclerosis of nonautologous biological bypass graft.** Code **414.04, Coronary atherosclerosis of artery bypass graft,** is assigned for an artery with arteriosclerosis. (Note: If there is no mention in the medical record of the patient having undergone a bypass, code **414.01, Arteriosclerosis of native coronary artery,** should be assigned.)

Heart revascularization is also performed by other techniques. Transmyocardial revascularization can be performed by open procedure (36.31), by other transmyocardial procedures (36.32), by robot-assisted or thoracoscopic procedures (36.33), and by percutaneous or endovascular procedures (36.34). A number of other procedures such as myocardial graft using omentum, mediastinal fat, or pectoral muscles are classified in code **36.39, Other heart revascularization.**

Exercise 24.8

Code the following diagnoses and procedures.

	Code(s)
1. A patient was admitted through the emergency department complaining of chest pain with radiation down the left arm increasing in severity over the past three hours. Initial impression was impending myocardial infarction, and the patient was taken directly to the surgical suite, where percutaneous transluminal angioplasty with insertion of coronary stent was carried out on the right coronary artery. Infarction was aborted, and the diagnosis was listed as acute coronary insufficiency.	411.89 00.66 00.40 00.45 36.06
2. Saphenous vein graft was used to bring blood from the aorta to the right coronary artery, the left coronary artery, and the left anterior descending artery. Intraoperative pacemaker was used during the procedure as well as extracorporeal circulatory assistance. Bypass	36.13 39.64 39.61
3. Right and left diagnostic cardiac catheterization with bundle of His study	37.23 37.29

Exercise 24.8 *(continued)*

4. Balloon <u>angioplasty</u> carried out on three coronary arteries with vessel bifurcation

<u>00.66</u>
36.06
00.42
00.44

<u>Insertion</u> of two stents
Extracorporeal <u>circulation</u>

00.46
39.61

5. Initial <u>insertion</u> of dual-chamber pacemaker device

37.72
37.83

6. Patient was <u>admitted</u> for replacement of single-chamber pacemaker device because the battery was expected to fail within a short time; device was <u>replaced</u> with single-chamber rate-responsive pacemaker device.

V53.31
37.86

7. Patient was admitted for <u>replacement</u> of displaced and protruding pacemaker device with single-chamber, rate responsive device.

996.01
37.86

<u>Complication, mechanical</u>

8. Catheter based invasive electrophysiological cardiac <u>study</u>

37.26

9. Patient with severe coronary arteriosclerotic disease was admitted for coronary <u>bypass</u> (no history of previous bypass surgery). The left internal mammary artery was taken down to the left anterior descending artery and a reverse saphenous Y graft was brought from the aorta to the distal LAD and diagonal, as well as a reverse saphenous vein graft to the obtuse marginal artery × two and distal right coronary artery.

414.01
36.14
36.15

HEART ASSIST DEVICES

There are two types of heart assist devices in use at present. One is a mechanical circulatory support system (for example, Heartmate) designed to provide temporary circulatory support for patients approved for heart transplantation. This portable system is intended for long-term use. The device is usually positioned in the abdomen and is attached parallel to the cardiovascular system, leaving the heart's natural pathway undisturbed while the assist system provides the energy to propel blood into the arteries. Code **37.66, Insertion of implantable heart assist system,** is assigned for the use of this device. The second type of heart assist device is an external pulsatile system used for patients with postcardiotomy ventricular dysfunction. The device remains outside the body but is connected to the heart. Code **37.65, Insertion of external heart assist system,** is assigned for the use of this device. A new code has been created for the insertion of a percutaneous external heart assist device (37.68).

IMPLANTABLE INFUSION PUMP AND VASCULAR ACCESS DEVICES

Implantable vascular access devices and implantable infusion pumps are two distinct catheter systems, each of which can be used to deliver drug therapy. The main difference between them is that the implantable infusion pump is self-contained and completely implanted in the body, whereas the implantable vascular access device is not a pump but a port implanted in the body to provide easy access to the vascular system. Code **86.06, Insertion of totally implantable infusion pump,** is assigned for the totally implantable infusion pump; code **86.07, Insertion of totally implantable vascular access device (VAD),** is assigned for the vascular access device.

The implantable infusion pump is surgically placed in the body, usually via laparotomy under general anesthesia. The laparotomy approach is not coded. In certain instances, a catheter is attached to the pump and inserted into an artery for direct infusion of a drug; in such cases, code **38.91, Arterial catheterization,** is also assigned. The pump is used to deliver intra-arterial drugs such as chemotherapeutic agents for patients with primary hepatomas or colon cancer with metastasis to the liver, as well as to deliver pain medication for terminal cancer patients. The pump allows the patient greater flexibility and freedom of movement while receiving treatment and also permits treatment on an outpatient basis once the pump has been inserted.

The use of an infusion pump that remains outside the body and infuses medication through a subcutaneous or venous needle is not coded. Only the procedure for placing a venous needle or catheter is coded (**38.93, Puncture of vessel, venous catheterization, NEC**). The application of this device includes the insertion of a permanent catheter.

An implantable VAD is a sterile catheter system implanted subcutaneously under local anesthesia and used for multiple purposes, such as infusion of total parenteral nutrition (TPN) and bolus injections of medication. The device is placed in central veins, such as the subclavian, rather than a peripheral vein. VADs are designed to provide repeated access to the vascular system without the trauma or complications of multiple venipuncture. The devices can be left in place for weeks or months as opposed to days and are generally placed in patients who require long-term access for chemotherapy, nutrition, or blood withdrawal.

Simple venous catheters are sterile catheter systems that provide repeated access to the vascular system for procedures such as blood withdrawal and medication or fluid administration. The catheter is inserted into a peripheral vein, such as the cephalic vein, by puncturing the skin and then taping the catheter in place. These catheters remain in place for a much shorter period of time than VADs. Examples of simple venous catheters (also called heparin locks) include Angiocaths, Abbott catheters, and Jelco catheters. Code **38.93, Venous catheterization NEC,** is assigned for insertion of a simple catheter system. Code **86.05, Incision with removal of foreign body from skin and subcutaneous tissue,** is assigned for the removal of a vascular access device.

IMPLANTABLE HEMODYNAMIC MONITOR

Codes 00.56 and 00.57 are assigned for the implantation of a hemodynamic monitoring system. The implantable hemodynamic monitoring system allows clinicians to identify early signs of volume overload before signs and symptoms of heart failure become apparent. Clinicians can then adjust treatment to prevent acute decompensated heart failure and the need for hospital admission. The device consists of two key components. A lead with a pressure sensor is placed within the right ventricle at the right ventricular outflow tract. The other component is the monitoring device, which includes pressure-sensing circuitry with memory to process and collect the data obtained by the sensor. The codes are as follows:

- 00.56 Insertion or replacement of implantable pressure sensor (lead) for intracardiac hemodynamic monitoring
- 00.57 Implantation or replacement of subcutaneous device for intracardiac hemodynamic monitoring

IMPLANTATION OF CARDIOMYOSTIMULATION SYSTEM

Code **37.67, Implantation of cardiomyostimulation system,** is used to report the use of a new surgical technique called dynamic cardiomyoplasty. It is a fairly complicated two-step open procedure that involves elevating the latissimus dorsi muscle, then wrapping it around the heart. A stimulator similar to a pacemaker is implanted and connected to both the heart and the wrapped muscle. There are a number of components to the procedure; all are included in code 37.67.

HEART TRANSPLANTATION

Heart transplantation is carried out when the heart is failing and doesn't respond to therapies. The main reasons for heart transplants are cardiomyopathy, severe coronary artery disease and congenital defects of the heart. Code **37.51, Heart transplantation,** is used to report the transplantation of a heart from a donor. There is an insufficient number of organs available for transplantation to meet the need. A patient may wait months for a transplant and many don't live long enough to receive the organ. With advances in new technology, there is now a completely implantable artificial heart available. Code **37.52, Implantation of total replacement heart system,** is used to report this procedure. Additional codes are also available to replace or repair the thoracic unit (37.53) or any other implantable component (37.54) of a total replacement heart system.

Review Exercise 24.9

Code the following diagnoses and procedures.

	Code(s)
1. Internal and external thrombosed <u>hemorrhoids</u>	455.1 455.4
Internal and external <u>hemorrhoidectomy</u> by cryosurgery	49.44
2. Varicose veins, right leg	454.9
Right greater saphenous <u>ligation</u> and <u>stripping</u> for varicosities	38.59
3. Mitral <u>stenosis</u> and aortic <u>insufficiency</u> Atrial <u>fibrillation</u> <u>Hypertension</u>	396.1 427.31 401.9
4. Abdominal aortic <u>aneurysm</u> <u>Hypertensive</u> cardiovascular disease essential	<u>441.4</u> 402.90
<u>Resection</u> of abdominal aortic aneurysm with graft replacement	38.44
5. Acute myocardial <u>infarction</u>, anterior wall (initial episode of care)	410.11

Review Exercise 24.9 *(continued)*

6. Renovascular <u>hypertension</u> secondary to   447.3
   fibromuscular <u>hyperplasia</u>, right renal artery   405.91

   Renogram   92.03

7. Congestive heart <u>failure</u> due to   402.91
   <u>hypertensive</u> heart disease   428.0

8. Congestive heart <u>failure</u>   428.0
   Permanent cardiac pacemaker in place   V45.01
   <u>Status</u>

9. Cerebral <u>occlusion</u>, thrombotic with   434.01
   cerebral <u>infarction</u>   402.90
   <u>Hypertensive</u> cardiovascular disease

10. <u>Hypertension</u>   403.90
    Chronic <u>kidney</u> disease   585.9

11. Iatrogenic pulmonary <u>infarction</u>   415.11

12. <u>Hypertensive encephalopathy</u> due to   437.2
    accelerated <u>hypertension</u>   401.0

13. <u>Insertion</u> of pacemaker leads: insertion of   37.72
    dual-chamber pacemaker device   37.83

Review Exercise 24.9 *(continued)*

---

14. Arteriosclerosis of coronary artery   414.02
    (four-vessel bypass graft with saphenous
    vein carried out two years ago)

---

15. Acute pulmonary edema with left   428.1
    ventricular failure

---

16. Cerebrovascular accident, acute, with thrombosis   434.00
    Residual hemiplegia, right, and aphasia   342.90
    (at discharge)   784.3
    Essential hypertension   401.9

---

17. Severe stenosis of left main coronary   414.01
    arteries in patient with no previous
    history of bypass surgery

    Aortocoronary bypass, left diagonal and   36.12
    left circumflex arteries with saphenous   39.61
    vein graft   39.64
    Cardiopulmonary bypass
    Insertion of intraoperative pacemaker

---

25 Neoplasms

A neoplasm is a new or abnormal growth. In the *ICD-9-CM* classification system, neoplastic disease is classified in categories 140 through 239.

BEHAVIOR CLASSIFICATION

The first axis for coding neoplasms is behavior; the second axis is the anatomical site. *ICD-9-CM* classifies neoplasms into five behavior groups:

- Malignant   140–208
- Benign   210–229
- Carcinoma in situ   230–234
- Uncertain behavior   235–238
- Unspecified nature   239

Malignant Neoplasms

Malignant neoplasms are tumor cells that extend beyond the primary site, attaching themselves to adjacent structures or spreading to distant sites. They are characterized by relentless growth and are difficult to cure. The term invasive is often used to describe the extension of the tumor cells to other adjacent sites. The resulting spread is called metastasis.

Certain types of malignant neoplasms are noted for their invasive properties (for example, malignant melanoma of the skin) and usually require excision beyond the primary site because of their potential microinvasiveness. In such cases, a biopsy finding of malignancy on tissue removed during outpatient surgery may indicate the need for more extensive surgery on an inpatient basis. When such further surgery is performed, however, the pathology report may or may not indicate further malignancy. When no further malignancy is found, the physician ordinarily documents the diagnosis as a malignancy in accordance with the findings of the initial biopsy, because that condition is the reason for admission and the primary neoplasm may, in fact, require further treatment. In this situation, the diagnosis provided by the physician should be coded even though the current pathology report does not confirm the diagnosis. A copy of the original pathology report should be obtained and filed with the current medical record if at all possible.

Benign Neoplasms

Benign neoplasms are not invasive and do not spread to either adjacent or distant sites. They may, however, cause local effects such as displacement, pressure on an adjacent structure, impingement on a nerve, or compression of a vessel and therefore require surgery. Uterine myomas, for example, may cause pressure on the urinary bladder, which results in urinary symptoms. Most benign tumors can be cured by total excision.

Carcinoma in Situ

Tumor cells in carcinoma described as in situ are undergoing malignant changes but are still confined to the point of origin without invasion of the surrounding normal tissue. Other terms that describe carcinoma in situ include intraepithelial, noninfiltrating, noninvasive, and preinvasive carcinoma. Severe cervical and vulvar dysplasia described as CIN III or

VIN III are classified as carcinoma in situ. (See chapter 17 of this handbook for more information.)

Neoplasms of Uncertain Behavior

The ultimate behavior of certain neoplasms cannot be determined at the time they are discovered, and a firm distinction between benign and malignant tumor cells cannot be made. Certain benign tumors, for example, may be undergoing malignant transformation; as a result, continued study is necessary to arrive at a conclusive diagnosis.

Neoplasms of Unspecified Nature

Category 239 is provided for those situations in which neither the behavior nor the morphology of the neoplasm is specified in the diagnostic statement or elsewhere in the medical record. This usually occurs when a patient is transferred to another medical care facility for further diagnosis and possible treatment before diagnostic studies are completed or when a patient is given a working diagnosis in an outpatient setting pending further study. A code from category 239 would not be used for a neoplasm treated in an acute-care facility because more definitive information should always be available. It is important not to confuse neoplasms of unspecified nature with those of uncertain behavior.

Unspecified Mass or Lesion

It is incorrect to select a code from category **239, Neoplasms of unspecified nature,** when only the terms "mass" or "lesion" are used. When coding diagnoses documented as mass or lesion of a particular site, and when that site is not listed under the main terms "Mass" or "Lesion," the coder should follow the cross-references under the main term representing the documented diagnosis. If a final diagnosis is documented as "lump," and there is no index entry for the affected organ or site under "lump" in the index, look up the main term "mass" as directed by the "see also" note under the main term "lump." If there is no index entry for the specific site under "mass," look up the main term "disease." The index directs the coder to see Disease of specified organ or site for "Mass, specified organ NEC."

   If a final diagnosis is documented as "lesion," and there is no index entry for the specified organ or site under the main term "Lesion," look up the main term "Disease." The index directs you to see Disease by site for "Lesion, organ or site NEC."

Exercise 25.1

By referring to the following subcategories in volume 1, match the codes in the left column with the descriptions listed in the right column. In some cases, more than one letter may be assigned to a code in the left column.

_c_	153.1 Transverse colon	a.	Benign
_d_	237.2 Adrenal gland	b.	Carcinoma in situ
_c_	172.0 Lip	c.	Malignant
_b + c_	231.1 Trachea	d.	Uncertain behavior
_e_	239.4 Bladder	e.	Unspecified nature
_a_	210.7 Nasopharynx		

MORPHOLOGY CLASSIFICATION

Morphology of neoplasms refers to the form and structure of tumor cells and is studied in order to classify a neoplasm by its tissue origin. The tissue of origin and the type of cells that make up a malignant neoplasm often determine the expected rate of growth, the severity of illness, and the type of treatment given. Metastatic neoplasms are identified at the metastatic site by their morphology, which is different from the normal tissue at that site but the same as that at the primary site.

Morphology codes consist of a capital letter "M," followed by four digits that identify the histological type, with a slash mark and a fifth digit indicating its behavior (M0000/0). Neoplastic disease is indexed by the morphological type as well as by other common terms, with the morphology code displayed in parentheses following the index entry. Many tumor-like conditions are not classified as neoplasms, however, and therefore no morphology code is provided. Examples of such conditions are adenomatous goiter, adenosis, mass, polyp, and leukoplakia.

Behavior identification for morphology codes parallels the behavior classification in *ICD-9-CM* as follows:

- 0   Benign
- 1   Uncertain behavior, borderline malignancy
- 2   Carcinoma in situ
- 3   Malignant, primary site
- 6   Malignant, secondary site

When the diagnostic statement or pathology report indicates a behavior other than that indicated by the morphology code, the medical record information prevails. For example, the morphology code for chordoma indicates that it is malignant (M9370/3), but a malignant neoplasm code should not be assigned when the record documents the neoplasm as benign.

Use of morphology codes is optional; they are rarely used except in tumor registries and pathology department indexes. *ICD-9-CM* provides a listing of morphology codes in appendix A of volume 1.

Exercise 25.2

Answer the following questions either true or false.

___T___ 1. Morphology of neoplasms refers to the study of the form and structure of the tissue and cells from which the neoplasm arises.

___F___ 2. Metastatic neoplasms can be identified by their morphology, which is identical to the morphology of the surrounding normal tissue and cells at the metastatic site.

___F___ 3. Morphology codes, such as M8090/3, are located in *ICD-9-CM,* volume 1, chapter 2, entitled Neoplasms.

___T___ 4. For morphology code M8090/3, the digit 3 identifies the behavior of the neoplasm as malignant.

___T___ 5. In hospitals and other health care settings, the use of the morphology codes (M codes) is optional, depending on the user's needs.

LOCATING OF CODES FOR NEOPLASTIC DISEASE

The first step in locating the code for a neoplasm is to refer to the main term for the morphological type in the Alphabetic Index of Diseases and Injuries and then to review the subentries. For some types, a specific diagnosis code is provided. For example, for a diagnosis of renal cell carcinoma, the Alphabetic Index lists the main term **Carcinoma** and the subterm renal cell as follows:

Carcinoma (M8010/3) . . .
    renal cell (M8312/3)   189.0

When the site is not listed as a subterm or when a specific code is not given in the index, a cross-reference to the neoplasm table in volume 2 appears. Cross-references should be followed closely; the following entries indicate the help the coder can receive when the type of neoplasm is referenced in the Alphabetic Index:

Sarcoma (M8800/3) . . .
 cerebellar (M9480/3) 191.6
 embryonal (M8991/3)—*see* Neoplasm, connective tissue, malignant . . .
 Ewing's (M9260/3)—*see* Neoplasm, bone, malignant

The neoplasm table (part of which is reproduced here as table 25.1) lists anatomical sites alphabetically on the far left. (The indention levels have the same significance as those used elsewhere in volume 2.) Columns to the right indicate the code for each behavior type for that site. To use the table, coders must first locate the anatomical site in the list, move across the page to the behavior type, and then select the appropriate code. Coders should work from the table only after taking the first step of referring to the main term for the morphological type because important information in the index could be missed, and an incorrect code could be assigned as a result. Codes from the neoplasm table should be verified in the Tabular List.

TABLE 25.1 Section of the Neoplasm Table in the Index of Diseases and Injuries

	Malignant				Uncertain	
	Primary	Secondary	Ca in situ	Benign	Behavior	Unspecified
Neoplasm, neoplastic—*continued*						
alveolar—*continued*						
ridge or process—*continued*						
mucosa	143.9	198.89	230.0	210.4	235.1	239.0
lower	143.1	198.89	230.0	210.4	235.1	239.0
upper	143.0	198.89	230.0	210.4	235.1	239.0
upper	170.0	198.5	—	213.0	238.0	239.2
sulcus	145.1	198.89	230.0	210.4	235.1	239.0
alveolus	143.9	198.89	230.0	210.4	235.1	239.0
lower	143.1	198.89	230.0	210.4	235.1	239.0
upper	143.0	198.89	230.0	210.4	235.1	239.0
ampulla of Vater	156.2	197.8	230.8	211.5	235.3	239.0

Exercise 25.3

Assign both diagnosis and morphology codes to the following diagnoses.

                    Code(s)

1. Bronchial <u>adenoma</u>   235.7
                    M8140/1

2. Burkitt's <u>lymphoma</u> of intrapelvic lymph   200.26
  nodes   M9750/3

Exercise 25.3 *(continued)*

3. Lipoma of breast

214.1
M8850/0

4. Giant cell leukemia

207.20
M9910/3

5. Endometrial sarcoma

182.0
M8930/3

6. Hodgkin's sarcoma

201.20
M9662/3

BASIC TYPES OF MALIGNANT NEOPLASMS

There are two basic types of malignant neoplasms:

- Solid   140–199
- Hematopoietic and lymphatic   200–208

Solid tumors have a single, localized point of origin and are considered to be primary neoplasms of that site. Solid tumors tend to spread to adjacent or remote sites, with such sites classified as secondary or metastatic neoplasms. For example, a diagnosis of carcinoma of the lung with metastasis to the brain indicates that a primary neoplasm of the lung has metastasized to a secondary site in the brain.

Lymphatic and hematopoietic neoplasms arise in the reticuloendothelial and lymphatic systems and the blood-forming tissues. These neoplasms differ from solid malignant neoplasms in several ways, including the following:

- They may arise in a single site or in several sites simultaneously.
- Tumor cells often circulate in large numbers in the bloodstream and the lymphatic system rather than remaining confined to a single site.
- Spreading to other sites in the hematopoietic and lymphatic system is not considered to be secondary but is also classified as primary neoplasm.

Because of the differences between solid and hematopoietic-lymphatic diseases, this handbook will deal with the two types of malignant neoplasms separately. Solid tumors will be discussed first and then the discussion will move on to tumors that arise in the hematopoietic and lymphatic systems.

CODING OF SOLID MALIGNANT NEOPLASMS

A solid malignant neoplasm may spread from its site of origin by either direct extension or metastasis. Direct extension is the invasion of adjacent sites; metastasis refers to the spread to distant sites and the establishment of a new center of malignancy. *ICD-9-CM* does not make a distinction between these two types of extension. The terms "metastatic" and "secondary" are generally used interchangeably.

Malignant Neoplasm of Esophagus

Category **150, Malignant neoplasm of esophagus,** presents a departure from usual *ICD-9-CM* classification principles in that the subcategories are not mutually exclusive. Because this modification appears in *ICD-9,* it has been retained in *ICD-9-CM* to maintain the compatibility of the two systems.

    The purpose of this dual-axis classification is to allow the classification to accommodate the differences in terminology often encountered in medical records. For example, the same neoplasm may be identified as being in either the cervical esophagus (150.0) or the upper third (150.3), in the thoracic esophagus (150.1) or the middle third (150.4), or in the abdominal esophagus (150.2) or the lower third (150.5). Depending on the terminology used by the physician, either code can be assigned, although it would be preferable for the facility to develop a coding policy that dictates which codes will be used.

Contiguous Sites

When the point of origin cannot be determined because the neoplasm overlaps the boundaries of two or more contiguous sites, it is classified with fourth digit 8, signifying other specified sites. For example, *ICD-9-CM* provides the following codes for certain malignant neoplasms whose point of origin cannot be established and whose stated sites overlap two or more three-digit category sites:

- 140.8   Neoplasm of overlapping sites of the lip whose point of origin cannot be assigned to any other code within category 140
- 151.8   Neoplasm of stomach whose point of origin cannot be assigned to any other code within category 151
- 162.8   Neoplasm of overlapping sites of lung, bronchus, and trachea whose point of origin cannot be assigned to any other code within category 162

Exercise 25.4

Code the following diagnoses. Do not assign M codes.

	Code(s)
1. Carcinoma of cervicothoracic esophagus	150.8
2. Carcinoma of oral cavity and pharynx	149.8

3. Adenocarcinoma of rectum and anus   154.8

Neoplasms Described as Metastatic

The terms "metastatic" and "metastasis" are often used ambiguously in describing neoplastic disease, sometimes meaning that the site named is primary and sometimes meaning that it is secondary. When the diagnostic statement is not clear in this regard, the coder should review the medical record for further information. When none is available, however, the following guidelines apply.

"Metastatic To"

The statement "metastatic to" indicates that the site mentioned is secondary. For example, a diagnosis of metastatic carcinoma to the lung is coded as secondary malignant neoplasm of the lung (197.0). A code for the primary neoplastic site should also be assigned when the primary neoplasm is still present; a history code from category **V10, Personal history of malignant neoplasm,** should be assigned when the primary neoplasm has been excised or eradicated. The fourth digit of category V10 indicates the body system where the prior neoplasm occurred, and the fifth digit indicates the specific organ or site involved.

Ordinarily, no history code is assigned when the patient has had a prior benign neoplasm. The one exception is that code **V12.41, Benign neoplasm of the brain,** is assigned for a personal history of a benign brain tumor, as these can recur, are often difficult to treat, and can be life-threatening.

"Metastatic From"

The statement "metastatic from" indicates that the site mentioned is the primary site. For example, a diagnosis of metastatic carcinoma from the breast indicates that the breast is the primary site (174.9). An additional code for the metastatic site should also be assigned.

Multiple Metastatic Sites

When two or more sites are described as "metastatic" in the diagnostic statement, each of the stated sites should be coded as secondary or metastatic. A code should also be assigned for the primary site when this information is available; it should be coded 199.1 when it is not.

Single Metastatic Site

When only one site is described as metastatic without any further qualification and no more definitive information can be obtained by reviewing the medical record, the following steps should be followed:

1. Refer first to the morphology type in the Alphabetic Index, and code to the primary condition of that site. For example, a diagnosis of metastatic renal cell carcinoma of

the lung indicates that the primary site is the kidney and the secondary site is the lung. The correct coding for this is **189.0, Renal cell carcinoma,** and **197.0, Secondary carcinoma of lung.**

When a specific site for the morphology type is not indicated in a code entry or is not indexed, assign the code for unspecified site within that anatomical site. For example, oat cell carcinoma is indexed to **162.9, Malignant neoplasm of bronchus and lung, unspecified,** when no more specific site is stated.

2. When the morphology type is not stated or the only code that can be obtained is either 199.0 or 199.1, code as a primary malignant neoplasm, unless the site is one of the following:

- Bone
- Brain
- Diaphragm
- Heart
- Liver
- Lymph nodes
- Mediastinum
- Meninges
- Peritoneum
- Pleura
- Retroperitoneum
- Spinal cord
- Sites classifiable to 195

Malignant neoplasms of these sites are classified as secondary when not otherwise specified, except for neoplasm of the liver. *ICD-9-CM* provides code **155.2, Malignant neoplasm of liver, not specified as primary or secondary,** for use in this situation.

Examples of coding by this two-step procedure include the following:

- Metastatic carcinoma of the lung, coded by step 2, with the primary site assigned to the lung: carcinoma of lung; secondary site not specified   162.9 + 199.1
- Metastatic carcinoma of bone, coded by step 2, with the primary site unknown and the bone as the secondary site: carcinoma, site unknown; secondary site bone 198.5 + 199.1

No Site Stated

When no site is indicated in the diagnostic statement but the morphology type is qualified as metastatic, the code provided for that morphological type is assigned for the primary diagnosis along with an additional code for secondary neoplasm of unspecified site. For example, a diagnosis of metastatic apocrine adenocarcinoma with no site specified is coded as a primary malignant neoplasm of the skin, site unspecified (173.9). An additional code of 199.1 is assigned for the secondary neoplasm. Code 173.9 is obtained by referring to the following main term and subterms in volume 2:

Adenocarcinoma (M8140/3) . . .
   apocrine (M8401/3) . . .
      unspecified site   173.9

Exercise 25.5

Code the following diagnoses. Do not assign M codes.

	Code(s)
1. Metastatic <u>carcinoma</u> from lung	<u>162.9</u> 199.1
2. Metastatic <u>carcinoma</u> to brain	<u>198.3</u> 199.1
3. Metastatic <u>carcinoma</u> from prostate to pelvic bone Previous prostatectomy <u>History</u>	198.5 V10.46
4. Metastatic <u>carcinoma</u> to brain from lung Previous resection of lung with no recurrence at primary site <u>History</u>	<u>198.3</u> V10.11
5. Metastatic <u>carcinoma</u> from prostate to pelvic bone	185 198.5
6. Metastatic <u>carcinoma</u> of brain and lung	198.3 197.0 199.1
7. Metastatic <u>carcinoma</u> of pancreas and <u>omentum</u>	197.8 197.6 199.1
8. Metastatic <u>adenocarcinoma</u> of transverse colon	<u>153.1</u> 199.1

Exercise 25.5 *(continued)*

9. Metastatic carcinoma of bronchus

162.9
199.1

10. Metastatic carcinoma of spinal cord

198.3
199.1

11. Metastatic carcinoma of femur

198.5
199.1

12. Metastatic carcinoma of brain

198.3
199.1

13. Metastatic serous papillary adenocarcinoma
    of bone

183.0
198.5

14. Metastatic infiltrating duct cell carcinoma

174.9
199.1

15. Metastatic odontogenic fibrosarcoma

170.1
199.1

16. Metastatic chondroblastic osteosarcoma

170.9
199.1

CODING OF MALIGNANCIES OF HEMATOPOIETIC AND LYMPHATIC SYSTEMS

Unlike solid tumors, neoplasms that arise in lymphatic and hematopoietic tissues do not spread to secondary sites. Instead, malignant cells circulate and may occur in other sites within these tissues. These sites are considered to be primary neoplasms rather than secondary.

Neoplasms of Lymph Nodes or Glands

Primary malignant neoplasms of lymph nodes or glands are classified in categories 200 through 202, with a fourth digit providing more specificity about the particular type of neoplasm and a fifth digit indicating the nodes involved. If the neoplasm involves lymph nodes or glands of additional sites, fifth digit 8 is assigned to indicate that the malignancy now involves multiple sites. For example, code **200.08, Reticulosarcoma-lymph nodes of multiple sites,** is assigned for a diagnosis of reticulosarcoma of intra-abdominal and intrathoracic lymph nodes; individual codes are not assigned.

When a solid tumor has spread to the lymph nodes, a code from category 196 is assigned. For example, adenocarcinoma of breast with metastasis to lymph nodes of the axilla is coded to **174.9, Malignant neoplasm of female breast,** and **196.3, Secondary metastatic neoplasm of axillary lymph nodes.** No code from categories 200 through 202 is assigned.

Lymphomas can be malignant or benign. Codes for benign lymphomas are located by referencing the site in the neoplasm table. Malignant lymphomas are located by referencing the subterms for the site under the main term **Lymphoma.** When a diagnostic statement of lymphoma does not match any subentry under **Lymphoma** in volume 2, the coder may find that the pathology report indicates the neoplasm's behavior.

Hodgkin's Disease

The same type of dual-axis classification used for esophageal neoplasms is provided for a diagnosis of **Hodgkin's disease (201.x)** and for the same reasons, that is, to maintain correlation with *ICD-9* and to take into consideration differences in terminology. One physician, for example, may describe Hodgkin's disease as **Hodgkin's paragranuloma (201.00),** whereas a pathologist may describe it as **Hodgkin's lymphoma of mixed cellularity (201.60).**

Multiple Myeloma, Other Immunoproliferative Neoplasms, and Leukemias

Multiple myeloma and other immunoproliferative neoplasms are classified in category 203, with a fourth digit indicating the particular type of neoplasm. Leukemias are classified in categories 204 through 208, with the fourth digit indicating the stage of the disease (acute, chronic, subacute). For all codes in categories 203 through 208, a fifth digit indicates whether the neoplastic disease is in remission. When the neoplasm is stated to be in remission, disease activity is reduced significantly but the disease is still present in its diminished form. The fifth digit indicating that the neoplasm is in remission is assigned only when the physician specifically describes it as such.

Exercise 25.6

Code the following diagnoses. Do not assign M codes.

	Code(s)
1. Aleukemic myelogenous leukemia, in remission	205.81
2. Reticulum cell sarcoma of the spleen	200.07
3. Reticulosarcoma, intrathoracic	200.02
4. Intrapelvic Hodgkin's granuloma	201.16
5. Chronic myeloid leukemia	205.10
6. Plasma cell leukemia	203.10
7. Carcinoma of lung with metastatic carcinoma of intrathoracic lymph nodes	162.9 196.1
8. Mycosis fungoides of intrathoracic and intra-abdominal lymph nodes	202.18

Exercise 25.6 *(continued)*

9. Castleman's <u>lymphoma</u>   785.6

10. Benign <u>lymphoma</u> of breast   217

SEQUENCING OF CODES FOR NEOPLASTIC DISEASES

The basic rule for designating principal diagnoses is the same for neoplasms as for any other condition; that is, the principal diagnosis is the condition found after study to have occasioned the current admission or encounter. There is no guideline that indicates that a code for malignancy takes precedence. Because the principal diagnosis is sometimes difficult to determine in a patient with a malignant neoplasm, however, the thrust of treatment can often be used as a guide to selecting the principal diagnosis.

Some neoplasms are functionally active in that they may affect the activity of endocrine glands. The code for these primary neoplasms is assigned first, followed by a code for the endocrine dysfunction. For example:

- Hyperestrogenism due to carcinoma of ovary   <u>183.0</u> + 256.0
- Carcinoma of ovary with hirsutism   <u>183.0</u> + 704.1

Treatment Directed at Primary Site

When the treatment is directed toward the primary site, the malignancy of that site is designated as the principal diagnosis unless the encounter or hospital admission is solely for the purpose of radiotherapy or chemotherapy, in which case the primary malignancy is coded and sequenced second. For example:

- Carcinoma of sigmoid colon with small metastatic nodules on the liver; sigmoid resection of the colon carried out: 153.3 + 197.7
- Carcinoma of sigmoid colon with prior resection; admitted for chemotherapy: <u>V58.11</u> + 153.3

Sometimes two primary sites are present; in this case, each is coded as a primary neoplasm. When treatment is directed primarily toward one site, the neoplasm of that site should be designated as the principal diagnosis. When treatment is directed equally toward both, either may be designated as the principal diagnosis.

Occasionally, a patient admitted for surgery to correct a nonneoplastic condition has a pathology report that indicates that a microscopic focus of malignancy is also present. In this situation, the condition that occasioned the admission remains the principal diagnosis, with an additional code assigned for the malignancy. For example:

- A patient with severe urinary retention due to hypertrophy of the prostate was admitted for prostatectomy. Transurethral resection of the prostate (TURP) was carried out, and the patient was discharged with a diagnosis of benign hypertrophy of the prostate. When the pathology report was received, this diagnosis was confirmed, but a microscopic focus of adenocarcinoma was also identified. **Code 600.01, Hypertrophy (benign) of prostate with urinary obstruction and other lower urinary tract symptoms (LUTS),** is assigned as the principal diagnosis with code **185, Malignant neoplasm of prostate,** assigned as an additional code.

- A patient was admitted for treatment of endometriosis of the uterus, and a total abdominal hysterectomy was carried out. The pathology report confirmed the endometriosis but indicated that carcinoma in situ of the cervix was also present. In this case, the endometriosis was the reason for admission and remains the principal diagnosis. An additional code is assigned for the cervical neoplasm.

Treatment Directed at Secondary Site

When a patient is admitted because of a primary neoplasm with metastasis and treatment is directed solely toward the secondary site, the secondary site is designated as the principal diagnosis even though the primary malignancy is still present. A code for the primary malignancy is assigned as an additional code.

When a patient is admitted because of a primary neoplasm with metastasis and treatment is directed equally toward the primary and the secondary sites, the primary malignancy should be designated the principal diagnosis, with an additional code assigned to the secondary neoplasm.

Admission for Complications Associated with a Malignant Neoplasm

Patients with malignant neoplasms often develop complications due to either the malignancy itself or the therapy that they have received. When admission is primarily for treatment of the complication, the following guidelines govern selection of the principal diagnosis:

- When the admission/encounter is for management of an anemia associated with the malignancy, and the treatment is only for anemia, the appropriate anemia code (such as code **285.22, Anemia in neoplastic disease**) is designated as the principal diagnosis and is followed by the appropriate code(s) for the malignancy. Code 285.22 may also be used as a secondary code if the patient suffers from anemia and is being treated for the malignancy.
- When the admission/encounter is for management of an anemia associated with chemotherapy, immunotherapy, or radiotherapy, and the only treatment is for the anemia, the anemia is sequenced first followed by code E933.1. The appropriate neoplasm code should be assigned as an additional code.
- When the admission/encounter is for management of dehydration due to the malignancy or the therapy or a combination of both, and only the dehydration is being treated (intravenous rehydration), the dehydration is sequenced first, followed by the code(s) for the malignancy.

Admission or Encounter Solely for Administration of Radiotherapy, Immunotherapy, or Chemotherapy

When a patient admission/encounter is solely for the administration of chemotherapy, immunotherapy, or radiation therapy, assign code **V58.0, Encounter for radiation therapy,** or **V58.11, Encounter for antineoplastic chemotherapy,** or **V58.12, Encounter for antineoplastic immunotherapy,** as the first-listed or principal diagnosis. When the patient receives more than one of these therapies during the same admission, more than one of these codes may be assigned, in any sequence. Because the patient is still under treatment for the malignancy even though it may have been removed surgically, an additional code for the malignancy is assigned, rather than a code from category V10.

Codes from category V10 are assigned only when the primary neoplasm has been totally eradicated and is no longer under any type of treatment. This guideline applies to both solid and hematopoietic or lymphatic neoplasms, including leukemia. Note, however, that patients with leukemia are often admitted for a variety of tests or other treatment in addition to chemotherapy. If there is any question about whether the admission is for the sole purpose of chemotherapy, immunotherapy, or radiotherapy, the physician should be consulted. Codes should also be assigned for the type of radiotherapy (92.2x), immunotherapy (99.28), or chemotherapy (99.25) provided.

When a patient is admitted for the purpose of radiotherapy, immunotherapy, or chemotherapy and develops complications such as uncontrolled nausea and vomiting or dehydration, the principal or first-listed diagnosis is **V58.0, Encounter for radiotherapy,** or **V58.11, Encounter for antineoplastic chemotherapy,** or **V58.12, Encounter for antineoplastic immunotherapy,** followed by any codes for the complications.

Chemoembolization is a variation of chemotherapy in which there is concurrent intra-arterial administration of a collagen particle with the chemotherapeutic agent. This arrests the vascular flow time of the chemotherapy and increases the target retention of the drug. Chemoembolization is included in code **99.25, Injection or infusion of cancer chemotherapeutic substance.** Code **38.91, Arterial catheterization,** is also assigned if the arterial line is placed during the episode of care.

New advancements in radiofrequency thermal ablation (RFA) have expanded treatment options for some cancer patients. Thermal ablative procedures utilize heat to destroy lung, liver, or renal malignancies. Minimally invasive, image-guided thermal ablation provides effective treatment of localized neoplastic disease and can also be used as an adjunct to traditional surgery, chemotherapy, and/or radiation treatment. Under radiological imaging, a needle-electrode is inserted at the site of the tumor; radiofrequency energy is then applied to destroy the tumor. Thermal ablation can be performed by three different methods: open, laparoscopic, and percutaneous. *ICD-9-CM* provides the following procedure codes to describe the various thermal ablative procedures:

- 32.23   Open ablation of lung lesion or tissue
- 32.24   Percutaneous ablation of lung lesion or tissue
- 32.25   Thoracoscopic ablation of lung lesion or tissue
- 32.26   Other and unspecified ablation of lung lesion or tissue
- 50.23   Open ablation of liver lesion or tissue
- 50.24   Percutaneous ablation of liver lesion or tissue
- 50.25   Laparoscopic ablation of liver lesion or tissue
- 50.26   Other and unspecified ablation of liver lesion or tissue
- 55.32   Open ablation of renal lesion or tissue
- 55.33   Percutaneous ablation of renal lesion or tissue
- 55.34   Laparoscopic ablation of renal lesion or tissue
- 55.35   Other and unspecified ablation of renal lesion or tissue

When a patient is admitted for the purpose of inserting a port for later administration of chemotherapy but no chemotherapy is given during the same episode of care, the malignancy is designated as the principal diagnosis and code **V58.11, Encounter for antineoplastic chemotherapy,** is not assigned. When insertion of the port is followed by chemotherapy during the same episode of care, code V58.11 is assigned as the principal diagnosis. If an intraperitoneal catheter is inserted for the chemotherapy access, code **54.99, Other operation on abdominal wall,** is assigned with code 99.25 added if chemotherapy is administered during the episode of care.

Bacille Calmette-Guerin (BCG) is a nonspecific immunotherapy agent (99.28) used in the treatment of melanoma, cancer of the lung, soft-tissue sarcoma, carcinoma of the colon, and carcinoma of the breast. Interferon is another nonspecific immunotherapy agent used in treating malignancy. Another type of immunotherapy is interleukin-2 (IL-2), which is used to treat patients with advanced renal cell carcinoma and advanced melanoma. There is a high-dose IL-2 and a low-dose IL-2 therapy. High-dose IL-2 therapy is a hospital inpatient-based regimen usually performed in specialized treatment settings such as the intensive care unit or bone marrow transplant unit. The administration of low-dose interleukin is coded to 99.28, while the high-dose IL-2 is assigned code 00.15. The high-dose IL-2 therapy requires highly specialized oncology professionals because of the severity of the predictable toxicities requiring extensive monitoring. The principal diagnosis code for a patient admitted for antineoplastic immunotherapy is **V58.12, Encounter for antineoplastic immunotherapy.**

An admission for radium implant or insertion or for treatment by radioactive iodine (I-131) is not considered an admission solely for a radiotherapy session. The code for the malignant neoplasm is designated the principal diagnosis; code V58.0 is not assigned. The Viadur (leuprolide acetate) implant is used as palliative treatment for advanced prostate cancer. The device is implanted subcutaneously in the arm and delivers leuprolide acetate continuously over a period of 12 months. Leuprolide acetate lowers testosterone, a hormone that is needed by prostate cancer cells. Assign code **99.24, Injection of other hormone,** for the insertion of the viadur implant. The code for the prostate malignancy is designated as the principal diagnosis.

When the reason for the admission/encounter is to determine the extent of the malignancy, or for a procedure such as paracentesis or thoracentesis, the primary malignancy or appropriate metastatic site is designated as the principal or first-listed diagnosis, even though chemotherapy or radiotherapy is administered. Because therapy such as radiotherapy and chemotherapy must be delivered at regularly scheduled intervals, it is often performed during an episode of care during which it is not the primary focus of treatment.

ENCOUNTER FOR PROPHYLACTIC ORGAN REMOVAL

For encounters specifically for prophylactic removal of breasts, ovaries, or another organ due to a genetic susceptibility to cancer or a family history of cancer, the principal or first-listed diagnosis should be a code from subcategory **V50.4, Prophylactic organ removal.** The appropriate genetic susceptibility and family history codes should be assigned as additional diagnoses.

If the patient has a malignancy of one site and is having prophylactic removal of another site to prevent either a new primary malignancy or metastatic disease, a code for the malignancy should also be assigned in addition to a code from subcategory V50.4. Code V50.4x should not be assigned if the patient is having organ removal for treatment of a malignancy, such as the removal of testes for the treatment of prostate cancer.

CODING OF ADMISSIONS OR ENCOUNTERS FOR FOLLOW-UP EXAMINATIONS

Once a malignant neoplasm has been excised or eradicated, periodic follow-up examinations are carried out to determine whether there is recurrence of the primary malignancy or any spread to a secondary site. When there is no evidence of recurrence at either a primary site or a metastatic site, the appropriate code from **V67.x, Follow-up examination,** is assigned as the principal diagnosis. The fourth digit should reflect the therapy most recently carried out. The appropriate code from category V10 should be assigned as an additional code. Codes should also be assigned for any diagnostic procedures (such as endoscopy and biopsy) that are carried out.

When there is evidence of recurrence at the primary site, the code for the malignancy is designated as the principal diagnosis. For example, a primary carcinoma of the anterior wall of the urinary bladder that was previously excised but has recurred in the lateral wall is coded to **188.2, Malignant neoplasm of lateral wall of urinary bladder.**

When there is no recurrence at the primary site but there is evidence of metastasis to a secondary site, a code for secondary neoplasm of that site is assigned along with a code from category V10. No code from category V67 is assigned.

Exercise 25.7

Answer the following questions either true or false.

___F___ 1. The recurrence of an original primary malignant neoplasm that was previously removed is classified to category **V10, Personal history of malignant neoplasm**.

___F___ 2. If a primary malignant neoplasm was excised previously and the original primary site has not recurred, assign the code for the previous primary malignant neoplasm, using the appropriate code from categories 140 through 195.

___T___ 3. Whenever secondary neoplasms are present, the V code for identifying personal history of malignant neoplasm can never be sequenced as the principal diagnosis code for Uniform Hospital Discharge Data Set (UHDDS) purposes.

Review Exercise 25.8

The following exercise provides a review of the material on neoplasms presented in this handbook. For this exercise, assign procedure codes where applicable, but do not assign M codes.

	Code(s)
1. Infiltrating papillary transitional cell carcinoma of urinary bladder (neck)	188.5
Suprapubic excision of bladder tumor	57.59
2. Carcinoma of mid-esophagus with spread to celiac lymph nodes	150.4 196.2
Permanent gastrostomy procedure High-voltage radiotherapy	43.19 92.22
3. Carcinoid small intestine	235.2

Review Exercise 25.8 *(continued)*

4. Carcinoma, scirrhous, left breast,   174.8
   outer portion

   Open biopsy with frozen section followed   85.45
   immediately by left radical mastectomy   85.12

5. Intramural leiomyoma of uterus   218.1

6. Multiple myeloma   203.00

7. Carcinoma of gallbladder with metastasis   156.0
   to abdominal lymph nodes and liver   196.2
   and peritoneal implants   197.7
                                                                              197.6

   Exploratory laparotomy with   51.22
   cholecystectomy and needle   54.24
   biopsy of peritoneal implant

8. Squamous cell carcinoma in situ,   230.0
   floor of mouth

   Resection of lesion, floor of mouth   27.49

Review Exercise 25.8 *(continued)*

---

9. Metastatic malignant <u>melanoma</u> from left
   lateral chest wall to axillary lymph node

   <u>172.5</u>
   196.3

                    <u>Neoplasm</u>

Radical <u>excision</u> of malignant melanoma
of chest wall with radical left
axillary <u>lymphadenectomy</u>

<u>34.4</u>
40.51

---

10. Metastatic <u>adenocarcinoma</u> of sacrum,
    prostatic in origin
    Previous prostatectomy

    <u>198.5</u>
    V10.46

                    <u>History</u>

---

11. A 33-year-old female admitted for prophylactic
    removal of both breasts, with documented genetic
    susceptibility to breast cancer due to extensive family
    history of breast carcinoma
    Bilateral mastectomy

    V50.41

    V84.01
    V16.3
    85.42

---

12. <u>Seminoma</u>, left testis
    Bilateral radical <u>orchiectomy</u>

    186.9
    62.41

---

13. <u>Lipoma</u>, right kidney

    214.3

---

14. Chronic lymphatic <u>leukemia</u>, in remission

    204.11

---

15. Admitted for <u>chemotherapy</u> following
    oophorectomy on previous admission for
    <u>carcinoma</u> of ovary

    <u>V58.11</u>
    183.0
    99.25

Coding of Injuries, Burns, Poisoning, and Complications of Care

26 | Injuries

Chapter 17 of *ICD-9-CM* classifies injuries, poisoning, other effects of external causes, complications of trauma, and complications of medical and surgical care not classified elsewhere. Because this chapter covers such a broad range of conditions, guidelines for the coding of burns, poisoning, adverse effects, and complications of medical and surgical care will be discussed in subsequent chapters of this handbook.

Injuries are classified in the following sections:

- Fractures   800–829
- Dislocations   830–839
- Sprains and strains   840–848
- Intracranial injuries   850–854
- Internal injuries   860–869
- Open wounds   870–897
- Blood vessel injuries   900–904
- Late effects of injuries   905–909
- Superficial injuries   910–919
- Contusions   920–924
- Crushing injuries   925–929
- Foreign body entering through orifice   930–939
- Burns   940–949
- Nerve and spinal cord injuries   950–957
- Early complications of trauma   958

The primary axis for classifying injuries is the type of injury as indicated in the preceding list; the second axis is determined by the anatomical site. Inclusion and exclusion notes are used extensively in this chapter, some of them long and complex, and it is important to give careful attention to these if correct code assignments are to be made. Fourth and fifth digits are provided for many categories to indicate a more detailed anatomical site or to provide more information regarding the injury. Examples of fifth-digit subclassifications found in chapter 17 of *ICD-9-CM* are shown in table 26.1.

TABLE 26.1   Fifth-Digit Subclassifications for Injuries

Category and Title		Fifth-Digit Axis
800	Fracture of vault of skull	Level of consciousness
805.0–805.1	Fracture of cervical vertebrae without mention of spinal cord injury	Cervical vertebrae involved
807.0–807.1	Fracture of rib(s)	Number of ribs involved
813	Fracture of radius and ulna	Anatomical site
864	Injury to liver	Type and severity of injury

MULTIPLE CODING OF INJURIES

Injuries classifiable in more than one subcategory should be coded separately unless a combination code is provided. General codes for multiple injuries are provided for use when there is insufficient detail in the medical record (such as trauma cases transferred promptly to another facility). Multiple injury codes should not be assigned when documentation permits more specific code assignment.

As discussed in chapter 2 of this handbook, the word "with" and the word "and" are used in a specific way in *ICD-9-CM*. They are used a great deal in chapter 17 of the *ICD-9-CM*. The word "with" means that both sites mentioned in the diagnostic statement are involved in the injury.

The word "and" is interpreted as meaning "and/or"—that is, that either or both sites are involved. In coding injuries, mention of fingers usually takes into account the thumb, but there are a few separate codes for injuries of the thumb. Terms such as "condyle," "coronoid process," "ramus," and "symphysis" refer to the portion of the bone involved in an injury, not to the bone itself.

SEQUENCING OF INJURY CODES

If admission is due to injury and several injuries are present, the code for the most severe injury is designated as the principal diagnosis. If the diagnostic statement is not clear on this point, the physician should be asked to make this determination.

EXTERNAL CAUSE OF INJURY

As mentioned earlier in chapter 8 of this handbook, E codes indicating the external cause of injury are used with injury and poisoning codes to provide information about how an injury occurred, the intent (accidental or intentional), and the place where the injury occurred.

Injuries are a major cause of mortality, morbidity, and disability, and the cost of care related to these conditions contributes significantly to the increased cost of health care. Reporting E codes provides data for injury research and evaluation of injury-prevention strategies. E codes capture how the injury or poisoning happened (cause), the intent (unintentional or accidental; or intentional, such as suicide or assault), and the place where the event occurred. Although reporting external cause is optional unless mandated by state or insurance carrier regulation, health care providers are strongly encouraged to report E codes for all initial treatment of injuries. Guidelines for reporting have been developed, and providers who do report E codes are urged to follow these guidelines so that there is consistency in the data.

The selection of appropriate E codes for injuries is guided by the Index to External Causes and by inclusion and exclusion notes in the Tabular List. The index is located in section 3 in volume 2; the tabular list follows the section on V codes in volume 1.

Sequencing of E Codes

An E code is never used as the principal diagnosis. If two or more events cause separate injuries, an E code should be assigned for each. If the injury is due to two or more external causes, the code for the proximal (direct) cause is listed first. For example:

- A patient was admitted with a fracture of the shaft of the left femur that he suffered during a fight when he stepped backwards and fell from the top of the stairs. The fall (E823.01) is the proximal cause of the fracture and the fight (E960.0) is the initiating event. The following codes should be assigned: **821.01 (Fracture, shaft of femur)**, **E880.9 (Fall on stairs or steps)**, and **E960.0 (Unarmed fight or brawl)**.
- A woman who had fractured her arm when the car she was driving hit a tree during a tornado was admitted. E908.1 is assigned for the tornado, with an additional code

for the collision. The proximal cause was the motor vehicle accident, but the code for tornado is listed first because a cataclysmic event takes precedence.

The E code listed first should correspond to the cause of the most serious diagnosis due to external cause. This sequencing hierarchy should be followed:

- E codes for child and adult abuse take precedence over all other E codes.
- E codes for cataclysmic events take priority over all E codes except those for child and adult abuse. Cataclysmic events include storms, floods, hurricanes, tornadoes, blizzards, volcanic eruptions, and earth surface movements and eruptions.
- Transport accidents take priority over all other E codes except those for abuse and cataclysmic events.

When a transportation accident involves more than one type of vehicle, the following order of precedence should be followed:

- Air and space transport accidents (E840–E845)
- Watercraft accidents (E830–E838)
- Motor vehicle traffic and nontraffic accidents (E810–E825)
- Other road vehicle accidents (E826–E829)
- Railway accidents (E800–E807)

For example, an accident involving both a motor vehicle and an aircraft is classified as an aircraft accident, and one that involves railway transportation equipment and a motor vehicle is classified as a motor vehicle accident. No general rule governs priority for other E codes. Exclusion notes should be followed carefully.

Transport and Vehicle Accidents

A transport accident (E800–E848) is one involving a device that is designed (or being used at the time) primarily for conveying goods or people from one place to another. A long note at the beginning of this section defines in detail just what is meant by each type of transportation and what vehicles are included.

The final digit in most of these categories indicates the role or activity of the person involved in the accident. For example, the injured person in a motor vehicle accident may be a passenger in the vehicle, a bicyclist, or a pedestrian. Definitions of these roles are provided at the beginning of each section. For example:

- Open fracture, shaft of femur (pedestrian struck by automobile)   <u>821.11</u> + E814.7

Accidents caused by machines such as agricultural equipment and earth-moving equipment are classified as transport accidents if the pieces of equipment were in operation as transport vehicles when the accidents occurred. Otherwise, they are classified in category E919, Accidents caused by machinery, with a fourth digit indicating the specific type of equipment.

External Cause of Injury Classified by Intent

Separate external cause codes are provided to classify the external cause of injuries resulting from accident, self-harm, or assault. If the intent is unknown, unspecified, suspected, possible, or probable, a code from categories E980 through E989, Undetermined whether accidentally or purposefully inflicted, should be assigned. When the intent of an injury or poisoning is known but the cause is unknown, use **E928.9, Unspecified accident, E958.9, Suicide and self-inflicted injury by unspecified means,** or **E968.9, Assault by other and unspecified means.** These E codes should rarely be used; medical record documentation usually provides enough detail to determine the cause of the injury.

Category E979, Terrorism, is used to identify injuries and illnesses acquired as a result of terrorism. These codes (E979.0–E979.9) follow the definition of terrorism established by the U.S. Federal Bureau of Investigation (FBI). Coders are not to classify a death or an injury as terrorist-related unless the federal government has designated the incident as terrorism.

LATE EFFECTS OF EXTERNAL CAUSES

When the condition code from the main classification is a late effect of injury, the associated E code must also indicate a late effect, as follows:

- E929.x   Late effect of accidental injury
- E959   Late effect of self-inflicted injury
- E969   Late effect of injury purposely inflicted by another person

For example, a diagnosis of extensive scarring of the face due to an old burn is coded **709.2, Scar conditions and fibrosis of skin,** + 906.5 + E929.4. In this example, code 906.5 indicates that the condition is a late effect of burn of eye, face, head, and neck, and code E929.4 indicates that it is a late effect of an accident caused by fire. Code **E897, Accident caused by controlled fire not in building or structure,** is not used because it identifies the external cause of a current injury rather than a late effect.

ICD-9-CM provides external cause category **E849, Place of occurrence,** for use as an additional code to indicate the place where an external event occurred when the place of occurrence is not implicit in the injury or poisoning code. When the place of occurrence is not specified, a code from E849 is not assigned. Note that codes from category E849 refer only to the location, not to the activity of the injured person. For example:

- Fall on escalator in airport building   E880.0 + E849.6
- Clothing caught fire while burning trash in backyard of home, causing burn E893.2 + E849.0

Exercise 26.1

Assign only the E codes in the following exercises.

	Code(s)
1. Closed fracture, right tibia and fibula, due to <u>fall</u> from bicycle	E826.1
2. Injury to delivery man who <u>jumped</u> from moving truck because he thought the driver was stopping	E825.1
3. Multiple facial lacerations to driver of automobile in <u>collision</u> with another vehicle on expressway	E812.0

Exercise 26.1 *(continued)*

4. Anoxic brain damage due to previous head injury, three years ago, when patient was accidentally struck by car while walking along highway

    Late effect of _____   E929.0

5. Injury received by crew member of commercial airline when he fell at takeoff

    Accident _____   E843.2

6. Injury received by guest passenger in hot-air balloon when balloon made unexpected descent

    Accident _____   E842.6

7. Passenger injured when he accidentally collided with another passenger while getting off a streetcar

    Accident _____   E817.4

8. Railway employee injured by accident involving collision with rolling stock

    Accident _____   E800.0

9. Railway employee injured when hit by rolling stock while unloading material

    Accident _____   E805.0

10. Passenger injured in accidental derailment of train

    Accident _____   E802.1

11. Motorcyclist injured in accidental collision with train _____   E810.2

CHILD AND ADULT ABUSE

Expanded codes for child and adult abuse facilitate the gathering of more specific data. Child abuse has become a major concern in the United States. National estimates indicate that approximately one to two million children in this country suffer abuse or neglect annually. Adult abuse is considered to be both underreported and underdiagnosed. Keep in mind that codes for child and adult abuse are assigned only when the physician documents abuse; coders should not interpret narrative descriptions as abuse without the physician's confirmation.

Codes for child abuse are found in subcategory 995.5, with the fifth digit indicating the type of abuse, as follows:

- Child emotional abuse   995.51
- Child physical abuse   995.54
- Child neglect   995.52
- Child sexual abuse   995.53
- Shaken infant syndrome   995.55

Adult abuse codes are provided in subcategory 995.8, with the fifth digit indicating the type of abuse:

- Adult physical abuse   995.81
- Adult emotional/psychological abuse   995.82
- Adult sexual abuse   995.83
- Adult neglect (nutritional)   995.84
- Other adult abuse and neglect   995.85

Abuse often results in physical injuries and other medical conditions. When this is the case, the abuse code is sequenced first, with an additional code for any associated injury or condition that has been documented by the physician.

When the cause of injury or neglect is intentional child or adult abuse, the E code from categories E960 through E966 and E968 through E969 should be listed as the first E code. An additional code from E967 should then be assigned to identify the perpetrator unless this information is not available. In cases of neglect, when the intent is determined to be accidental, code **E904.0, Abandonment or neglect of infants and helpless persons,** should be the first listed external injury code.

Examples of child and adult abuse include the following:

- A patient was seen in the emergency department with a diagnosis of battered woman syndrome and with a laceration of the right forehead. She reported that her husband hit her in the face because he was angry when she was late getting ready to go out to dinner. The following codes should be assigned: **995.81, Adult physical abuse, 873.42, Open wound of forehead, E960.0, Unarmed fight or brawl,** and **E967.3, Adult battering by spouse or partner.**
- A four-month-old infant was seen in the emergency department with a diagnosis of shaken infant syndrome. The baby had been unconscious for approximately two hours after being shaken vigorously by the father when he was unable to make the infant stop crying. The diagnostic statement also included diagnoses of subdural hematoma and retinal hemorrhage. The following codes should be assigned: **995.55, Shaken infant syndrome, 852.23, Subdural hematoma without mention of open intracranial wound, 362.81, Retinal hemorrhage,** and **E967.0, Battering or other maltreatment by father.**
- An elderly woman was brought to the hospital in a state of severe malnutrition. She had been living in an unlicensed care home, where she was fed only one meal per

day for several months. In the hospital, a gastric feeding tube was placed and high-protein supplements were given for severe caloric deficiency malnutrition. The following codes should be assigned: **995.84, Adult neglect, 261, Nutritional marasmus, E904.1, Lack of food, E967.8, Abuse by non-related caregiver,** and **96.35, Gastric gavage.**

- A six-month-old infant with heat prostration was brought to the hospital by her parents, who had left her alone in their car while they did their grocery shopping. The parents stated that the child was asleep and they had felt that she would be all right for the short time they would be gone. The following codes should be assigned: **995.52, Child neglect, 992.53, Heat prostration,** and **E904.0, Abandonment or neglect of infant.**

Codes from category V15 are also available to indicate that a patient has a past history of psychological trauma:

- History of physical abuse, including rape   V15.41
- History of emotional abuse or neglect   V15.42
- History of other psychological trauma   V15.49

Counseling codes have been expanded to provide more specificity regarding the person receiving counseling:

- V61.11   Counseling for the victim of spousal and partner abuse
- V61.12   Counseling for the perpetrator of spousal and partner abuse
- V61.21   Counseling for victim of child abuse
- V61.22   Counseling for perpetrator of parental child abuse
- V62.83   Counseling for perpetrator of physical/sexual abuse (to be used only when the perpetrator is a person other than spouse/partner or parent)

FRACTURES

Fractures are classified in categories 800 through 829 as follows:

- Fractures of skull   800–804
- Fractures of neck and trunk   805–809
- Fractures of the upper extremity   810–819
- Fractures of the lower extremity   820–829

Three-digit categories indicate more specific sites within these broad groupings, fourth digits usually indicate whether the fracture is open or closed, and fifth digits usually indicate a more specific bone within the general site.

In an open fracture, an open wound that communicates with the bone is present. Terms that indicate open fracture include the following: compound, infected, missile, puncture, and with foreign body.

Closed fractures do not produce an open wound. They are described by terms such as comminuted, depressed, elevated, greenstick, spiral, and simple. A more complete listing can be found in the note at the beginning of the coding manual's section on fractures. Any fracture not specified as open is classified as closed in *ICD-9-CM*. Occasionally, a diagnostic statement contains terms that relate to both open and closed fractures. In this case, the code for the open fracture always takes precedence. For example, a diagnosis of compound comminuted fracture uses terms that can indicate both open and closed fractures. However, such a fracture would be coded as open because the term "compound" always carries this meaning, even though the term "comminuted" by itself would refer to a closed fracture.

Skull Fractures and Intracranial Injuries

Categories 800–804 classify skull fractures by site. Fourth digits indicate whether the fracture is open or closed, whether there is associated intracranial injury, and the type of intracranial injury. Intracranial injury not associated with skull fracture is classified in categories 850 through 854, with an additional digit providing more specificity as to the type of injury and whether it was associated with an open wound.

Codes for skull fractures and intracranial injuries without skull fracture use another digit to indicate whether a loss of consciousness was associated with the injury, how long the unconscious state lasted, and whether there was a return to the preexisting level of consciousness. Because this information is rarely included in the diagnostic statement, it usually must be obtained through a review of the medical record, particularly the emergency department record and admitting note. Fifth digit 5 (with prolonged loss of consciousness without returning to consciousness) is used when an unconscious patient dies before regaining consciousness, regardless of the duration of the unconscious state.

Concussion (category 850) refers to cerebral bruising that sometimes leads to a transient unconsciousness, often followed by brief amnesia, vertigo, nausea, and weak pulse. Fourth digits (and in some instances fifth digits), provide additional specificity regarding the length of time the patient was unconscious, if any. The patient may experience severe headache and blurred vision after regaining consciousness. Recovery usually takes place within 24 to 48 hours. Patients with this type of head injury are often dazed, and the physician may have to rely on clinical findings alone to make a diagnosis of concussion.

Postconcussion syndrome (310.2) includes a variety of symptoms that may occur for a variable period of time following a concussion, sometimes as long as a few weeks. The symptoms most often associated with postconcussion syndrome are headache, dizziness, vertigo, fatigue, difficulty in concentrating, depression, anxiety, tinnitus, heart palpitations, and apathy. Any of these may cause the patient to seek treatment. Code 310.2 is ordinarily not assigned on the initial admission for treatment of the concussion. When the patient is treated for symptoms within 24 to 48 hours of injury and the physician lists a diagnosis as postconcussion syndrome, the coder should ask the physician whether the concussion is still in the current state. If it is, it should be coded to 850.x rather than 310.2.

When the head injury is further described as a cerebral laceration or a cerebral contusion or when it is associated with subdural, subarachnoid, other intracranial hemorrhage, or other specified condition classifiable in categories from 851 through 854, the code for concussion is not assigned.

Vertebral Fractures

Separate subcategories are provided to distinguish fractures of the vertebra that involve spinal cord injury (806.x) from those that do not (805.x). Spinal cord injury not associated with vertebral fracture is classified into category 952. Fourth digits with categories 805, 806, and 952 indicate the vertebral site; fifth digits for categories 806 and 952 indicate the type of spinal cord injury. For example:

- 806.03   Fracture of cervical vertebral column at C1–C4 level with central cord syndrome
- 952.16   Spinal cord lesion, dorsal T7–T12, with complete lesion of spinal cord, without vertebral fracture
- 952.2   Spinal cord injury, lumbar, without vertebral fracture

Fractures of the Extremities

Category codes 810 through 829 classify fractures of the extremities; the fourth digit indicates whether the fracture is open or closed, and the fifth digit provides more specificity as to the portion of the bone involved. Combination codes are provided for certain sites as follows:

- Category **813, Fracture of radius and ulna,** uses a fifth digit to indicate which bone had the fracture and when both bones are involved.
- Category **811, Fracture of scapula,** uses a fifth digit to include both the glenoid cavity and the neck of the scapula.
- Category **823, Fracture of tibia and fibula,** uses a fifth digit 2 for fracture of the same site involving both tibia and fibula.

Multiple fractures of the same bone(s) classified with different fourth-digit subdivisions (bone part) within the same three-digit category are coded individually by site. For example:

- Comminuted fracture of the shaft of the right humerus with closed fracture-dislocation of right shoulder involving the greater tuberosity is coded **812.21, Shaft of humerus,** and **812.03, Greater tuberosity.**
- Closed fractures of the olecranon process of the ulna and the head and neck of the radius are coded **813.01, Olecranon process of ulna, 813.05, Head of radius,** and **813.06, Neck of radius.**

ICD-9-CM makes no provision for distinguishing between unilateral and bilateral fractures of the same site in the upper or lower limbs. The procedure code is reported twice, however, when bilateral fracture procedures are carried out to reflect more accurately the resources used.

Exercise 26.2

Code the following diagnoses. Do not assign E codes.

	Code(s)
1. Comminuted fracture, upper end of left tibia	823.00
2. Fracture, left ischium	808.42
Fracture, left second, third, fourth, fifth, and sixth ribs	807.05
3. Closed fracture of vault of skull with subdural hemorrhage; 3-hour loss of consciousness	800.23

Exercise 26.2 *(continued)*

4. Open Monteggia <u>fracture</u>	813.13

5. Cerebral concussion Brain stem <u>contusion</u> without open wound Patient unconscious for almost two hours	851.43

6. Trimalleolar <u>fracture</u>, left ankle	824.6

7. Closed <u>fracture</u>, lateral condyle, left humerus	812.42

8. Compound <u>fracture</u> coronoid process of mandible	802.33

9. Compound <u>fracture</u>, shaft of tibia and fibula, left	823.32

10. Bilateral compound depressed skull <u>fractures</u> Massive cerebral <u>contusion</u> and <u>laceration</u>	803.60

Pathological Fractures

Bones weakened by conditions such as osteoporosis or neoplastic disease often develop pathological fractures that occur with no trauma or only minor trauma that would not result in fracture in a healthy bone. This type of fracture is classified with musculoskeletal conditions, rather than injuries, and is discussed in chapter 19 of this handbook.

Compression Fractures

Compression fractures may be due either to disease or to trauma. The coder should search the medical record for any recent significant trauma or for any indication of concurrent bone disease that might point to pathological fracture. If the diagnosis cannot be clarified, the physician should be asked to provide further specificity.

Fractures Due to Birth Injury

Fractures due to birth injury are not classified in the injury chapter of *ICD-9-CM* but instead are classified as perinatal conditions (767.2–767.4), and are discussed in chapter 23 of this handbook.

PROCEDURES RELATED TO FRACTURES

In the treatment of fractures, the primary goal is to achieve correct bone alignment and maintain alignment until healing is completed and normal function can be restored. Procedures include open and closed reduction, simple manipulation, and application of various types of fixation and traction devices. The type of treatment depends on the general condition of the patient, the presence of any associated injuries, and the type and location of the fracture.

Reduction of Fractures

The most common fracture treatment involves moving bone fragments into as nearly normal an anatomic position as possible, with stabilization to maintain the bone in this position until it is sufficiently healed to prevent displacement. Although orthopedic surgeons now prefer to use the term "manipulation" for this procedure, the term "reduction" is still used in *ICD-9-CM*.

The first axis for coding reduction of fractures is whether the reduction is open or closed. The second axis is whether internal fixation is applied. Fourth digits indicate the bone involved.

In an open reduction, the surgeon exposes the bone by extending the open wound over the fracture or making a further incision to work directly with the bone for the purpose of restoring correct alignment. Debridement is often necessary to remove debris or other material that has entered an open fracture site. A code from category **79.6, Debridement of open fracture site**, is assigned as an additional code for debridement carried out in connection with reduction of open fracture of bones of the upper and lower extremities. Debridement is included in the codes for reduction of open fractures involving the skull, nasal and orbital bones, other facial bones, and vertebral bones.

In a closed reduction, alignment is achieved without incision to the fracture site. Debridement of the bone is not needed.

Internal Fixation

Internal fixation includes the use of pins, screws, staples, rods, and plates that are inserted into the bone to maintain alignment. When the fractured bone is in good alignment so that no manipulation is necessary, internal fixation may be used to stabilize the bone without any fracture reduction being performed. Internal fixation is also used without reduction when it is necessary to reinsert an internal fixation device because the original is either displaced or broken. An incision is made for the purpose of inserting the internal fixation wires or pins; a code from category **78.5, Internal fixation of bone without fracture reduction,** is assigned for fixation that is not associated with fracture reduction. Internal fixation can also be used with closed fracture reduction. The small incision necessary to insert the fixation device does not warrant considering the procedure to be an open reduction. Internal fixations associated with bone grafts and shortening or lengthening of bone are included in the codes for these procedures.

External Fixation

Unlike internal fixation, external fixation is ordinarily noninvasive and includes traction or immobilization by the use of casts or splints. Additional codes should be assigned for the application of an external fixator device (78.10–78.19). In addition, if the type of fixator device is known, adjunct codes should be assigned. The classification essentially recognizes three types of external fixator devices: monoplanar (84.71); ring system (84.72); and hybrid system (84.73), which includes both ring and monoplanar devices. When reduction is not carried out, however, a code from category **93.4, Skeletal traction and other traction,** is used for application of traction or a code from category 93.5 for **Other immobilization, pressure, and attention to wounds.** Code 97.88 is assigned for removal of such external immobilization devices. Although traction devices are usually applied by means of Kirschner wires or Steinmann pins, the use of these materials is not considered an internal fixation. Traction devices include the following:

- Skin traction such as tape, foam, or felt traction devices applied directly to the skin, with longitudinal force applied to the limb
- Skeletal traction into or through the bone that applies force directly to the long bones (the wires or pins are drilled transversely through the bone and exit through the skin)
- Cervical spinal traction, such as Baron's tongs, Crutchfield tongs, and halo skull traction
- Upper extremity traction, such as Dunlap's skin traction
- Lower extremity traction, such as Buck's extension skin traction, Charnley's traction unit, Hamilton-Russell's traction, balanced suspension traction, and fixed skeletal traction

A separate code is assigned for the application of the external fixator device called a minifixator. This complex type of external stabilization is performed under anesthesia. Holes are drilled into both proximal and distal portions of the bone, and pins are inserted through the bone and attached to the metal frame of the fixator. The pins are located internally except for the portion to which the external frame is connected. A code from subcategory **78.1, Application of external fixator device,** is assigned for this procedure in addition to any code for fracture reduction. A code from category **78.6, Removal of implanted devices from bone,** is assigned for removal of the minifixator.

ADMISSIONS OR ENCOUNTERS FOR ORTHOPEDIC AFTERCARE

Patients who have had fracture reduction usually require aftercare for removal of wires, pins, plates, or external fixation devices. In addition, patients with orthopedic injuries still in the healing stage may be seen primarily for conditions not related to the injury but with some monitoring or clinical evaluation of the injury carried out during the episode of care. V codes are provided for admissions or encounters for these situations, as follows:

- V53.7   Admission for fitting or adjustment of orthopedic device, such as the adjustment of an orthopedic brace or cast, or the removal or replacement of an orthopedic device
- V54.01   Encounter for removal of internal fixation device
- V54.02   Encounter for lengthening/adjustment of growth rod
- V54.89   Other orthopedic aftercare

Codes V54.10–V54.29 are available to provide greater specificity in identifying the fracture site being treated, as well as differentiate between traumatic (V54.1x) and pathologic fractures (V54.2x). For example:

- V54.11   Aftercare for healing traumatic fracture of upper arm
- V54.23   Aftercare for healing pathologic fracture of hip

> Example 1: A patient who suffered a traumatic fracture of the left humerus a month earlier was admitted with fever and pain secondary to diverticulitis. The healing fracture was treated minimally. Principal diagnosis: 562.11, Diverticulitis; additional diagnosis: V54.11, Aftercare for healing traumatic fracture of upper arm.

> Example 2: A young man who fractured the lateral malleolus of the left fibula six weeks previously was admitted for removal of the internal pins under local anesthesia. Principal diagnosis: V54.01, Encounter for removal of internal fixation device; additional diagnosis: V54.16, Aftercare for healing traumatic fracture of lower leg.

V codes are also provided to indicate an orthopedic status when it is significant for the episode of care. Orthopedic status codes include **V43.6x, Joint replacement, complete or partial, any joint,** and **V45.4, Arthrodesis status.**

Exercise 26.3

Code the following procedures; do not code diagnoses.

	Code(s)
1. Thomas splint traction	93.45
2. Open reduction and debridement of Monteggia fracture, right upper extremity, with Rush pin (internal) to stabilize ulna	79.32 79.62
3. Open reduction of fracture, ankle, with Knowles pins (internal) and two-inch screw Below-the-knee cast applied	79.36

Exercise 26.3 *(continued)*

---

4. Open reduction and Kirschner wire   79.31
   fixation (internal) of distal to main
   fragment, fracture of left humerus

---

5. Open reduction of fracture, left hip,   79.35
   with Jewett nail fixation

---

6. Reduction, fracture right humerus, with cast   79.01

---

7. Open reduction and internal fixation,   76.76
   fracture of mandible

---

8. Open reduction, fracture of left maxilla and   76.74
   left zygomatic arch   76.72
   Closed reduction, nasal bone fracture   21.71

---

9. Bifrontal craniotomy with elevation and
   debridement of compound skull fractures   02.02
   Open reduction, orbital fracture   76.79
   Tracheostomy (temporary)   31.1

DISLOCATIONS

Dislocation associated with fracture is included in the fracture code, and reduction of the dislocation is included in the code for the fracture reduction. Dislocation of a joint without associated fracture is classified in categories 830 through 839. The first axis is the general site, such as wrist, and the fifth digit indicates a more specific site such as midcarpal dislocation of the wrist; the fourth-digit axis indicates whether the dislocation is open or closed. Open dislocation is described by such terms as "compound," "infected," or "with foreign body;" closed dislocation is described as "complete," "partial," "simple," or "uncomplicated." When the dislocation is not specified as either open or closed, a code for closed dislocation is assigned. Reduction of dislocation not associated with fracture is coded under subcategory **79.7x, Closed reduction of dislocation,** or subcategory **79.8x, Open reduction of dislocation.**

INTERNAL INJURIES OF THE CHEST, ABDOMEN, AND PELVIS

Internal injuries of the chest, abdomen, and pelvis are classified in categories 860 through 869, and the fourth digit indicates whether there is an associated open wound. A fifth-digit subclassification is used for certain categories within this series to provide more specificity regarding the type of injury or site. For example:

- Pneumothorax (traumatic) without mention of open wound   860.0
- Hemothorax with open wound into thorax   860.3
- Injury of duodenum without mention of open wound into cavity   863.21
- Contusion of heart without mention of open wound into the thorax   861.01

BLOOD VESSEL AND NERVE INJURIES

When a primary injury results in minor damage to peripheral nerves or blood vessels, the primary injury is sequenced first, with additional codes from categories 950 through 957, Injury to nerves and spinal cord, and/or categories 900 through 904, Injury to blood vessels.

When the primary injury is to a blood vessel or nerve, however, the code for that injury should be sequenced first. For example, an open wound of the anterior abdominal wall with rupture of the aorta would be coded 902.0, Injury to abdominal aorta; an additional code for open wound of abdominal wall, anterior, without mention of complication, 879.2, or open wound of abdominal wall, anterior, complication, 879.3, may be assigned.

OPEN WOUNDS

Open wounds such as lacerations, puncture wounds, cuts, animal bites, avulsions, and traumatic amputations that are not associated with fracture, dislocation, internal injury, or intracranial injury are classified in categories 870 through 897. Fourth digits for categories 870 and 871, which classify open wounds of the eyeball and ocular adnexa, indicate whether the wound was a laceration or a penetrating wound. Codes for penetrating injury of these sites indicate whether a foreign body is present. The fourth digit for other codes of open wounds indicates whether a complication is present and may also indicate a more specific site. An open wound is considered to be complicated when any of the following conditions is present:

- Delayed healing
- Delayed treatment
- Foreign body in wound
- Major infection

Both cellulitis and osteomyelitis sometimes occur as complications of open wounds. Sequencing of codes for open wounds with these major infections depends on the circumstances of admission. It is important to determine whether it is the wound that is being addressed or only the resulting infection. For example, a patient who had an open wound of the hand six weeks ago might be seen because osteomyelitis has developed. In this situation, the osteomyelitis would ordinarily be designated as the principal diagnosis, with an additional code for the open wound and a fourth digit indicating that the wound is complicated. A patient who had a slight puncture wound earlier in the week might show evidence of cellulitis at the site. The wound itself did not require any attention; the reason for the encounter would be the cellulitis. In this case, cellulitis would be the principal diagnosis.

AMPUTATIONS

When listed as a diagnosis, traumatic amputation is classified as an open wound in *ICD-9-CM*. For example:

- 887.2   Traumatic amputation of arm at or above elbow
- 887.0   Traumatic amputation of arm below elbow
- 897.2   Traumatic amputation of leg at or above knee

The term "amputation" is also used for an amputation procedure, which can be performed for a variety of reasons other than the treatment of trauma. Amputation is performed by either disarticulation or cutting through the bone. Amputation procedures are classified in category 84, Other procedures on musculoskeletal system; the third digit indicates whether amputation is of the upper or lower limb, and the fourth digit indicates the portion of the limb involved and the type of amputation. Sample codes include the following:

- Disarticulation of wrist   84.04
- Amputation through foot   84.12
- Amputation above knee   84.17
- Amputation through forearm   84.05

A below-the-knee amputation of the lower limb is through the tibia and fibula (84.15); an above-the-knee amputation is through the femur (84.17). Code 84.17 is also assigned when a below-the-knee amputation is converted into an above-the-knee amputation. A metatarsal amputation is classified as an amputation of the toe; a transmetatarsal amputation is classified as an amputation through the foot.

A revision of an amputation involves transecting the entire circumference of the bone. The length of bone transected or resected does not matter as much as the fact that the entire circumference of bone is cut through, and the revision is carried out through an existing wound (site of previous amputation). Revision of the amputation stump is coded 84.3 except for revision of a current traumatic amputation, which is classified as further amputation of the current traumatic amputation site (84.1x).

OTHER INJURIES

Superficial injuries such as blisters, abrasions, and friction burns are classified to categories 910 through 919. The fourth digit indicates a more specific site or type of injury and/or whether infection is present. When such injuries are associated with a major injury such as fracture of the same site, a code for the superficial injury is usually not assigned. Note that the term "superficial" does not refer to the severity of the injury but to the superficial structures affected, those pertaining to or situated near the surface.

The presence of a foreign body entering through an orifice is classified in categories 930 through 939. When the foreign body is associated with an open wound, it is coded as an open wound, complicated, by site. A foreign body accidentally left during a procedure in an operative wound is considered to be a complication of a procedure and is coded 998.4.

EARLY COMPLICATIONS OF TRAUMA

Certain early complications of trauma that are not included in the code for the injury are classified in category 958, Certain early complications of trauma. The fourth-digit axis indicates the type of complication, such as air or fat embolism, traumatic shock, or traumatic anuria. Ordinarily, codes from category 958 are assigned as secondary codes, with the code for the injury sequenced first. With today's shorter lengths of stay and increased emphasis on outpatient care, however, the complication itself may occasionally be the reason for an outpatient encounter or admission and would be the principal diagnosis in such cases.

A new subcategory, **958.9, Traumatic compartment syndrome,** classifies compartment syndrome secondary to trauma. Acute traumatic compartment syndrome is usually a sequelae of a serious injury to the lower or upper extremities and can lead to significant motor and sensory deficits, pain, stiffness, and deformity when untreated. Acute traumatic compartment syndrome is always associated with fractures, dislocations, and/or crush injuries. Other risk factors for the development of acute traumatic compartment syndrome include vascular injuries and coagulopathy. The diagnosis is established by multiple compartment pressure readings. Traumatic compartment syndrome is coded as follows:

- 958.90   Compartment syndrome, unspecified
- 958.91   Traumatic compartment syndrome of upper extremity
- 958.92   Traumatic compartment syndrome of lower extremity
- 958.93   Traumatic compartment syndrome of abdomen
- 958.99   Traumatic compartment syndrome of other sites

Exercise 26.4

Code the following diagnoses. Do not assign E codes.

	Code(s)
1. Stab wound of abdominal wall, infected	879.3
2. Lacerations, left foot, infected	892.1
3. Traumatic amputation of left arm and hand above the elbow	887.2
4. Traumatic anuria due to injury to kidney	866.00 958.5

OTHER EFFECTS OF EXTERNAL CAUSE

Categories 990 through 995 classify other and unspecified effects of external causes resulting from exposure to heat, cold and a variety of other conditions due to external causes that are not classifiable elsewhere in *ICD-9-CM*. Codes from these categories are not assigned when a more specific code for the effect is available. For example, colitis due to radiation therapy is coded **558.1, Gastroenteritis and colitis due to radiation,** because the effect is identified. A diagnosis of complication of radiation therapy not otherwise specified and with no further information documented in the medical record would be coded **990, Effects of radiation, unspecified.**

Category **995, Certain adverse effects not elsewhere classified,** is used to classify a variety of adverse effects such as anaphylactic shock, shock due to anesthesia, and angioneurotic edema. Anaphylactic shock due to an adverse food reaction is coded **995.6,** with a fifth digit indicating the type of food involved. Anaphylactic shock due to drugs or medicinal substances used correctly is classified to **995.0, Other anaphylactic shock,** with an additional code from the E930 through E949 series to indicate the responsible medicine. When the shock is due to an incorrect use of a drug, a medicinal or biological substance, or a toxic material not chiefly medicinal, anaphylactic shock is classified as a poisoning, with the poisoning code sequenced first and an additional code of 995.0 assigned to indicate the shock.

Code 991.6 is assigned for hypothermia with several exceptions. If it is due to anesthesia, code 995.89 is assigned; code 995.86 is used for malignant hyperthermia. When the hypothermia is not due to low temperature, code 780.99, Other general symptom, is assigned. Two codes are provided for hypothermia of the newborn, 778.2, Cold injury of newborn, and 778.3, Other hypothermia of newborn.

Exercise 26.5

Code the following diagnoses and assign E codes.

	Code(s)
1. Heat prostration due to salt and water depletion	992.4 E904.2
2. Frostbite, toes	991.2 E901.0
3. Radiation cataract	366.46 E926.9
4. Anaphylactic shock due to eating peanuts	995.61

LATE EFFECTS OF INJURIES

In coding late effects of injuries, the residual condition (such as malunion, nonunion, deformity, or paralysis) is sequenced first, followed by a cause of late effect code from categories 905–909; a late effect E code is also assigned. A current injury code is never used with a late effect code for the same type of injury.

Malunion (733.81) implies that bony healing has occurred but that the fracture fragments are in poor position. Treatment of malunion ordinarily involves surgical cutting of the bone (osteotomy), repositioning the bone, and adding some type of internal fixation device with or without bone graft. Malunion is frequently diagnosed while the fracture is still in a healing state, but sometimes no surgical intervention is used in the hope that the patient may not have any functional problems as a result of the malunion.

Nonunion (733.82), on the other hand, implies that healing has not occurred and that there is still separation of the bony structures involved in the fracture. Treatment of nonunion usually involves opening the fracture, scraping away intervening soft tissue (usually scar tissue), doing a partial debridement of the bone end, and repositioning the bone. Treating nonunion of a fracture is more complicated and difficult to perform than treating a malunion.

Exercise 26.6

Code the following diagnoses and assign E codes; sequence the codes according to the principles for coding late effects.

		Code(s)
1. Paralysis of right wrist due to previous		354.9
laceration of right radial nerve		907.4
	Late	E929.8
2. Esophageal stricture due to old lye burn		530.3
of esophagus		906.8
	or Late	E929.8
3. Nonunion fracture of neck of femur		733.82
suffered in a bar brawl three months ago		905.3
	or Late	E969
4. Posttraumatic scars of face due to old		709.2
accidental lacerations		906.0
	Late	E929.8

Review Exercise 26.7

Code the following diagnoses and procedures. Assign E codes where information is provided.

	Code(s)
1. Anterior dislocation of shoulder,	831.01
patient thrown from horse she was riding	E828.2

Review Exercise 26.7 *(continued)*

Dislocation <u>reduction</u>	79.71

2. <u>Fracture</u> dislocation left humerus,		812.01
surgical neck; patient caught in avalanche		E909.2
while skiing at mountain resort	or <u>Dislocation</u>	E849.4

Open <u>reduction</u> and internal fixation with Rush pin and screws	79.31

3. Colles <u>fracture</u>	813.41
Patient <u>fell</u> from chair at home	E884.2
	E849.0

Closed <u>reduction</u> with anterior-posterior plaster splints	79.02

4. Intracapsular <u>fracture</u>, neck of femur, right	820.00
Patient fell from in-line skates	E885.1

Closed <u>reduction</u> with insertion of Smith-Petersen nail	79.15

5. Closed <u>fractures</u> of right femur and left ilium		808.41
Fat <u>emboli</u>, posttraumatic		821.00
Patient driving motorcycle on highway		958.1
lost control and overturned		E816.2
	<u>Loss of control</u>	

Review Exercise 26.7 *(continued)*

	Open reduction with plate fixation, right	79.35
	femur, with skeletal traction	93.44
	for ilium fracture	

6.	Fracture of base of skull, with right	801.20
	subdural hemorrhage; patient fell from	E842.7
	parachute during voluntary descent	

7.	Posttraumatic shortening of left radius	736.09
	due to previous comminuted fracture of	905.2
	distal end of left forearm, broken in	E929.0
	accidental crash of snowmobile	
	Late effect of	

8.	Ruptured spleen, traumatic	865.04
	Severe crush injury to left kidney	866.00
	Traumatic shock	958.4
	Patient caught in heavy farm machinery	E919.0
	that he was operating on his farm	E849.1

	Excretory urography	41.5
	Splenectomy	87.73

9.	Cerebral cortex contusion; patient died	851.05
	without regaining consciousness;	E882
	patient had fallen from skyscraper	E849.6
	observation tower while sightseeing	

10.	Battered wife syndrome due to severe	995.81
	beating of chest wall by husband	922.1
	Multiple contusions over trunk	E960.0
		E967.3

11.	Anoxic brain damage due to previous	348.1
	intracranial injury three years ago,	907.0
	when patient was accidentally struck by	E929.0
	car while walking along highway	
	Late effect of	

27 | Burns

Codes from categories 940 through 949 are assigned for current unhealed burns except sunburn and friction burns, which are classified as dermatitis and superficial injury, respectively. Nonhealing burns and necrosis of burned skin are coded as acute current burns. Sequelae (such as scarring or contracture) that remain after a burn has healed are classified as late effects (906.5–906.9). Because burns heal at different rates, a patient may have both healed and unhealed burns during the same episode of care. For this reason, it is possible to use current burn codes as well as late effect burn codes on the same record (when both a current burn and sequelae of an old burn exist).

ANATOMICAL SITE OF BURN

The first axis for classifying burns is the general anatomical site, with a fifth digit to indicate a more specific site. Category **940, Burn confined to eye and adnexa,** is an exception in that the fourth digit indicates the more specific site as well as whether the burn was due to the use of acid chemical, alkaline chemical, or other cause.

Categories 941–945 have a fifth digit for multiple specified sites; category 946 provides only codes for multiple specified burns. When coding burns, assign separate codes for each burn site. Codes for multiple sites and category 946 should only be used if the location of the burns is not documented. Category **949, Burn, unspecified,** is extremely vague and should rarely be used.

DEPTH OF BURN

For categories 941–946, the fourth digit axis indicates the type of burn according to depth or degree as follows:

- First degree (erythema)
- Second degree (blistering)
- Third degree (full-thickness involvement)
- Deep necrosis (deep third degree) without loss of body part
- Deep necrosis (deep third degree) with loss of body part

First Degree

Damage from first-degree burns is limited to the outer layer of the epidermis, with erythema and increased tenderness. First-degree burns have good capillary refill and do not represent significant injury in terms of fluid replacement needs.

Second Degree

Second-degree burns represent a partial-thickness injury to the dermis, which may be either superficial or deep. Deep second-degree burns heal much more slowly than first-degree burns and are prone to developing infection. The end result of second-degree burns may be hypertrophic scarring.

Third Degree

In third-degree burns, the dermal barrier is lost, and the presence of necrotic tissue creates fluid volume loss with systemic effects on capillaries well away from the burn site. In addition, the burn site establishes an ideal culture medium for infection, which may be life-threatening. The critical factor in healing of third-degree burns is blood supply. Areas rich in blood supply, such as hair follicles and sweat glands, have a better chance for re-epithelialization.

Deep third-degree burns are characterized by an underlying necrosis with thrombosed vessels and are identified by fourth digit 5 when there is an associated loss of a body part and by fourth digit 4 when no such loss is mentioned. Codes for burns of this depth are assigned only on the basis of a specific diagnosis made by the physician.

SEQUENCING OF CODES FOR BURNS AND RELATED CONDITIONS

Burns of the same local site at the three-digit category level but of different degrees (depth) are classified according to the highest degree recorded in the diagnostic statement. A third-degree burn takes precedence over a second-degree burn, and a second-degree burn takes precedence over a first-degree burn. For example, first-degree and second-degree burns of the leg are classified as second-degree burn of limb (945.20); no code is assigned for the first-degree burn.

When coding multiple burns, sequence first the code that reflects the burn of the highest degree (most severe) with additional codes for the burns of other sites. For example, a patient is admitted with third-degree burns of the lower leg and first-degree and second-degree burns of the forearm. The following codes should be assigned:

- 945.34   Third-degree burn of leg
- 943.21   Second-degree burn of forearm

The circumstances of the admission will determine the principal diagnosis or first-listed diagnosis if a patient has both internal and external burns.

Encounters for the treatment of the late effects of burns (i.e., scars or joint contractures) should be coded to the residual condition (sequelae) followed by the appropriate late effect code (906.5–906.9). A late effect E code is also used. Code E929.4 indicates that the condition is a late effect of an accident caused by fire. Code **E897, Accident caused by controlled fire not in building or structure,** is not used because it identifies a current cause rather than a late effect.

Note that using code **V51, Aftercare involving the use of plastic surgery,** is inappropriate for burn patients admitted for repair of scar tissue, skin contracture, or other sequela. For such patients, a code should be assigned for the condition being treated. Code V51 is used only for an admission for plastic surgery when there is no residual condition that can be classified elsewhere in *ICD-9-CM*, such as plastic repair of a mastectomy site.

EXTENT OF BURN

Category 948 classifies burns according to the extent of body surface involved. The fourth digit indicates the total percentage of body surface involved in all types of burns, including third-degree burns. The fifth digit indicates the percentage of the body surface involved in third-degree burns only. Because the fourth digit refers to total body surface, the fifth digit can never be greater than the total amount. For example, code 948.73 indicates that 70–79% of the body surface was involved in some type of burn; the fifth digit indicates that third degree burns were involved in 30–39% of the body surface. The fifth-digit zero (0) is assigned when less than 10 percent of body surface (or when no body surface) is involved in a third-degree burn.

The extent of body surface involved in a burn injury is an important factor in burn mortality, and hospitals with burn centers need this information for evaluating patient care management and for preparing statistical data. In addition, third-party payment is often influenced by the extent of burn. When more than 20 percent of the body surface is involved in third-degree burns, it is advisable to assign an additional code from category 948. Burn centers sometimes use a code from category 948 as a solo code because many of their patients present with such extensive and severe burns involving many sites that coding them individually is difficult.

Category 948 is based on the "rule of nines" for estimating the amount of body surface involved in a burn. Physicians may modify the percentage assignments for head and neck in infants and small children because young children have proportionately larger heads than adults. The percentage may also be modified for adults with large buttocks, abdomens, or thighs. The rule of nines establishes estimates of body surface involved as follows:

- Head and neck, 9 percent
- Each arm, 9 percent
- Each leg, 18 percent
- Anterior trunk, 18 percent
- Posterior trunk, 18 percent
- Genitalia, 1 percent

For example, based on this rule, a physician can calculate that first-degree burns involve 9 percent of the body surface, second-degree burns involve 18 percent, and third-degree burns involve 36 percent. Adding these together, 63 percent of the body was involved in some type of burn. Code 948.63 (burn of any degree involving 60–69 percent of body surface, with 30–39 percent involved in third-degree burn) could then be assigned. Coders are not expected to calculate the extent of burn, but understanding the rule of nines may help the coder recognize when burns are so extensive that the physician should be asked for additional information.

SUNBURN

Sunburn and other ultraviolet radiation burns are classified in the dermatitis category. Historically, code 692.71 was assigned for first-, second-, or third-degree sunburns. Unique codes are now available to identify more severe sunburns: code 692.75 for second-degree sunburns, and code 692.76 for third-degree sunburns. Sunburn due to other ultraviolet radiation exposure, such as a tanning bed, is classified to code 692.82.

EXTERNAL CAUSES OF BURNS

E codes, including codes from category E849, **Place of occurrence**, are assigned for burns, as discussed in the previous chapter on other injuries. The most commonly used E codes for burns are:

- E890–E899   Accident caused by fire and flames
- E924.x   Accident caused by hot substance or object, caustic or corrosive material, or steam
- E925.x   Accident caused by electric current
- E968.0   Assault by fire
- E968.3   Assault by hot liquid
- E958.1   Suicide and self-inflicted injuries by burns, fire
- E958.2   Suicide and self-inflicted injuries by scald
- E929.4   Late effects of accident caused by fire
- E926.2   Visible and ultraviolet light sources, tanning beds

ASSOCIATED INJURIES AND ILLNESSES

When a burn is described as infected, two codes are required. The code for the burn is sequenced first, with code **958.3, Posttraumatic wound infection, not elsewhere classified,** assigned as an additional code. For example:

- Infected second-degree burn of abdominal wall   942.23 + 958.3

Other injuries frequently occur with burns, and other conditions are sometimes caused by burns. Examples of such injuries include the following:

- Smoke inhalation often occurs in cases of burns due to combustible products (987.0–987.9). Certain toxic substances from plastic products may produce hydrocyanic acid gas inhalation (987.7). When a patient presents with a burn injury and another related condition, such as smoke inhalation or respiratory failure, the circumstances of admission determine the selection of the principal or first-listed diagnosis.
- Electrical burns, such as those caused by high-tension wires, may cause ventricular arrhythmias (427.4x) that require immediate attention.
- Traumatic shock (958.4) is often present at the time of admission or may occur later.

Pre-existing conditions may also have an impact on the burn patient's prognosis and on care management and therefore should be coded as additional diagnoses when they otherwise meet criteria for reportable diagnoses. Examples of potentially harmful pre-existing conditions that should be reported include the following:

- Cardiovascular disorders (such as angina, congestive heart failure, or valvular disease) may increase ischemia and precipitate myocardial infarction in a patient with extensive second-degree or third-degree burns. Pulmonary wedge monitoring (Swan-Ganz) (89.64) may be necessary in these cases.
- Asthma, chronic bronchitis, and other chronic obstructive pulmonary diseases may require ventilation therapy.
- Peptic ulcers, either gastric or duodenal, and ulcerative colitis are pre-existing conditions that may lead to gastrointestinal bleeding and require treatment along with the burn.
- Pre-existing kidney disease increases the risk of tubular necrosis and renal failure in patients with third-degree burns or extensive second-degree burns.
- Alcoholism may pose a threat of alcohol withdrawal syndrome, requiring prophylactic treatment for delirium tremens.
- Diabetes mellitus slows the healing process, and diabetes mellitus with stated manifestations can further complicate the management of burn cases.

Review Exercise 27.1

Code the following diagnoses, including E codes.

	Code(s)
1. First-degree burn of lower left leg and	945.22
second-degree burns of left foot when	945.14
adding wood to bonfire at beach resort	E897
	E849.4

Review Exercise 27.1 *(continued)*

2. First-degree burns of face and both eyes, involving cornea, eyelids, nose, cheeks, and lips, due to lye spill at home	941.12 E924.1 E849.0
3. Burns over 38% of body, with 10% of body involved in third-degree burns and 28% involved in second-degree burns; firefighter burned in forest fire	948.31 E892 E849.8
4. Acid burns to left cornea from nitric acid	940.3 E924.1
5. Nonhealing first- and second-degree burns of back that occurred five weeks ago when patient's clothing caught fire in kitchen accident in his home	942.24 E893.0 E849.0
6. First-degree and second-degree burns, thumb and two fingers, right, from kitchen fire in nursing home	944.24 E896 E849.7
7. Severe shock due to third-degree burns of back due to uncontrolled barn fire	942.34 958.4 E891.3 E849.1
8. First-, second-, and third-degree burns of trunk; 10% first degree, 15% second degree, and 32% third degree; patient was crew member of steamship on which boiler exploded	942.30 948.53 E921.0 E837.2
9. Severe sunburn of face, neck, and shoulders; patient spent most of the day at the beach	692.71 E926.2 E849.8

Review Exercise 27.1 *(continued)*

10. Infected <u>friction burn</u> of left thigh due to	<u>916.1</u>
rope burn while water skiing at	E838.4
Lake Berryessa	E849.8

11. First-degree <u>burns</u> of back of left hand	<u>944.16</u>
due to hot tap water in home where	E924.2
patient was visiting	E849.0

28 Poisoning and Adverse Effects of Drugs

Conditions due to drugs and medicinal and biological substances are classified as either poisoning or adverse effects. The condition is classified as an adverse effect when the correct substance was administered as prescribed. When the substance was used incorrectly, it is classified as a poisoning (960–979). The condition may be exactly the same and the drug may be the same; the determination is based on the manner in which the substance was used. *ICD-9-CM* makes the distinction between adverse effects of drugs administered correctly and poisoning to facilitate the collection of data on adverse effects that result from the correct use of drugs and the extent to which incorrect use results in patient care problems. Note that using the prescribed medication as frequently as prescribed or in smaller amounts is not coded as poisoning.

When the drug was correctly prescribed and properly administered, a code for the adverse effect is sequenced first, followed by an E code indicating the responsible drug or drugs (E930–E949). When the condition results from the interaction of two or more therapeutic drugs, each used correctly, it is classified as an adverse effect, and an E code is assigned for each drug involved. When the condition is a poisoning, the poisoning code is sequenced first, followed by a code for the manifestation and an E code to indicate the circumstance of the poisoning.

The adverse effects of therapeutic substances correctly prescribed and properly administered (toxicity, synergistic reaction, side effect, and idiosyncratic reaction) may be due to (1) differences among patients, such as age, sex, disease, and genetic factors, and (2) drug-related factors, such as type of drug, route of administration, duration of therapy, dosage, and bioavailability.

Harmful substances ingested or coming into contact with a person are classified as toxic effects. These are assigned to categories 980–989, Toxic effects of substances chiefly nonmedicinal as to source, except for certain localized effects that are classified to 001 through 799. For example:

- Chronic manganese toxicity   985.2 + E866.4
- Toxicity due to exposure to arsenical pesticide   985.1 + E863.4
- Toxicity due to asbestos exposure   989.81 + E866.8

Toxic effect codes should be sequenced first, followed by the appropriate code(s) to identify the result of the toxic effect. An external cause code should be assigned to indicate intent—accidental exposure (categories E860–E869), intentional self-harm (codes E950.6 or E950.7), assault (E962), or undetermined (categories E980–E9872).

A diagnostic statement of toxic effect, toxicity, or intoxication due to a prescription drug such as digitalis or lithium without any further qualification usually refers to an adverse effect of a correctly administered prescription drug. The adverse effect should be coded as such unless medical record documentation indicates otherwise. The following terms in the medical record usually indicate correct usage and identify the condition as an adverse effect:

- Allergic reaction
- Cumulative effect of drug (toxicity)
- Hypersensitivity to drug
- Idiosyncratic reaction
- Paradoxical reaction
- Synergistic reaction

When the medical record documents an error in dosage or administration, the condition should be coded as a poisoning. Terms that usually identify the condition as a poisoning include the following:

- Wrong medication given or taken
- Error made in drug prescription
- Wrong dosage given or taken
- Intentional drug overdose
- Nonprescribed drug taken with correctly prescribed and properly administered drug

Category codes 960–979 classify poisoning due to drugs, medicinal and biological substances. Subcategory code 965.6 is assigned to separately identify antirheumatics drugs that are propionic acid derivatives (965.61) and other antirheumatics drugs (965.69). The propionic acid derivatives have become widely used since they became available as over-the-counter medications.

When a condition is the result of the interaction of a therapeutic drug used correctly with a nonprescription drug or with alcohol, it is classified as poisoning. Poisoning codes are also assigned for each drug. For example, a diagnosis of coma identified as an adverse reaction to Valium taken correctly but associated with the intake of two martinis is coded as follows:

- Poisoning due to alcohol   980.0
- Poisoning due to Valium   969.4
- Coma   780.01
- Accidental poisoning by ethyl alcohol   E860.0
- Accidental poisoning by benzodiazepine tranquilizers   E853.2

Note that taking a lower amount or discontinuing the use of a prescribed medication is not classified as either a poisoning or an adverse reaction. Taking a larger or more frequent dosage than prescribed would be classified as a poisoning.

Figure 28.1 illustrates a process for coding poisoning and adverse effects of drugs.

FIGURE 28.1   Decision Tree for Coding Adverse Effects of Drugs or Poisoning Due to Drugs or Medicinal or Biological Substances

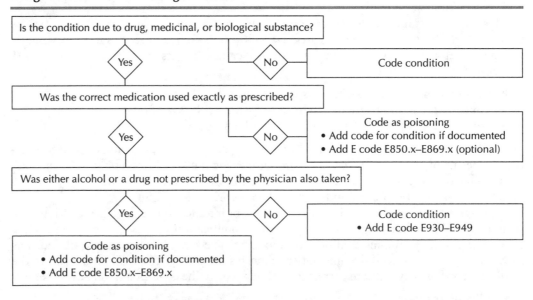

LOCATION OF POISONING CODES AND E CODES ASSOCIATED WITH POISONING AND ADVERSE EFFECTS

Codes for poisoning and E codes associated with poisonings or adverse effects are located most easily by referring to the Table of Drugs and Chemicals in section 2 of volume 2 of

ICD-9-CM. Drugs and other chemicals are listed in alphabetical order at the far left of the table, with the first column on the right listing the poisoning code for that substance and the remaining columns providing E codes for the external circumstance (accident, suicide, assault). A code from the therapeutic use column is selected for coding an adverse effect.

If a specific drug cannot be located in the table, it can usually be found by referring to the American Hospital Formulary Service (AHFS). As an example of how to use the AHFS number in locating codes in the table, consider the drug Elavil, which is not listed as such in the Table of Drugs and Chemicals. Through reference to the AHFS index, the number 28:16:04 is located and Elavil can then be located in the table under the main term drug by referring to this number. AHFS numbers are listed in numerical order in the table. A list of AHFS numbers with the associated *ICD-9-CM* poisoning codes is also available in appendix 3 of volume 1. They are listed only by the function of the drug, not the name of the specific drug.

The American Hospital Formulary is published by the American Society of Hospital Pharmacists. It consists of a collection of monographs on various drugs and a drug index, which is the section that will be most useful to the coder. If this publication is not available in the medical records department, it is usually available in the hospital pharmacy. The hospital pharmacist can also be a valuable source of information.

Neither a poisoning code nor an E code from the table should be assigned without verification in the Tabular List. The Table of Drugs and Chemicals is extensive and very detailed, but it does not take into account the instructional notes in the Tabular List. For example, the table lists codes from category **960, Poisoning by antibiotics,** but the exclusion note at category 960 indicates that codes from category 976 should be used for local (topical) applications or for treating eyes, ears, nose and throat.

GUIDELINES FOR ASSIGNMENT OF EXTERNAL CAUSE CODES FOR POISONING AND ADVERSE EFFECTS

When the same E code describes the causative agent for more than one adverse reaction, assign the E code only once. When two or more drugs or medicinal or biological substances are reported as being responsible for an adverse effect, code each individually unless a combination code is listed in the therapeutic use column in the Table of Drugs and Chemicals, in which case the combination code should be assigned. For example:

- Supraventricular premature beats secondary to use of digitalis and Valium, both used as prescribed   427.61 + E942.1 + E939.4
- An infant with a high fever due to correct administration of DPT vaccine 780.6 + E948.6
- Patient suffering from dry mouth and itching as a result of taking phenobarbital as prescribed by his physician   527.7 + 698.9 + E937.0

When the external cause for a poisoning is not stated, a code for poisoning undetermined whether accidental or purposely inflicted (E980–E982) is assigned. For example, a diagnosis of coma due to codeine is coded as follows:

- Coma due to accidental poisoning due to codeine   965.09 +780.01 + E850.2
- Coma due to codeine taken in a suicide attempt   965.09 + 780.01 + E950.0
- Coma due to overdose of codeine, cause unknown   965.09 + 780.01 + E980.0

The coder should assign as many E codes as needed to completely describe all responsible substances for either an adverse effect or a poisoning. However, if the reporting format limits the number of E codes that can be used, the one most closely related to the principal diagnosis should be assigned. If complete coding would require different E codes in the same three-digit category, use the code for other specified in that category; if there is no other specified code in that category, use the appropriate unspecified code in that category. If the codes are from different three-digit categories, assign the appropriate E code for other multiple drugs and medicinal substances. For example, a poisoning that resulted from ingestion of aspirin, phenobarbital, and antihistamines taken in a suicide attempt would ordinarily require E codes from three different three-digit categories. If the reporting form does not allow for assignment of all three, code **E950.4, Suicide and self-inflicted poisoning by other specified drugs and medicinal substances,** would be assigned.

Exercise 28.1

Code the following diagnoses, assuming that the drug involved was taken correctly unless otherwise specified. Assign E codes where appropriate.

	Code(s)
1. Coma due to acute barbiturate intoxication, attempted suicide	967.0 780.01 E950.1
2. Two-year-old patient ingested an unknown quantity of mother's Enovid	962.2 E858.0
3. Syncope due to hypersensitivity to antidepressant medication Table	780.2 E939.0
4. Hypokalemia resulting from reaction to Diuril given by mistake in physician's office	974.3 276.8 E858.5
5. Diplopia due to allergic reaction to antihistamine, taken as prescribed Table	368.2 E933.0
6. Lethargy due to unintentional overdose of sleeping pills	967.9 780.79 E852.9
7. Electrolyte imbalance due to interaction between lithium carbonate and Diuril, both taken as prescribed Table	276.9 E939.8 E944.3

Exercise 28.1 *(continued)*

---

8. Parkinsonism, secondary to correct use   332.1
   of haloperidol   E939.2
                                Table

---

9. Cerebral anoxia resulting from   967.0
   barbiturate overdose, suicide attempt   348.1
                                      E950.1

---

10. Toxic encephalopathy due to   965.1
    excessive use of aspirin   349.82
                                      E980.0

---

11. Ataxia due to Valium (taken as prescribed)   969.4
    consumed with three martinis   980.0
              Table, Valium; Table, alcohol   781.3
                                      E853.2
                                      E860.0

---

12. Allergic dermatitis due to bovine insulin   693.0
                                      E932.3
                                Table

---

13. Coumadin intoxication due to accumulative   599.7
    effect resulting in gross hematuria   E934.2
                                Table

---

14. Severe bradycardia due to accidental   972.1
    double dose of digoxin   427.89
                   Table, digoxin   E858.3

---

15. Generalized convulsions due to accidental   965.8
    Darvon overdose   780.39
                                      E850.8

Exercise 28.1 *(continued)*

16. Light-headedness resulting from   780.4
    interaction between Aldomet and   E942.6
    peripheral vasodilating agent (both   E942.5
    taken as prescribed)

Table

UNSPECIFIED ADVERSE EFFECT OF THERAPEUTIC USE

ICD-9-CM provides subcategory **995.2, Other and unspecified adverse effect of drug, medicinal and biological substance,** to identify adverse reactions when the nature of the reactions are not specified. Subcategory 995.2 was expanded to provide additional codes to describe an array of nonspecific drug allergies, hypersensitivities, and/or adverse reactions. An additional code from the E930 through E949 series is also assigned to indicate the responsible drug or biologic substance. These codes may be used in the outpatient setting, but their use for inpatient reporting is inappropriate. If the patient is exhibiting symptoms or signs, the code for that condition should be assigned. If the adverse condition cannot be identified, code **796.0, Nonspecific abnormal toxological findings,** should be assigned. This code includes abnormal levels of heavy metals or drugs in blood, urine, or other tissues. An additional code from categories E930–E949 should be assigned to indicate the responsible substance. The code assignments are as follows:

- 995.20   Unspecified adverse effect of unspecified drug, medicinal and biological substance
- 995.21   Arthus phenomenon
- 995.22   Unspecified adverse effect of anesthesia
- 995.23   Unspecified adverse effect of insulin
- 995.27   Other drug allergy
- 995.29   Unspecified adverse effect of other drug, medicinal and biological substance

POISONING DUE TO SUBSTANCE ABUSE OR DEPENDENCE

An acute condition due to alcohol or a drug involved in abuse or dependence is classified as a poisoning. Additional codes are assigned for both the acute manifestation of the poisoning and the dependence or abuse. An E code to indicate the circumstances of the episode should be assigned. For example:

- Acute pulmonary edema due to accidental heroin overdose in a patient who is heroin dependent   965.01 + 518.4 + 304.00 + E850.0

Chronic conditions related to alcohol or drug abuse or dependence are not classified as poisoning. The code for the chronic condition is sequenced first, followed by a code for the abuse or dependence. For example:

- Alcoholic cirrhosis of the liver; chronic alcohol dependence   571.2 + 303.90
- Alcoholic hepatitis; chronic alcohol dependence, episodic   571.1 + 303.90
- Drug-induced depressive state due to cocaine abuse   292.84 + 305.60

Exercise 28.2

Code the following diagnoses. Assign E codes where appropriate.

		Code(s)
1. Muscle cramps of leg due to occupational use of arsenic pesticide		985.1
		729.82
	Table, arsenic	E863.4
2. Systemic hypocalcemia and hypokalemia due to use of lye in household chores		983.2
		275.41
		276.8
	Table, lye	E864.2
		E849.0
3. Bradycardia due to ingestion of oleander leaves		988.2
		427.89
	Table, oleander	E980.9

LATE EFFECTS OF POISONING

The rules discussed earlier in relation to coding late effects also apply to coding late effects of poisoning. The code for the residual condition is sequenced first, with code **909.0, Late effect of poisoning due to drug, medicinal or biological substance,** or **909.1, Late effect of toxic effects of nonmedicinal substance,** assigned as an additional code. Code E929.2 is also assigned for late effects of poisoning.

LATE EFFECTS OF ADVERSE REACTIONS TO DRUGS

ICD-9-CM does not provide a late effect E code for adverse reactions to drugs correctly administered. A code is assigned for the residual condition, with code **909.5, Late effect of adverse effect of drug, medicinal or biological substance,** assigned as an additional code. An E code (E930–E949) for the responsible drug is also assigned.

Long-term chronic effects of a prescription drug taken over a period of time—and still being taken at the time the chronic effects arise—are coded as current adverse effects. For example, steroid-induced diabetes in a patient currently taking steroids as prescribed is coded as an adverse effect (251.8 + E932.0). If the patient suffers delayed effects that arose or remain long after the medication was discontinued, code **909.5, Late effect of adverse effect of drug, medicinal or biological substance,** would be assigned as an additional code to indicate that it is a late effect. For example:

- Brain damage due to allergic reaction to penicillin (current medication)
  348.9 + E930.0
- Brain damage due to allergic reaction to penicillin (use of medication discontinued six months ago) 348.9 + 909.5 + E930.0

Review Exercise 28.3

Code the following diagnoses, sequencing the codes correctly. Assign E codes.

	Code(s)
1. Extrapyramidal <u>disease</u> resulting from previous overdose of Thorazine in an attempted suicide six months ago <u>Late</u> or <u>Late effect of</u>	<u>333.90</u> 909.0 E959
2. Neural <u>deafness</u> resulting from accidental overdose of streptomycin administered in physician's office two years ago <u>Late</u> or <u>Late effect of</u>	<u>389.12</u> 909.0 E929.2
3. Anoxic brain <u>damage</u> secondary to previous accidental overdose of Nembutal nine months ago <u>Late</u> or <u>Late effect of</u>	<u>348.1</u> 909.0 E929.2
4. Secondary <u>Parkinsonism</u> due to poisoning by lithium four years ago <u>Late</u> or <u>Late effect of</u>	<u>332.1</u> 909.0 E929.2

29 Complications of Surgery and Medical Care

Categories 996 through 999 are provided in *ICD-9-CM* for complications of medical and surgical care that are not classified elsewhere. Note that all conditions that occur following surgery or other patient care are not classified as complications. First, there must be more than a routinely expected condition or occurrence. For example, a major amount of bleeding is expected with joint replacement surgery; hemorrhage should not be considered a complication unless such bleeding is particularly excessive. In addition, there must be a cause-and-effect relationship between the care provided and the condition, and some indication that it is a complication, not a postoperative condition in which no complication is present, such as an artificial opening status or absence of an extremity. In some cases, this is implicit, as in a complication due to the presence of an internal device, an implant or graft, or a transplant. In other situations, the fact that the problem is a complication due to a procedure must be documented by the physician; the coder cannot make this determination. Note that the term complication as used in *ICD-9-CM* does not imply that improper or inadequate care is responsible for the problem.

No time limit is defined for the development of a complication. It may occur during the hospital episode in which the care was provided, shortly thereafter, or even years later. When it occurs during the episode in which the operation or other care was given, it is assigned as an additional code. When it develops later and is the reason for the hospital admission, it is designated as the principal diagnosis. Complications of surgical and medical care are classified in *ICD-9-CM* as follows:

- Complications that occur only in other specified body sites are classified in that chapter of *ICD-9-CM*.
- Complications that affect multiple sites or body systems are generally classified in categories 996–999.
- Complications of abortion, pregnancy, labor, or delivery are reclassified in chapter 11 of *ICD-9-CM*.

It is imperative that the coder use the index carefully and follow all instructional notes. Exclusion notes are fairly extensive in this section and often direct the coder elsewhere. There are several basic exclusions that must be observed:

- Complications of medicinal agents, such as adverse effects, complications of anesthesia, and poisoning due to medicinal or toxic agents
- Burns from local applications and irradiation
- Complications of anesthesia and other drugs
- Complications of the condition for which surgery was performed
- Specified conditions classified elsewhere, such as serum hepatitis or electrolyte imbalance
- Any condition classified elsewhere in the Alphabetic Index when described as being due to a procedure or medical care, such as postoperative psychosis or postlaminectomy syndrome. (Note that the adjective iatrogenic is often used to indicate that the condition is a result of treatment.)

LOCATING COMPLICATION CODES IN THE ALPHABETIC INDEX

The coder should first refer to the main term for the condition and look for a subterm indicating a postoperative or other iatrogenic condition. For example:

Adhesion(s) . . .
    postoperative (gastrointestinal tract) . . .   568.0
        eyelid   997.9 . . .
        urethra   598.2
Colostomy . . .
    malfunction   569.69

When no entry can be found under the main term for the condition, the coder should refer to the main term **Complications** and look for an appropriate subterm, such as one of the following:

- Nature of complication, such as foreign body, accidental puncture, or hemorrhage
- Type of procedure, such as colostomy, dialysis, or shunt
- Anatomical site or body system affected, such as respiratory system
- General terms such as mechanical, infection, or graft

Examples include the following entries from the Alphabetic Index:

Complications
    postmastoidectomy . . .   383.30
Complications
    cardiac . . .   429.0
        device . . .   996.72
            infection . . .   996.61
            long-term effect   429.4
            mechanical . . .   996.00

POSTOPERATIVE CONDITIONS NOT CLASSIFIED AS COMPLICATIONS

Certain conditions resulting from medical or surgical care are residual conditions of a procedure, but no complicating factor is involved. For example, postlaminectomy syndrome often occurs following laminectomy, but it is a sequela of the procedure, not a complication. The extensive exclusion list at the beginning of the 996 through 999 series is helpful in making some of these distinctions. Other examples include:

- Postoperative intestinal or peritoneal adhesions with obstruction   560.81
- Infection of enterostomy, due to group C Streptococcus   569.61 + 041.03
- Postoperative pelvic adhesions   614.6

Some conditions that occur postoperatively are neither classified as complications nor have special codes to indicate that they are postoperative in nature. Pain, for instance, is coded only to the site of the pain when a code is warranted at all. Patients are frequently admitted from outpatient surgery with pain and/or nausea and vomiting, but these are common symptoms during postoperative recovery and are not coded to categories 996 through 999 unless the physician identifies them specifically as complications of the surgery. The principal diagnosis is the symptom or other condition that occasions the postoperative admission. Sometimes the patient is admitted because of a general concern rather than because of specific symptoms. Although physicians may state that the admission is for observation, this type of situation is ordinarily not coded to **V71.x, Observation and evaluation for suspected conditions not found.** If no specific condition is identified, the principal diagnosis would be admission for surgical aftercare (V58.4x).

Postoperative anemia is rarely considered to be a complication of surgery. When the physician documents postoperative anemia, code **285.1, Acute posthemorrhagic anemia,** is assigned, but no complication code is assigned unless the physician documents excessive bleeding as a complication. The fact that blood is administered during a surgical procedure does not indicate a postoperative anemia. Transfusions are sometimes given as a prophylactic replacement in order to avoid postoperative anemia. Anemia is not assigned solely because the patient received a transfusion; the physician must document the condition.

A diagnosis of postoperative hypertension often means only that the patient has a preexisting essential hypertension or only that the patient has an elevated blood pressure. If the physician clearly identifies it as a postoperative complication, code **997.91, Complications affecting other specified body systems not elsewhere classified, Hypertension,** is assigned.

Exercise 29.1

Code the following diagnoses. Do not assign E codes.

	Code(s)
1. Postoperative pulmonary embolism	415.11
2. Postoperative pulmonary edema	518.4
3. Colostomy malfunction	569.62
4. Postleukotomy syndrome	310.0
5. Postoperative peritoneal adhesions	568.0
6. Postoperative blind loop syndrome	579.2

COMPLICATIONS DUE TO PRESENCE OF INTERNAL DEVICE, IMPLANT, OR GRAFT

Category **996, Complications peculiar to certain specified procedures,** classifies conditions that occur only because an internal device, implant, or graft is present. Complications of this type are classified first according to whether they are mechanical or nonmechanical in nature. A mechanical complication is one that results from a failure of the device, implant, or graft, such as displacement or malfunction. These are classified in subcategories 996.0 through 996.5, with a fifth digit indicating the body system and/or type of device involved. For example:

- Perforation of uterus by intrauterine contraceptive device   996.32
- Protrusion of intramedullary nail in left femur   996.40
- Mechanical complication of peritoneal dialysis catheter   996.56
- Mechanical complication of arteriovenous dialysis catheter   996.1
- Malfunction of transjugular intrahepatic portosystemic shunt (TIPS)   996.1
- Defective automatic implantable cardiac defibrillator (AICD)   996.04

Subcategory **996.4, Mechanical complication of internal orthopedic device, implant, and graft,** has been expanded to fifth-digit subclassification. The specific mechanical complications are indicated as follows:

- 996.40   Unspecified mechanical complication of internal orthopedic device, implant, and graft
- 996.41   Mechanical loosening of prosthetic joint
- 996.42   Dislocation of prosthetic joint
- 996.43   Prosthetic joint implant failure
- 996.44   Peri-prosthetic fracture around prosthetic joint
- 996.45   Peri-prosthetic osteolysis
- 996.46   Articular bearing surface wear of prosthetic joint
- 996.47   Other mechanical complication of prosthetic joint implant
- 996.49   Other mechanical complication of other internal orthopedic device, implant, and graft

Infection and inflammatory reactions due to the presence of a device, implant, or graft that is functioning properly are classified in subcategory **996.6x, Infection and inflammatory reaction due to internal prosthetic device, implant, and graft.** Code **996.64, Infection or inflammation due to indwelling urinary catheter,** should have additional codes for the specific infection, such as cystitis or sepsis, and for the responsible organism if that information is available. Subcategory 996.7x classifies other complications due to the presence of internal prosthetic device, implant, and graft such as nonmechanical complications, such as embolism, thrombosis, fibrosis, stenosis, or pain. An additional code is used to identify the complication, such as pain due to presence of device, implant, or graft (338.18–338.19, 338.28–338.29). Fifth digits indicate the site and/or type of complication. For example:

- Infected pacemaker pocket   996.61
- E. coli infection due to peritoneal dialysis catheter   996.68 + 041.4
- Chronic interstitial cystitis due to indwelling catheter   996.64 + 595.1

Code 996.72 is assigned for occlusion of a coronary bypass graft unless it is identified by the physician as being due to arteriosclerosis. Arteriosclerotic occlusions of a coronary artery bypass graft are classified as codes 414.02 through 414.05, Coronary atherosclerosis. The fifth digit indicates the type of graft. Occlusion of the coronary artery when there is no history of bypass graft is classified as arteriosclerosis of native coronary arteries (414.01).

Subcategory **996.8, Complications of transplanted organ,** is reserved for transplant complications or rejections, with the fifth digit indicating the organ involved. When infection is present, a code from category 041 or 079 should be assigned as an additional code. A transplant complication code is only assigned if the complication affects the function of the transplanted organ. Two codes are required to fully describe a transplant complication: the appropriate code from subcategory 996.8 and a secondary code that identifies the complication. Preexisting conditions or conditions that develop after the transplant are not coded as complications unless they affect the function of the transplanted organs.

Post-transplant surgical complications that do not relate to the function of the transplanted organ are classified to the specific complication. For example, a postsurgical infection is coded as a postoperative wound infection, not as a transplant complication. Post-transplant patients who are seen for treatment unrelated to the transplanted organ are assigned a code from category **V42, Organ or tissue replaced by transplant,** to capture the transplant status of the patient. A code from category V42 should never be used with a code from subcategory 996.8.

Patients with chronic kidney disease (CKD) following a transplant should not be assumed to have transplant failure or rejection unless it is documented by the provider. If documentation supports the presence of failure or rejection, then it is appropriate to assign code **996.81, Complications of transplanted organs, kidney,** followed by the appropriate CKD code (585.1–585.9).

Exercise 29.2

Code the following diagnoses. Do not assign E codes.

	Code(s)
1. Leakage of breast prosthesis	996.54
2. Intrauterine contraceptive device imbedded in uterine wall	996.32
Imbedding	
3. Erosion of skin by pacemaker electrodes	996.01
Complication	
4. Bone marrow transplant with rejection syndrome	996.85
Complication	
5. Displaced lens implant, right eye	996.53
Complication	
6. Complication of transplanted intestine	996.87

COMPLICATIONS AFFECTING SPECIFIC BODY SYSTEMS NOT CLASSIFIED ELSEWHERE

Titles for most of the codes from category **997, Complications affecting specified body systems, not elsewhere classified,** are general in nature and offer little specificity. These codes are not assigned when the Alphabetic Index provides another code, and they should not be assigned without specific documentation by the physician that the condition is a complication of the surgery. When a code from category 997 is assigned, an additional code for the condition is ordinarily assigned to provide specificity.

Complications of an amputated stump are classified in subcategory 997.6 with the addition of a fifth digit indicating the type of amputated stump complication. A code from subcategories V49.6 through V49.7 is assigned to indicate the site of the amputation. Amputation stump complications are classified as follows:

- 997.60   Amputation stump complication, Unspecified complication
- 997.61   Amputation stump complication, Neuroma of amputation stump
- 997.62   Amputation stump complication, Infection (chronic)
- 997.69   Amputation stump complication, Other

ICD-9-CM differentiates between cardiac complications that occur during the immediate postoperative period following any type of surgery (997.1) and long-term functional effects following cardiac surgery (429.4). Originally, the immediate postoperative period was defined as the time between the surgery and the patient's discharge from the hospital. With current changes in medical practice resulting in earlier discharges, this definition is no longer viable, and code 997.1 may be assigned for complications that occur reasonably soon after surgery, even though the patient may have been discharged. Code **429.4, Functional disturbance,** also classifies long-term functional effects that result from the presence of a cardiac prosthesis.

Pacemaker syndrome (429.4) sometimes occurs when a patient fitted with a ventricular pacemaker experiences decreased cardiac output during paced rhythm. This syndrome can overshadow any improvement resulting from pacemaker therapy and may actually lead to a worsening of the symptoms that were present before the pacemaker was implanted.

- Acute cholecystitis; postoperative cardiac arrhythmia (same admission)
  575.0 + 997.1 + 427.9
- Heart failure following cardiac surgery performed during previous admission; patient discharged one month ago   429.4
- Heart failure on second postoperative day following surgery   997.1

OTHER COMPLICATIONS OF PROCEDURES NOT CLASSIFIED ELSEWHERE

Category **998, Other complications of surgery, not elsewhere classified,** is used to classify a miscellaneous group of postoperative complications. For the most part, additional codes are not required because the complication code itself provides sufficient specificity. For example:

- 998.32   Disruption of external operation wound
- 998.82   Cataract fragments in eye following cataract surgery
- 998.0   Postoperative shock

Subcategory **998.1, Hemorrhage or hematoma or seroma complicating a procedure,** classifies the specific complication with a fifth digit as follows:

- 998.11   Hemorrhage complicating a procedure
- 998.12   Hematoma complicating a procedure
- 998.13   Seroma complicating a procedure

Code **998.2, Accidental puncture or laceration during a procedure,** classifies inadvertent rents, tears, or lacerations that occur during surgery. For example:

- Dural tear occurring during spinal fusion surgery   998.2

Patients are frequently seen for continued care for postsurgical wounds that are either healing slowly or not healing at all. Code **998.83, Non-healing wound,** is assigned for such admissions or encounters.

COMPLICATIONS OF MEDICAL CARE NOT CLASSIFIED ELSEWHERE

Category **999, Complications of medical care,** provides codes for classifying a number of specific conditions that may occur following almost any type of procedure. Codes from category 999 classify conditions that result from medical care, rather than surgery. For example:

- Rh incompatibility reaction following transfusion   999.7
- Anaphylactic shock due to serum   999.4

COMPLICATIONS VS. AFTERCARE

As discussed earlier, it is important to differentiate between an admission for a complication of surgery or medical care and one for aftercare. An admission for aftercare is usually planned in advance to take care of an expected residual or to carry out follow-up activity, such as removal of pins or plates placed during earlier orthopedic surgery. Aftercare is classified into categories V50 through V58. Subcategory **V58.3, Attention to dressing and sutures,** has been expanded to describe an encounter for change or removal of nonsurgical wound dressing (V58.30), encounter for change or removal of surgical wound dressing (V58.31), and encounter for removal of sutures (V58.32). The coder must be careful not to assign complication codes for routine aftercare encounters. For example:

- Admitted for removal of pins from femur   V54.01
- Patient visit for removal of cast   V53.7

Exercise 29.3

Code the following diagnoses, some of which identify complications and some of which identify aftercare. Do not assign E codes or procedure codes.

	Code(s)
1. Admitted for removal of internal fixation nail that has extruded into surrounding tissue, causing severe pain	996.40
Complication, orthopedic	
2. Admitted for closure of colostomy	V55.3

Exercise 29.3 *(continued)*

3. Admitted for <u>adjustment</u> of   V52.4
   breast prosthesis

4. Admitted for removal of displaced breast   996.54
   prosthesis

   Complication, surgical, internal

STATUS POST

The term "status post" used in diagnostic statements is sometimes interpreted by coders to mean that there is a postoperative complication; however, the term is rarely intended to carry this meaning. It usually indicates that the patient underwent the procedure at some time in the past. The condition ordinarily would be classified in the V10 through V19 series, but only when it is significant for the current episode of care.

SURGICAL OR MEDICAL CARE AS EXTERNAL CAUSE

ICD-9-CM provides two sets of E codes to indicate medical or surgical care as the cause of a complication. Codes from categories E870 through E876 are used only when the condition is stated to be due to a misadventure of medical or surgical care. Codes from categories E878 through E879 are used when the condition is described as due to medical or surgical care but without mention of misadventure. Examples include the following:

- Radiation pneumonitis due to adverse reaction to radiotherapy   508.0 + E879.2
- Sponge inadvertently left in abdomen during laparotomy   998.4 + E871.0

Because of the potential legal problems that may develop from reporting these codes, the facility should give careful thought to formulating policies and guidelines for their use. Coders should never make an assumption that there has been a misadventure; such codes should be assigned only when there is a clear-cut diagnostic statement to this effect by the physician.

Review Exercise 29.4

Code the following diagnoses. Do not assign E codes, V codes, or procedure codes.

	Code(s)
1. <u>Infected</u> injection site, left buttock	999.3
or Complications	

Review Exercise 29.4 *(continued)*

2. Sloughing of skin graft due to rejection of   996.52
   pedicle graft to right arm

3. Headache due to lumbar puncture   349.0

4. Postoperative cardiac arrest occurring in   997.1
   recovery room during closure of abdomen,   427.5
   with successful resuscitation

5. Persistent vomiting following   564.3
   gastrointestinal surgery

6. Air embolism resulting from   999.1
   intravenous infusion

7. Thrombophlebitis of antecubital vein of the   999.2
   upper arm resulting from intravenous infusion   451.82
                                    Postoperative

8. Hypovolemic shock due to surgery   998.0
   this morning
                                    Postoperative

9. Persistent postoperative vesicovaginal fistula   998.6
                                                        619.0

Review Exercise 29.4 *(continued)*

10. Cardiac insufficiency resulting from
    mitral valve prosthesis, in place
    for three years   429.4

11. Perforation of coronary artery by   998.2
    catheter during cardiac catheterization

                                            Complication

12. Displacement of cardiac pacemaker   996.01
    electrode

                                    Complication, mechanical

13. Phantom limb following surgical amputation   353.6

14. Neuroma of stump following surgical   997.61
    amputation of left leg

15. Staphylococcus aureus infection of   996.81
    transplanted kidney   041.11

                                Complication, transplant, organ

Preview of *ICD-10-CM* and *ICD-10-PCS*

30 Introduction to the *ICD-10-CM* and *ICD-10-PCS* Classifications

Nelly Leon-Chisen, RHIA

The *International Classification of Diseases, Tenth Revision, Clinical Modification* (ICD-10-CM) and the *International Classification of Diseases, Tenth Revision, Procedure Classification System (ICD-10-PCS)* have been developed as a replacement for *ICD-9-CM*. *ICD-10-CM* consists of a clinical modification of the World Health Organization's *ICD-10*. *ICD-10-CM* consists of diagnosis codes, while *ICD-10-PCS* consists of procedure codes. **The United States implementation date for either one of these systems has not yet been announced.** A federal regulatory update to the Health Insurance Portability and Accountability Act (HIPAA) is required for a change to either *ICD-10-CM* or *ICD-10-PCS*.

RATIONALE FOR CHANGE

ICD-9-CM has been in use in the United States since 1979. Many improvements in medical practice and technology have taken place since *ICD-9-CM* was first implemented. Although *ICD-9-CM* is updated on a regular basis, the classification is limited in its ability to expand enumeration because of the physical numbering constraints contained in the current system. Some categories have vague and imprecise codes. This lack of specificity creates problems such as the inability to collect accurate data on new technology, increased requirements for submission of documentation to support claims, lack of quality data to support health outcomes, and less accurate reimbursement.

Over the years, many of the *ICD-9-CM* categories have become full, making it difficult to create new codes. Once a category is full, several types of similar diagnoses or procedures are combined under one code, or a place is found in another section of the classification for a new code. Due to a lack of space in the classification, several distinct procedures performed in different parts of the body, and with widely different resource utilization, may be grouped together under the same procedure code. The structural integrity of the *ICD-9-CM* procedure classification has already been compromised with new code numbers being assigned to "chapter 00" when new numbers were not available within the appropriate body system chapter. More importantly, many other countries have already converted to *ICD-10*, making it difficult to compare United States health data with international data. Thus far, 138 countries have implemented *ICD-10* for mortality and 99 countries have implemented it for morbidity reporting.

THE RAND COST-BENEFIT STUDY

A cost-benefit study commissioned by the National Committee on Vital and Health Statistics (NCVHS) from the RAND Corporation in 2003 identified the following expected benefits from the implementation of *ICD-10-CM* and *ICD-10-PCS:*

- Improvements to the quality of care and patient safety
- Fewer rejected or questionable reimbursement claims
- Improved information for disease management
- More accurate reimbursement rates for emerging technologies, and
- Better understanding of the value of new procedures

INTERNATIONAL DEVELOPMENT OF *ICD-10*

ICD-10 was released by the World Health Organization (WHO) in 1993. The WHO authorized development of an adaptation of the *ICD-10* for use in the United States. All modifications to the *ICD-10* need to conform to the WHO conventions for the *ICD.* *ICD-10* contains only diagnosis codes. Each country needs to develop its own procedure coding system.

UNITED STATES DEVELOPMENT OF *ICD-10*

In the United States, a clinical modification of the WHO diagnosis coding system has been developed *(ICD-10-CM),* while a new, unique procedure classification system was created: *ICD-10-PCS.*

ICD-10-CM was developed under the leadership of the National Center for Health Statistics, a federal agency under the Centers for Disease Control. *ICD-10-CM* is intended as a replacement for volumes 1 and 2 of the *ICD-9-CM* (diagnosis codes).

ICD-10-PCS was developed by 3M Health Information Systems under contract to the Centers for Medicare & Medicaid Services (CMS, formerly the Health Care Financing Administration, or HCFA). The *ICD-10-PCS* was designed to replace volume 3 of the *ICD-9-CM* for reporting hospital inpatient procedures.

ESTIMATED IMPLEMENTATION DATE

As mentioned earlier, a United States implementation date for *ICD-10-CM* or *ICD-10-PCS* has not been set at this time. The NCVHS, the advisory committee to the Secretary of Health and Human Services, has been studying the problems with the existing *ICD-9-CM* classification system since the 1980s. During 2002 and 2003, the NCVHS held public hearings on *ICD-10-CM* and *ICD-10-PCS.* Hospitals, health information professionals, software vendors, health researchers, and device and technology manufacturers supported migrating to *ICD-10-CM* and *ICD-10-PCS.* In November 2003, after reviewing public testimony, the results of the RAND cost-benefit study, and *ICD-10-CM* field testing, the NCVHS issued a recommendation to the Secretary to implement *ICD-10-CM* and *ICD-10-PCS.*

The NCVHS has issued the following recommendations:

- The regulatory process should be initiated for the concurrent adoption of *ICD-10-CM* and *ICD-10-PCS.*
- The implementation period should be at least two years following the issuance of a final rule.

- The Notice of Proposed Rulemaking (NPRM) should specifically invite comments on key issues presented in testimonies and letters before the Committee:
  —What could be done to minimize the costs of a transition to *ICD-10-CM* and *ICD-10-PCS*?
  —What could be done to maximize the benefits of implementing *ICD-10-CM* and *ICD-10-PCS*?
  —What are the potential unintended consequences of such a migration, and how could they be mitigated?
  —What timeframes would be adequate for implementation?
  —What additional steps would be required to ensure a realistic and smooth migration?

At the time of publication, draft legislation contained a provision to implement *ICD-10*. If passed, HR 4157, The Health Information Technology Promotion Act, would require the Secretary to implement *ICD-10-CM* and *ICD-10-PCS* on October 1, 2009.

31 | *ICD-10-CM*

Nelly Leon-Chisen, RHIA

The *International Classification of Diseases, Tenth Revision, Clinical Modification (ICD-10-CM),* is the United States modification to the World Health Organization's diagnosis coding system. In this chapter we discuss its development and field testing, as well as the structure, format, and conventions of *ICD-10-CM*.

DEVELOPMENT OF *ICD-10-CM*

In 1994 the National Center for Health Statistics (NCHS) determined that a clinical modification of the *ICD-10* would be a significant improvement worth implementing in the United States. A clinical modification was needed to include emerging diseases and more recent medical knowledge, as well as to include new concepts and expand distinctions for ambulatory and managed care encounters.

The clinical modification for *ICD-10* was developed in three phases, with the first phase being the development of a prototype with the assistance of a technical advisory panel (TAP). The next two phases consisted of enhancements to the prototype based on minutes of the ICD-9-CM Coordination and Maintenance Committee and public comments. Development of the *ICD-10-CM* was done in consultation with physician groups, professional associations (e.g., the American Hospital Association, or AHA) and other users of *ICD-9-CM*. Future improvement is expected as a result of problems identified during the field testing.

The *ICD-10-CM* is in the public domain. However, neither the codes nor the code titles may be changed except through the Coordination and Maintenance process overseen jointly by NCHS and the Centers for Medicare & Medicaid Services (CMS).

ICD-10-CM consists of twenty-one chapters. The classification of external causes of injury and poisoning (E codes), and the classification of factors influencing health status and contact with health services (V codes), are incorporated within *ICD-10-CM* instead of being considered supplementary classifications, as in *ICD-9-CM*.

Major modifications in the *ICD-10-CM* include:

- Identification of trimesters to obstetrical codes
- Expanded diabetes, injury, alcohol/substance abuse, and postoperative complication sections
- Ability to report laterality (to specify whether a medical condition occurred on the right or left side)
- Standard definitions for "excludes" notes
- Combination diagnosis/symptoms codes
- Identification of initial encounter, subsequent encounter, and sequelae of injuries
- Expanded external causes of injuries
- Improved clinical detail
- Addition of a sixth character
- Addition of a seventh character extension in some chapters (from a maximum of five character codes in *ICD-9-CM)*

Table 31.1 provides a quick overview of the major differences between *ICD-9-CM* (volumes 1 and 2) and *ICD-10-CM*.

TABLE 31.1   Major Differences Between *ICD-9-CM* and *ICD-10-CM*

Feature	ICD-9-CM	ICD-10-CM
Minimum number of digits/characters	3	3
Maximum number of digits/characters	5	7
Number of chapters	17	21
Supplemental classification	V codes and E codes	No, incorporated into classification
Laterality (right vs. left)	No	Yes
Alphanumeric vs. numeric	Numeric, except for V codes and E codes	Alphanumeric, with all codes starting with an alpha character and some codes with alpha 7th character extension
Excludes notes	Yes	Exclude 1
		Exclude 2
Dummy placeholders	No	Yes: "x"

FIELD TESTING

The AHA and the American Health Information Management Association (AHIMA) conducted the world's first field test of *ICD-10-CM* over the summer of 2003. The Web-based data collection process, results tabulation, and assistance with data analysis were provided by the Health Information Management & Systems Division, School of Allied Medical Professions, and by the Medical Media Design Department, College of Medicine and Public Health, both at the Ohio State University. The field testing was conducted with the help of hundreds of health information management volunteers across the United States. The primary purpose of the study was to assess the functionality and utility of applying *ICD-10-CM* to actual medical records in a variety of health care settings and to assess the level of education and training required by professional, credentialed coders to implement *ICD-10-CM*.

For detailed information on the study's design and a complete report of the field study, visit the American Hospital Association's Web site: www.aha.org. The complete report is available for download at: http://www.ahacentraloffice.org/ahacentraloffice/html/icd10/icd10resources/index.html.

Results of Field Testing

Over six thousand completed medical records were coded using both *ICD-9-CM* and *ICD-10-CM*. The records were obtained from a variety of settings, including: short-term acute care hospital inpatient settings, short-term acute care hospital outpatient settings, post–acute care settings (home health, hospice, nursing homes, long term care hospitals, and rehabilitation units or facilities), physician practices, clinics, community health centers, freestanding ambulatory surgery centers, and freestanding diagnostic facilities. More than 23,000 *ICD-10-CM* codes were assigned, and all chapters were represented in the test.

There was no time difference between assigning *ICD-9-CM* and *ICD-10-CM* codes for 3,616 records, or more than half of the sample. Taking longer to code with *ICD-10-CM* was expected because participants were basically unfamiliar with the coding system, had received minimal training, and lacked user-friendly coding tools. None of the participants had the opportunity to gain significant *ICD-10-CM* coding proficiency. On the other hand, the vast majority of them were highly proficient in *ICD-9-CM*.

Considering the barriers to coding productivity, it is particularly surprising that the time required to code records in *ICD-10-CM* was not greater. The availability of much-improved coding tools, more training, and increased familiarity with *ICD-10-CM* will significantly reduce the amount of time needed to code records in *ICD-10-CM*, possibly to the point whereby *ICD-10-CM* may actually require less coding time than *ICD-9-CM*.

The clinical descriptions of the *ICD-10-CM* codes were thought to be better than *ICD-9-CM*. Respondents thought the notes, instructions, and guidelines in *ICD-10-CM* were clear and comprehensive.

The testing participants favored migration to *ICD-10-CM* and thought the system should be implemented in three years or less. *ICD-10-CM* was seen to be an improvement over *ICD-9-CM*. Participants in some nonhospital settings indicated that they believed *ICD-10-CM* was much more applicable to those settings than *ICD-9-CM*. *ICD-10-CM* codes can be applied to today's medical records in a variety of health care settings, without having to change documentation practices, although improved documentation would result in higher coding specificity, and therefore higher data quality, in some cases.

Participants felt that a maximum of sixteen hours of training would be necessary to adequately prepare coding professionals for *ICD-10-CM* coding. Participants suggested training should be provided relatively close to the implementation date (three to six months before the date).

Study Conclusion

The study concluded that the results of this field-testing project, and independent data analysis, support *ICD-10-CM* as an appropriate replacement for the *ICD-9-CM* diagnosis coding system. *ICD-10-CM* represents an improvement over *ICD-9-CM* in that it reflects advances in medical care and knowledge that have occurred since the implementation of *ICD-9-CM* in 1979. *ICD-10-CM* is sufficiently flexible to accommodate medical advances, and it ensures that the systems will remain useful well into the future. Significantly, *ICD-10-CM* meets criteria established under the Health Insurance Portability and Accountability Act (HIPAA) for code set standards as well as National Committee on Vital and Health Statistics criteria for a diagnosis coding system.

Exercise 31.1

Without referring to the handbook material, answer the following questions either true or false.

_____F_____ 1. The *ICD-10-CM* field testing estimated forty hours of training would be required for experienced coders.

_____T_____ 2. Testing included a variety of records, including hospitals, clinics, physician offices, and post–acute care settings.

_____F_____ 3. *ICD-10-CM* codes have a maximum of five digits.

_____T_____ 4. A major modification to *ICD-10-CM* includes the ability to identify trimesters with obstetrical codes.

_____T_____ 5. The *ICD-10-CM* has improved clinical detail.

ICD-10-CM STRUCTURE, FORMAT, AND CONVENTIONS

ICD-10-CM has many similarities to *ICD-9-CM*, especially with regard to the classification format and conventions. The code structure has changed slightly to accommodate code expansion and improvements to the classification.

Code Structure

All *ICD-10-CM* codes have an alphanumeric structure, with all codes starting with an alphabetic character. The basic code structure consists of three digits. A decimal point is used to separate the basic three-digit category code from its subcategory and subclassifications. Most *ICD-10-CM* codes contain a maximum of six characters, with a few chapters having a seventh character code extension.

Format

The *ICD-10-CM* is divided into the Index and the Tabular List. The Index is an alphabetical list of terms and their corresponding code. The Tabular List is a chronological list of codes divided into chapters based on body system or condition.

Alphabetical Index

The Alphabetical Index is divided into the Index to Diseases and Injuries and the Index to External Causes of Injury. Similar to *ICD-9-CM*, there is also a Neoplasm Table and a Table of Drugs and Chemicals.

The Alphabetical Index includes entries for main terms, subterms, and more specific subterms. An indented format is used for ease of reference. It is expected that a variety of vendors will develop user-friendly printed versions, as well as computer encoding programs, as they currently exist for *ICD-9-CM*.

Tabular List

The Tabular List contains categories, subcategories, and codes. The basic code used to classify a particular disease or injury consists of three digits and is called a category. The first character of a category is a letter, while the second and third characters are numbers (e.g., K29, Gastritis and duodenitis). If a three-character category has no further subdivision, it is considered a code. Subcategories may be made up of four or five characters. These subcategory characters may be letters or numbers. Codes are three, four, five, or six characters long, depending on whether they are further subdivided. Each level of subdivision after a category is a subcategory. The final level of subdivision is a code. The final character in a code may be either a letter or a number. For example:

- K29 Gastritis and duodenitis   *(category)*
    - K29.0 Acute gastritis   *(subcategory)*
        - K29.00 Acute gastritis without bleeding   *(code)*
- R10 Abdominal and pelvic pain   *(category)*
    - R10.8 Other abdominal pain   *(subcategory)*
        - R10.81 Abdominal tenderness   *(subcategory)*
            - R10.811 Right upper quadrant abdominal tenderness   *(code)*

The *ICD-10-CM* uses the letter "x" as the fifth character dummy place holder for certain six character codes. This was done to allow for future expansion without disrupting the sixth character structure for codes where the sixth character has a specific use. An example of this may be seen with the poisoning (T36–T50) and the toxic effects (T51–65) codes. For these categories, the sixth character represents the intent: accidental, intentional self-harm, assault, undetermined, adverse effect, or underdosing. For example:

T37.5x1   Poisoning by antiviral drugs, accidental (unintentional)
T37.5x2   Poisoning by antiviral drugs, intentional self-harm
T52.0x1   Toxic effect of petroleum products, accidental (unintentional)
T52.0x2   Toxic effect of petroleum products, intentional self-harm

Certain categories have an additional seventh character extension. The extension must always be the seventh character in the code. If a code is not a full six characters long, a dummy placeholder "x" must be used to fill in the empty characters when a seventh character extension is required. Seventh character extensions can be seen in chapter 19, Injury, poisoning and certain other consequences of external causes (S00–T98).

An example of the use of the dummy place holder "x" and the seventh character extension is shown here with an excerpt from the Tabular List:

T16 Foreign body in ear
     Includes: auditory canal
     The following 7th character extensions are to be added to each code for category T16
          a   initial encounter
          d   subsequent encounter
          q   sequela
T16.1 Foreign body in right ear
T16.2 Foreign body in left ear
T16.3 Foreign body in ear, unspecified ear

A child presents to the emergency department with a bean in the right ear. The mother has brought the child because she was not able to remove the bean at home. This encounter would be assigned code **T16.1xxa**. The Tabular List showed subcategory T16.1 as the descriptor best fitting this scenario. Category T16 requires a seventh character extension. Since the code subcategory has only four characters (T16.1), the dummy placeholder "x" is inserted twice to preserve the code structure before the seventh character "a" is added to report this as the initial encounter.

Exercise 31.2

Using the excerpt from the Tabular List above, select an *ICD-10-CM* code for the following scenarios:

1. A child goes to the physician's office as a referral from the emergency department after having had a bean removed from the right ear.   T16.1xxd

2. A child is seen by an audiologist for an evaluation for hearing loss after having had a pen tip removed from the left ear.   T16.2xxq

Conventions

ICD-10-CM has retained several conventions already familiar to users of *ICD-9-CM*, such as instructional notes, abbreviations, cross-reference notes, punctuation marks, and relational terms ("and"). Where conventions are similar to *ICD-9-CM*, they are not further explained in this chapter.

INSTRUCTIONAL NOTES

Several different instructional notes appear in the Tabular List and the Index. These include: "inclusion" and "exclusion" notes, "code first" notes, "use additional code" notes, and "code also" notes.

Inclusion Notes

Inclusion notes are similar to their counterparts in *ICD-9-CM* in terms of the location of the notes, as well as their application. The notes may include conditions for which the code number may be used. It is important to remember that the list of inclusion terms is not meant to be exhaustive.

Exclusion Notes

One of the more significant changes for *ICD-10-CM* is the clarification of the exclusion notes. There are two types of "excludes" notes—each one with a different use; but both indicate that codes excluded are independent of each other.

"Excludes1"

An "excludes1" note means "not coded here." An "excludes1" note instructs the user that the code excluded should never be used at the same time as the code above the "excludes1" note. This instruction is used when two conditions cannot occur together, and therefore both codes cannot be used together. For example:

> **Q03 Congenital hydrocephalus**
> Excludes1: acquired hydrocephalus (G91.-)

In this example the congenital form of the condition cannot be reported with the acquired form of the same condition.

"Excludes2"

An "excludes2" note means "not included here." An "excludes2" note instructs the user that the condition excluded is not part of the condition represented by the code. However, a patient may have both conditions at the same time. When an "excludes2" note appears under a code, it is acceptable to use both the code and the excluded code together. For example:

> **F90 Attention-deficit hyperactivity disorders**
> Excludes2: anxiety disorders (F40.-, F41.-)
>   mood [affective] disorders (F30–F39)

In this example, the "excludes2" note serves as a warning that if a patient has an anxiety disorder, rather than attention-deficit hyperactivity disorder, the user should go to categories F40–F41, rather than remain in category F90. However, if the patient has both attention-deficit hyperactivity and an anxiety disorder, a code from category F90 could be used along with a code from categories F40–F41.

"Code First" and "Use Additional Code"

"Code first" and "use additional code" notes are similar to their counterparts in *ICD-9-CM*. Certain conditions have both an underlying etiology and multiple body system manifestations. *ICD-10-CM* "code first" and "use additional code" instructional notes indicate the proper sequencing order of these conditions: etiology (underlying condition), followed by manifestation. The "use additional code" note is found at the etiology code as a clue to identify the manifestations commonly associated with the disease. The "code first" note is found at the manifestation code to provide instructions that the underlying condition should be sequenced first.

The manifestation codes usually have the phrase "in diseases classified elsewhere" as part of the code title. Codes with this phrase are never used as a first-listed or principal diagnosis code. They must be used with the underlying condition code sequenced first. An example of this convention is category F02, Dementia in other diseases classified elsewhere.

"Code Also"

"Code also" notes in *ICD-10-CM* are similar to the "use additional code" instruction found in *ICD-9-CM*. This note indicates that two codes may be required to describe a condition fully. The sequencing order will depend on the reason for the encounter and the severity of the conditions.

ABBREVIATIONS

The following abbreviations familiar to *ICD-9-CM* users are found in *ICD-10-CM*:

- NEC—Not elsewhere classified. This represents "other specified" in the *ICD-10-CM*.
- NOS—Not otherwise specified. This represents "unspecified" in the *ICD-10-CM*.

CROSS-REFERENCE NOTES

Cross-reference notes are used in the Alphabetical Index to advise the coder to look elsewhere before assigning a code. These notes are similar to their counterparts in *ICD-9-CM*. The cross-reference instructions include:

- "See"
- "See also"
- "See condition"

PUNCTUATION MARKS

The following punctuation marks are used, and their use is similar to *ICD-9-CM:*

- Parentheses
- Square brackets
- Colons

THE RELATIONAL TERM *AND*

The use of the term *and* is similar to *ICD-9-CM*, and it means "and" or "or."

GUIDELINES

Draft guidelines have been developed and were used for the AHA-AHIMA field-testing project. The guidelines were developed by NCHS and reviewed by the remaining *ICD-9-CM* cooperating parties (AHA, AHIMA, and CMS). The guidelines were arranged similarly to the *ICD-9-CM* Official Guidelines. Section 1 includes *ICD-10-CM* conventions. Section 2 covers general guidelines, while section 3 is devoted to chapter-specific guidelines. The chapter-specific guidelines are sequenced in the same order they appear in the Tabular List.

The complete guidelines may be found by visiting the following Web site: http://www.cdc.gov/nchs/data/icd9/draft_i10guideln.pdf.

32 ICD-10-PCS

Nelly Leon-Chisen, RHIA

The *International Classification of Diseases, Tenth Revision, Procedure Classification System* (*ICD-10-PCS*) is the procedure classification system developed as a replacement for volume 3 of the *ICD-9-CM*. In this chapter we discuss its development and field testing, as well as the structure, format, and conventions of *ICD-10-PCS*.

DEVELOPMENT OF *ICD-10-PCS*

In 1992 the United States Health Care Financing Administration (HCFA, now the Centers for Medicare & Medicaid Services, or CMS) funded a preliminary design project for a replacement for volume 3 of the *ICD-9-CM*. In 1995 HCFA awarded a three-year contract to 3M Health Information Systems (HIS) to complete the development of a procedure coding replacement system. The new system was called *ICD-10 Procedure Coding System* (*ICD-10-PCS*). The first year of the 3M contract involved the completion of the first draft of the system. The second year was devoted to external review and limited informal testing, while the third year consisted of formal independent review and testing. *ICD-10-PCS* was completed in 1998 and has been updated annually by 3M HIS since then. The goal of the revisions is to keep current with medical technology and coding needs.

A Technical Advisory Panel (TAP) was convened to provide extensive input into the development process. The TAP included representatives from the American Health Information Management Association (AHIMA), the American Hospital Association (AHA), and the American Medical Association. Many other medical specialty organizations also contributed to the development of *ICD-10-PCS*.

The four main objectives in the development of *ICD-10-PCS* were:

- *Completeness:* All substantially different procedures should have a unique code.
- *Expandability:* The structure of *ICD-10-PCS* should allow for the easy incorporation of unique codes as new procedures are developed.
- *Multi-axial:* The structure of *ICD-10-PCS* should be multi-axial, with each code character having the same meaning within a specific procedure section and across procedure sections, whenever possible.
- *Standardized methodology:* *ICD-10-PCS* should include unique definitions for the terms used, with each term having a specific meaning.

The guiding principles that were followed in the development of *ICD-10-PCS* are:

- Diagnostic information is not included in the procedure description.
- Explicit "not otherwise specified" (NOS) options are not provided.
- "Not elsewhere classified" (NEC) options are provided on a limited basis.
- All possible procedures are defined regardless of the frequency of occurrence. If a procedure could be performed, a code was created.

The initial drafts of *ICD-10-PCS* were widely distributed to all major physician specialty societies, as well as being made available to the general public. Feedback from the extensive review was used to modify *ICD-10-PCS*. The lack of NOS codes was one of the most frequent concerns raised by the reviewers. It was felt that the medical record documentation might lack sufficient specificity to support the detail required by *ICD-10-PCS*. Modifications were made to the classification to address this concern.

There are fifteen sections in *ICD-10-PCS* representing nearly eighty-eight thousand codes. *ICD-10-PCS* uses a grid structure that permits the specification of a large number of codes on a single page in the Tabular division. The combined Tabular and Index divisions of *ICD-10-PCS* represent nearly half the size of the Tabular List and Index in the World Health Organization's *ICD-10* diagnosis coding manual.

Major modifications in the *ICD-10-PCS* include:

- All codes have a unique definition.
- *ICD-10-PCS* affords users the ability to aggregate codes across all essential components of a procedure.
- *ICD-10-PCS* provides users with extensive flexibility.
- New procedures and technologies are easily incorporated.
- Code expansions do not disrupt systematic structure.
- *ICD-10-PCS* makes limited use of the NOS and NEC categories.
- All terminology is precisely defined and used consistently across all codes.
- No diagnostic information is included in the code.

Table 32.1 provides a quick overview of the major differences between *ICD-9-CM* (volume 3) and *ICD-10-PCS*.

TABLE 32.1   Major Differences Between *ICD-9-CM* and *ICD-10-PCS*

Feature	ICD-9-CM	ICD-10-PCS
Minimum number of digits/characters	3	7
Maximum number of digits/characters	4	7
Decimal point	Yes	No
Alphanumeric or numeric	Numeric	Alphanumeric
Includes notes	Yes	No
Excludes notes	Yes	No
Embedded meaning of characters	No	Yes, multi-axial structure, with each code character having the same meaning within the specific procedure section and across procedure sections, to the extent possible

FIELD TESTING

There have been two field-testing projects—a formal one and an informal one. An informal test was conducted in October 1996 with the assistance of the AHA and the AHIMA. Health information professionals volunteered for training and then coded a sample of records from their institutions using *ICD-10-PCS*. Problems, questions, and suggestions were addressed to the *ICD-10-PCS* project staff at 3M Health Information Systems.

The formal testing of *ICD-10-PCS* was conducted in 1997–98 by HCFA (now CMS) using contractors. The contractors were two Clinical Data Abstraction Centers (CDACs): DynKePRO in York, Pennsylvania, and FMAS in Columbia, Maryland. The CDACs coded a sample of five thousand medical records using *ICD-10-PCS*. Any questions or concerns noted by the CDAC coders were forwarded to the 3M project staff. This interaction resulted in revisions to the final draft of *ICD-10-PCS*. The second phase of the test included a subset of one hundred medical records recoded blindly with both *ICD-9-CM* and *ICD-10-PCS*. The systems were compared on ease of use, time needed to identify codes, number of codes required, problems identifying codes, and strengths and weaknesses of each system.

For detailed information on the development of *ICD-10-PCS* and a complete report of the testing study, visit the CMS Web site: http://www.cms.hhs.gov/ICD9ProviderDiagnostic Codes/08_ICD10.asp.

Results of Field Testing

The CDAC coders were able to use *ICD-10-PCS* easily. They found that a medical dictionary or anatomy textbook were occasionally needed because of the added detail in *ICD-10-PCS*. The CDACs felt that the initial *ICD-10-PCS* training manual would need to be strengthened with additional examples before it could be used on a national level. Both CDACs felt that, once coders were familiar with *ICD-10-PCS*, the result would be improved accuracy and efficiency of coding. The users found the system to be so well organized and well structured that codes could easily be found in the correct section of the Tabular List without using the Index. It was felt that *ICD-10-PCS* was an improvement over *ICD-9-CM* because of its greater specificity. The major strength identified was the system's detailed structure. This level of detail would allow users to more precisely recognize and report the procedures performed.

ICD-10-PCS STRUCTURE, FORMAT, AND CONVENTIONS

ICD-10-PCS is an entirely new classification system bearing little resemblance to *ICD-9-CM* volume 3 classification format or conventions.

Code Structure

All *ICD-10-PCS* codes have an alphanumeric structure, with all codes made up of seven characters and no decimal points. Each character has up to thirty-four different values. Each character is made up of digits 0–9, or the letters A–H, J–N, and P–Z. The letters "O" and "I" are not used so as not to be confused with the digits "0" and "1."

The classification is divided into fifteen sections relating to the general type of procedure. The first character of each *ICD-10-PCS* code specifies the section. Within each section, the second through seventh characters have a standard meaning—but may have different meanings across sections. *ICD-10-PCS* is divided into the sections displayed in table 32.2.

TABLE 32.2 *ICD-10-PCS* Sections and Their Corresponding Character

Character	Section	Character	Section
0	Medical and Surgical	8	Osteopathic
1	Obstetrics	9	Rehabilitation and Diagnostic Audiology
2	Placement	B	Extracorporeal Assistance and Performance
3	Administration		
4	Measurement and Monitoring	C	Extracorporeal Therapies
		F	Mental Health
5	Imaging	G	Chiropractic
6	Nuclear Medicine	H	Miscellaneous
7	Radiation Oncology		

The majority of the procedures that would normally be reported in an inpatient setting can be found in the Medical and Surgical section. Therefore, the following discussion regarding the component characters of a code refers strictly to the Medical and Surgical section. Within this section, the seven characters have the following meaning (see also figure 32.1, "Structure of Codes in the Medical and Surgical Section"):

FIGURE 32.1   Structure of Codes in the Medical and Surgical Section

Section: The first character in the code always refers to the section. The number "0" represents the Medical and Surgical section.

Body System: The second character indicates the general body system (e.g., gastrointestinal). For additional detail, some traditional body systems have been assigned multiple categories. For example, the circulatory system has been subdivided into heart and great vessels, upper arteries, lower arteries, upper veins, and lower veins.

Root Operation: The third character refers to the root operation. The root operation specifies the objective of the procedure (e.g., resection). In the Medical and Surgical section, there are thirty different root operations. Each root operation is precisely defined in the classification. Mastering the definitions of these root operations is the key to "building" a code in *ICD-10-PCS*. Root operations include terms such as *alteration, bypass, change, creation, dilation, excision, resection, fusion, insertion, occlusion,* and *repair.* As part of the continuous updating of the classification, revisions were made in 2006 to streamline the root operations Change, Removal, and Revision.

Body Part: The fourth character indicates the specific part of the body system where the procedure was performed (e.g., appendix). In 2006, new body part values were added to some body systems, while others were updated, such as the vertebral values being subdivided by number of vertebral joints.

Approach: The fifth character refers to the approach used to reach the procedure site (e.g., open). In the 2006 release of *ICD-10-PCS*, the number of approaches in the Medical and Surgical section was reduced from fifteen to seven. The approaches are:

- Open
- Open endoscopic
- Percutaneous
- Percutaneous endoscopic
- Via natural or artificial opening
- Via natural or artificial opening endoscopic
- External

As with root operations, each approach is precisely defined in the classification.

Device: The sixth character is only used to specify devices that remain after the procedure is completed. They do not include materials that are incidental to a procedure, like sutures or clips. When there is no device involved in the procedure, the letter "Z" representing "none" is used as the sixth character to complete the code structure.

Qualifier: The seventh character indicates a qualifier. A qualifier has a unique meaning within individual procedures. This position within the code is used to provide additional information. When there is no qualifier, the seventh character is the letter "Z" to complete the code structure.

Format

The *ICD-10-PCS* is divided into Index, Tabular List, and List of Codes. Codes can be located in alphabetical order within the Index. The Index will refer to a specific location within the Tabular List, but the Index will not specify the complete code. The complete code can only be obtained by referring to the Tabular List. The List of Codes allows for direct lookup of each code, with a short description of each code being provided.

Alphabetical Index

The Index is arranged in alphabetical order based on the type of procedure being performed. Unlike *ICD-9-CM,* the *ICD-10-PCS* Index does not provide a complete code, but it will point to the Tabular List by specifying the first three or four characters of the code, followed by periods.

For example, *appendectomy* may be looked up by "appendectomy," by "resection, appendix," or "excision, appendix." The term *appendectomy* has two reference notes as follows:

> **Appendectomy**
> —*see* Excision, Gastrointestinal System 0DB. . . .
> —*see* Resection, Gastrointestinal System 0DT. . . .

The first three characters of the code (in this example, "0DB" or "0DT") can be used to locate the corresponding table in the Tabular List to find the remaining four characters to complete the code. The difference between the two entries above is that a partial appendectomy would be the "excision" entry and a total appendectomy would be the "resection."

Tabular List

The *ICD-10-PCS* Tabular List, unlike the *ICD-9-CM* Tabular, is composed of grids specifying the valid combinations of characters that make up a procedure code. Figure 32.2 shows a portion of the Tabular List.

FIGURE 32.2   Excerpt from Tabular List

O: Medical and Surgical
D: Gastrointestinal System
T: Resection: Cutting out or off, without replacement, all of a body part

Body Part Character 4	Approach Character 5	Device Character 6	Qualifer Character 7
1 Esophagus, Upper 2 Esophagus, Middle 3 Esophagus, Lower 4 Esophagogastric Junction 6 Stomach 7 Stomach, Pylorus 8 Small Intestine 9 Duodenum A Jejunum B Ileum C Ileocecal Valve D Large Intestine F Large Intestine, Right G Large Intestine, Left H Cecum J Appendix K Ascending Colon L Transverse Colon M Descending Colon N Sigmoid Colon P Rectum Q Anus	0 Open 2 Open Endoscopic 4 Percutaneous Endoscopic 7 Via Natural or Artificial Opening 8 Via Natural or Artificial Opening Endoscopic	Z No Device	Z No Qualifier
R Anal Sphincter S Greater Omentum T Lesser Omentum	0 Open 4 Percutaneous Endoscopic	Z No Device	Z No Qualifier

The top portion of each grid contains a description of the first two or three characters of the procedure code. In this particular example "0DT" refers to the Medical and Surgical section (0) of the gastrointestinal body system (D), and a root operation of resection (T). The root operation (resection) is followed by its definition.

The lower portion of the grid has four columns representing the valid combinations of characters for the four through seven positions. Basically, the user "builds" a code based on the characters across each row on the grid. Each of the columns represents the body part, approach, device, and qualifier for the code. The Tabular List contains only combinations representing valid procedures.

Using the sample grid to build a code for an appendectomy would result in the combination of characters shown in figure 32.3.

FIGURE 32.3   Sample Grid for Building a Code for an Appendectomy

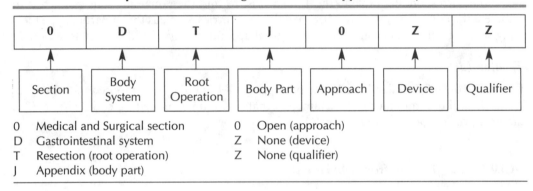

| 0 | D | T | J | 0 | Z | Z |

| Section | Body System | Root Operation | Body Part | Approach | Device | Qualifier |

0   Medical and Surgical section   0   Open (approach)
D   Gastrointestinal system   Z   None (device)
T   Resection (root operation)   Z   None (qualifier)
J   Appendix (body part)

In other words, the code for an open appendectomy is 0DTJ0ZZ. Conversely, if this were a laparoscopic appendectomy, instead of open, then the code would be 0DTJ4ZZ. The difference between the two procedures is the approach, which is represented by the fifth character. An open approach is reported with the character "0" in the fifth position, while a laparoscopic approach is reported with the character "4" (percutaneous endoscopic) in the fifth position.

Exercise 32.1

Using the excerpt of the grid from the Tabular List above (figure 32.2), select the appropriate *ICD-10-PCS* code for the following procedures:

1. Open resection of the upper esophagus   0DT10ZZ

2. Laparoscopic assisted resection of descending colon   0DTM4ZZ

3. Sigmoidectomy   0DTN0ZZ

List of Codes

The actual codes that can be generated from the grids are incorporated into the List of Codes. Each code has a complete and easy-to-read description.

GUIDELINES

Draft guidelines have been developed by the cooperating parties (AHA, AHIMA, CMS, and the National Center for Health Statistics), in collaboration with the 3M Health Information Systems *ICD-10-PCS* project staff. The guidelines can be found on the CMS Web site as appendix B of the *Training Guide on ICD-10-PCS*. This training guide may be downloaded from http://www.cms.hhs.gov/ICD9ProviderDiagnosticCodes/Downloads/traingd.pdf.

The guidelines are divided into three categories: General, Medical and Surgical section (section 0), and Other medical- and surgical-related sections (sections 1–9). Guidelines within the Medical and Surgical section are further grouped by character (e.g., body system, root operation, and so on). The guidelines are numbered sequentially within each category for ease of reference. For 2006, new coding clarification has been further provided in several sections of the draft guidelines, such as when to code multiple procedures, fusion of multiple joints, distinguishing between division and release, and bilateral body part values.

ICD-9-CM AND *ICD-10-PCS* MAPPING

To facilitate the transition from *ICD-9-CM* to *ICD-10-PCS*, mapping between the two coding systems has been developed. New for 2006 is an *ICD-9-CM* to *ICD-10-PCS* basic map in a text file format. The previously available basic map from *ICD-10-PCS* to *ICD-9-CM* has been updated and is available in a text file format.

33 Preparing for *ICD-10-CM* and *ICD-10-PCS*

Nelly Leon-Chisen, RHIA

Although a decision regarding national implementation of *ICD-10-CM* or *ICD-10-PCS* has not yet been made, it is not too early to start preparing. Health information management (HIM) professionals will be expected to take a leadership role in their respective organizations in the transition process. In this chapter we list preparations as individuals. The next chapter discusses implementation issues to be considered by provider organizations.

CHECKLIST

Preparations for HIM/coding staff:

✔ Take advantage of the lead time to brush up on or expand your knowledge of anatomy and physiology. *ICD-10-CM* and *ICD-10-PCS* have the ability to provide greater specificity, and you need to be ready to select the more specific code.

✔ Keep current on the status of *ICD-10* issues by reading articles, attending conferences, or visiting the Web sites of the *ICD-9-CM* cooperating parties:

American Hospital Association: www.ahacentraloffice.org

American Health Information Management Association: www.ahima.org

National Center for Health Statistics (NCHS):
www.cdc.gov/nchs/about/otheract/icd9/abticd10.htm

Centers for Medicare & Medicaid Services (CMS):
http://www.cms.hhs.gov/ICD9ProviderDiagnosticCodes/08_ICD10.asp

✔ It may be too early to take a full-blown *ICD-10* coding seminar, but you can get an overview of the system and familiarize yourself with the coding structure.

✔ Review the coding system by downloading the classification from the NCHS and CMS Web sites.

✔ Review the draft *ICD-10-CM* and *ICD-10-PCS* guidelines and become familiar with new concepts such as definitions of root operations.

✔ If you are really ambitious, work your way through the *ICD-10-PCS* training manual available from CMS. While this is a preliminary draft, and while it is very likely to change before actual implementation, it will give you a basic knowledge of the classification as well as allow you a chance to practice code assignment.

34 Implementation Issues for *ICD-10-CM* and *ICD-10-PCS*

Nelly Leon-Chisen, RHIA

For organizational providers, implementation of new coding systems involves primarily two types of costs: coder training and information system changes. Hospitals need to plan for the transition to *ICD-10-CM* for both inpatient and outpatient services, and to *ICD-10-PCS* for inpatient services. All other providers, such as physicians, home health agencies, skilled nursing facilities, and post–acute care settings, will be affected by a change to *ICD-10-CM* only—since *ICD-10-PCS* is only being contemplated for reporting inpatient services by hospitals.

PERSONNEL TRAINING

The bulk of the costs for implementing *ICD-10-CM* and *ICD-10-PCS* will be incurred for the training of coding personnel. Training will need to include support staff, such as coders and billers, as well as any others involved in coding or reviewing coding information. Users will need to attend training seminars to familiarize themselves with the new coding guidelines, rules, and definitions. Hospitals will need to work with their medical staff to ensure that the appropriate documentation is available to support the new coding system. *ICD-10-PCS* code selection requires that more specific and detailed physician documentation be available in the health record. This greater level of specificity may also require that coders and billers expand their knowledge of medical terminology, anatomy and physiology, and disease process.

There will be expected loss-of-productivity issues as coders take time away from coding to familiarize themselves with the new coding system. Many hospital coders already attend approximately sixteen hours of training during the year to keep their coding skills current. It is assumed that these training costs will be replaced by costs associated with learning to use *ICD-10-CM* and *ICD-10-PCS*. However, current training for *ICD-9* is spread throughout the year, while training for *ICD-10* is likely to require bigger blocks of time. Coding productivity will also suffer until coders become proficient in the new system.

INFORMATION SYSTEM ISSUES

A change to *ICD-10-CM* and *ICD-10-PCS* also requires extensive modifications to information systems. Issues vary from software changes to data-field expansion, timing, and data-conversion planning. Hospitals and other providers will need to perform an inventory of existing databases and information systems to determine the impact on their operations. Collaboration among departments will be necessary to identify these systems. A systems inventory should be conducted to determine where databases exist, what software is available, and whether the software is from a commercial vendor or a homegrown or proprietary program unique to the provider facility. Senior management and information systems staff should be made aware of the imminent transition to a new coding system so that future expansions in software and hardware may be made while taking into consideration the needs of a coding change. Some providers have started making changes to their systems, and some of their commercial vendors have already done the work. Others are waiting to have more formal direction from the Department of Health and Human Services before making plans. However, taking advantage of the lead time will ease the transition process once a migration decision is published.

Commercial Software

Hospitals use a combination of purchased software and in-house developed applications. Physician offices also rely on purchased software, although some may have homegrown programs. The software applications that will require modification encompass functions such as code assignment, health records abstraction, aggregate data reporting, utilization management, clinical systems, billing, claim submission, groupers, and other financial functions. In essence, every electronic transaction requiring an *ICD-9-CM* code would need to be changed. These changes include software interfaces, field-length formats on screens, report formats and layouts, table structures holding codes, expansion of flat files, coding edits, and significant logic changes.

A migration to new coding systems such as *ICD-10-CM* and *ICD-10-PCS* would be a regulatory change. Most large health information system (HIS) vendors build the costs of regulatory changes into their user maintenance fees, so providers do not expect to incur additional costs for programming changes related to *ICD-10*. However, providers anticipate that, as a result of increased maintenance costs, they will see maintenance fees go up in the future.

Most maintenance contracts have a clause that covers regulatory changes. Some proactive providers have already been working with their commercial vendors to determine their system's capability for accepting new codes. Many large HIS vendors have indicated that they are ready to accept *ICD-10-CM* codes (because of Canadian or other international implementations), or that the field lengths have already been increased in anticipation of a migration to *ICD-10-CM* and *ICD-10-PCS*.

Homegrown/Proprietary Software

There is some variation across hospitals and other providers in the area of homegrown/ proprietary software. The majority of hospitals have been moving away from homegrown systems in the last few years because of the expense and lack of sufficient information systems and technology personnel to maintain a homegrown system. University-based or large research centers may have more proprietary systems built for a specific application or research project than would be found in small- or medium-sized urban or rural hospitals.

Large hospital systems may have commercial applications, but they may also have proprietary billing systems or billing edits specific to their hospitals. Some of the homegrown systems may have smaller databases built by a department using a PC-based application and using Excel or Access.

Several different software applications use *ICD-9-CM* codes. Examples of hospital software applications that would be affected by a change to *ICD-10-CM* and *ICD-10-PCS* may be found in figure 34.1.

FIGURE 34.1   Examples of Hospital Applications Affected by the Migration to *ICD-10-CM* and *ICD-10-PCS*

- Advanced Beneficiary Notice (ABN) Software
- Billing System
- Birth Defect Registries
- Case Management System
- Clinical Data Reporting
- Clinical Department Systems (including Lab, EKG, Radiology, Surgical Scheduling, Physical Therapy, Occupational Therapy, Speech Therapy, etc.)
- Compliance Checking Systems
- Decision Support Systems
- Diagnostic Related Groupings (DRG) Grouper
- Electronic Processing Systems (to submit claims to clearinghouse)
- Encoder Software
- Hospital Information System (HIS)
- Interface Engines
- Inpatient Rehabilitation Facility-Patient Assessment Instrument (IRFPAI) Data Collection System

- Managed Care (HEDIS) Reporting Systems
- Medical Necessity System
- Medical Record Abstracting System
- Minimum Data Set (MDS) Collection System
- OASIS System
- Outpatient Code Editor (OCE)
- Pharmacy Systems
- Physician Credentialing System
- Research Databases
- State Birth Registration Systems
- State Death Registration Systems
- State Reporting Systems (e.g., California hospitals, which report all their *ICD-9-CM* codes to the state of California)
- Test Ordering System
- Utilization Management

Hardware

During the transition period, information systems software will have to support both *ICD-9-CM* and *ICD-10-CM* and *ICD-10-PCS* coding systems, therefore potentially requiring additional data storage space. Some hospitals have already started expanding the field size for the diagnosis and procedure fields based on the HIPAA Transaction Standard Notice of Proposed Rulemaking that mentioned *ICD-10* as a possibility for the future.

Neither the field-size expansion nor the larger number of codes is considered to be a problem with today's systems. It would not be a huge increase since it is a small pocket compared to the rest of the database. Validation rules may take up more room in the system, but experts don't anticipate requiring more CPU or disk space. From a technology perspective, it is considered that twenty years ago the larger field size and more codes would have been a problem; but disk capacity is inexpensive now, and CPUs are cheaper, too.

DATA CONVERSION ISSUES

Providers will have to make decisions regarding the need to convert existing *ICD-9-CM* data. After conducting an inventory of the applications utilizing *ICD-9-CM* codes, a cost/benefit analysis should be performed to determine which databases would need to be converted. More than likely, a combination of old data conversion on an as-needed basis, with some up-front conversion immediately before implementation of *ICD-10*, would work best.

Other providers may consider it easier to run a report in *ICD-9-CM* and a separate report in *ICD-10-CM* or *ICD-10-PCS*, and then to add up both reports manually—therefore negating the need to perform a full conversion of the database.

Although a decision regarding national implementation of *ICD-10-CM* or *ICD-10-PCS* has not been made, a facility may start to prepare for the transition. The items in the following checklist should be considered in anticipation of this change. Once a notice of proposed rulemaking is published, a smoother transition can be accomplished if the following activities have already been performed.

CHECKLIST

- ✔ Start working with your medical staff to improve medical record documentation. There are tangible benefits that can be gained even with *ICD-9-CM.*

- ✔ Inform senior management regarding the potential budgetary, administrative, and operational implications of making the transition to *ICD-10.*

- ✔ Identify key players in your organization who should be part of your *ICD-10* implementation team.

- ✔ Identify an *ICD-10* team leader.

- ✔ Obtain a senior management level "sponsor" for *ICD-10*–related activities.

- ✔ Develop an inventory of existing databases and systems likely to be affected by a transition to *ICD-10-CM* and *ICD-10-PCS.*

- ✔ Determine which systems use homegrown, proprietary, or custom-made software.

- ✔ Consult with your existing software vendors to determine their awareness of *ICD-10* and their plans for upgrades.

- ✔ Determine whether your current contractual agreements with vendors will cover a change to *ICD-10.*

- ✔ Ensure that any future system improvements, such as plans for an electronic health record, take into consideration *ICD-10* readiness.

Final Review Exercise, Appendix, and Index

Final Review Exercise

The final review exercise draws on concepts presented throughout this handbook. Read each brief summary below and assign codes for all diagnoses and procedures, including E codes for external causes and locations of occurrence as needed. For purposes of this assignment, accept narrative statements (for example, conditions, procedures, or other therapy) as though listed in a diagnostic statement.

1. A patient was admitted with complaint of a dull ache and occasional acute pain in the right calf. Examination revealed swelling and redness of the calf as well as a slight fever. The patient gave a history of having been on Premarin therapy for the past 20 years and stated that she has always followed the doctor's instructions for its use. Venous plethysmography revealed the presence of a thrombus. The estrogen therapy dosage was modified, and the patient was discharged with a diagnosis of deep vein thrombosis and thrombophlebitis due to supplemental estrogen therapy. She will be seen in the office in one week and will be followed regularly over the next several months.

2. A patient was admitted to the hospital because he was suffering acute abdominal pain. He was also found to be intoxicated, and his medical history indicated that he has been alcohol dependent for several years with binging every three to four months. The current binge apparently started three days ago. The abdominal pain proved to be due to acute pancreatitis, and he was treated with nasogastric suction, administration of IV fluids, and pain control. The patient was observed for possible withdrawal reaction with standby orders; multiple vitamins were given.

3. A patient with a four-year history of anorexia nervosa was seen in the physician's office because of significant weight loss over the past three months, going from 82 pounds down to 53 pounds. She was admitted to increase body weight and to be given nutritional counseling because of her severe malnutrition.

4. A patient was admitted through the emergency department following a fall from a ladder while painting his house. He had contusions of the scalp and face and an open intertrochanteric fracture of the femur. The fracture site was debrided, and an open reduction with internal fixation was carried out.

5. A patient who underwent a modified radical mastectomy of the left breast six months earlier because of carcinoma now has metastasis to the bone. She was admitted for a transfusion of packed cells to treat aplastic anemia, probably due to her treatment by chemotherapy. She was discharged with a hemoglobin of 11.5 and will be followed as an outpatient.

6. A patient was admitted for cholecystectomy because of chronic cholecystitis. Before she went to the operating room the next morning, nursing personnel noted that she had apparently developed a urinary infection, and laboratory tests confirmed a diagnosis of urinary tract infection due to E. coli. Because of the infection, the surgery was canceled, antibiotic therapy was instituted, and the patient was discharged on the third hospital day to continue antibiotic therapy at home. She will be seen in the physician's office in three weeks, and surgery will be rescheduled.

7. A patient who recently underwent an oophorectomy because of adenocarcinoma of the ovary was admitted to the hospital for chemotherapy. Shortly after administration of the therapy, the patient developed a fever and chills and on the second day she had a productive cough. Chest X-rays indicated an acute pneumonia, and sputum culture was positive for Klebsiella. Antibiotics were administered, and the patient was discharged on the fifth hospital day.

8. A patient who had noticed significant abdominal enlargement over a period of several weeks without a change in her dietary habits was admitted for exploratory laparotomy. Surgery revealed a large ovarian tumor, and the left ovary was resected. The pelvic cavity was explored thoroughly for any evidence of metastatic spread, but none was noted. Chemotherapy treatments were started on the day prior to discharge, and the patient was scheduled to continue therapy on an outpatient basis.

9. A patient who had undergone surgery for carcinoma of the breast two months earlier has since been on a program of chemotherapy. On a routine office visit yesterday, the physician noted that she had become severely dehydrated as a result of this program and she was admitted for IV therapy for rehydration. Her regular chemotherapy session was carried out on the third day.

10. A patient was admitted with abdominal pain and complaints of melena noted for the past two days. Examination revealed an acute diverticulitis of the colon. Laboratory studies reported a significant hypokalemia, and the patient was placed on oral potassium. Bleeding subsided within a few days on conservative treatment, and the patient was discharged to be followed on an outpatient basis.

11. A patient was admitted with complaints of severe joint pain affecting the hands and hips. The physician's diagnosis indicated rheumatoid arthritis with sympathetic inflammatory myopathy.

12. A patient who was two months pregnant contracted rubella. On her next prenatal visit to the doctor's office, it was decided to admit the patient for therapeutic abortion because of the probability of abnormality of the fetus. Complete abortion was carried out by D & C.

13. Increasing fetal distress was noted during labor. The patient was transferred to the surgical suite, where a classical cesarean delivery was performed. A full-term normal male was delivered.

14. A patient was admitted with congestive heart failure and unstable angina. The unstable angina was treated with nitrates, and IV Lasix was administered to manage the heart failure. Both conditions improved, and the patient was discharged to be followed on an outpatient basis.

15. A patient was admitted for observation and evaluation for possible intracranial injury following a collision with another car while he was driving to work. Patient had minor bruises on the upper back and abrasions of the skin of the upper extremity. The bruises did not appear to need any treatment; the abrasions were swabbed with disinfectant and Neosporin was applied. Intracranial injury was ruled out.

16. A patient was brought to the emergency department following a burn injury experienced in a fire at the garage where he works. He was admitted and treated for first-degree and second-degree burns of the forearm and third-degree burn of the back.

17. A patient was admitted because of suspected carcinoma of the colon. Exploratory laparotomy was carried out, and a significant mass was discovered in the sigmoid colon. The sigmoid colon was resected and end-to-end anastomosis accomplished. Small nodules were noted on the liver, and a needle biopsy of the liver was performed during the procedure. The pathology report confirmed adenocarcinoma of the colon with metastasis to the liver.

18. A patient was discharged following prostate surgery with an indwelling catheter in place. He was readmitted with urinary sepsis due to Staphylococcus aureus due to the presence of the catheter. The physician confirmed the diagnosis of sepsis. The catheter was removed and the patient started on antibiotic therapy. The patient's condition improved over several days, and he was discharged without an indwelling catheter.

19. A patient six months pregnant was diagnosed as having an iron-deficiency anemia and was admitted for packed-cell transfusion.

20. A patient was admitted with occlusion of the carotid artery, and carotid endarterectomy was carried out with extracorporeal circulation used throughout the procedure.

21. A patient was admitted in a coma due to acute cerebrovascular thrombosis with cerebral infarction; the coma cleared by the fourth hospital day. Aphasia and hemiparesis were also present. The aphasia had cleared by discharge, but the hemiparesis was still present.

22. A patient was admitted with severe abdominal pain that began two days ago and progressed in severity. Esophagogastroduodenoscopy (EGD) revealed an acute gastric ulcer, but no signs of hemorrhage or malignancy were noted. The patient was put on a medical regimen that included an ulcer diet and was advised not to take aspirin.

23. A patient with type 1 diabetes mellitus seriously out of control was admitted for regulation of insulin dosage. The patient had been in the hospital four weeks earlier for an acute ST elevation myocardial infarction of the inferoposterior wall, and an EKG was performed to check its current status.

24. A patient who was treated seven weeks ago at Community Hospital for an acute antero-lateral myocardial infarction is now admitted to University Hospital for surgical repair of an atrial septal defect resulting from the previous infarction. Following thoracotomy, the defect was repaired with a tissue graft; cardiopulmonary bypass was used during the procedure. The patient was discharged in good condition, to be followed as an outpatient.

25. A patient with both conductive and sensorineural deafness was admitted for cochlear implantation. A multiple-channel implant was inserted, and the patient was discharged, to be followed as an outpatient.

26. A patient who underwent a kidney transplant three months ago is admitted for biopsy because of an increased creatinine level discovered on an outpatient visit. Percutaneous biopsy revealed chronic rejection syndrome. The patient was discharged on a modified medication regimen, to be followed closely as an outpatient.

27. A patient was admitted with a fracture of the shaft of the right femur. Closed reduction was carried out and skeletal traction applied.

28. A patient who has had recurrent attacks of angina pectoris was seen in his physician's office because he felt that the anginal attacks seemed to be occurring more frequently and to be more severe and more difficult to control. He had not had a thorough evaluation previously and bypass surgery had not been recommended in the past. He was admitted to the hospital for diagnostic studies to determine the underlying cause of this unstable angina. He underwent combined right- and left-heart catheterization, which revealed significant atherosclerotic heart disease. He was advised that coronary artery bypass surgery was indicated, but he did not want to make a decision without further discussion with his family. He was discharged on antianginal medication and will be seen in the doctor's office in one week.

29. The patient discussed in the preceding case returned to the hospital for bypass surgery. Reverse saphenous vein grafts were brought from the aorta to the obtuse marginal and the right coronary artery; the internal mammary artery was loosened and brought down to the left anterior descending artery to bypass this obstruction. The gastroepiploic artery was used to bypass the circumflex. Extracorporeal circulation and intraoperative pacemaker were used during the procedure.

30. A patient was brought to the hospital by ambulance after a fall from the scaffolding while working on the construction of a new bank building. He had struck his head and experienced a brief period of unconsciousness (less than one hour). On examination, he was found to have an open skull fracture with cerebral laceration and contusion. The skull fracture was reduced after debridement and the patient was transferred to the intensive care unit, where he stayed for four days. He was discharged on the tenth day in good condition, advised to avoid any strenuous activity and to see his physician in one week.

31. A patient was admitted for corrective surgery for a keloid of the left hand due to a burn experienced in a brush fire one year ago. Radical excision of the scar was carried out, and the defect was covered with a full-thickness graft taken from the upper arm. The patient was discharged in good condition, to be seen in the physician's office in two weeks.

32. A patient was brought to the emergency department by ambulance at 1 a.m. by her husband, who stated that they had been to a dinner party at a friend's home earlier in the evening. His wife had two martinis before the meal and several glasses of wine with the meal. At bedtime she took Valium that her physician had ordered prn for nervousness and inability to sleep. Shortly thereafter, the husband noticed that she appeared to be somewhat stuporous and became worried about her condition and brought her to the emergency department.

33. A patient was admitted to the hospital with an admitting diagnosis of acute hip pain. There was no history of trauma; she stated that she had simply stood up from her chair, immediately experienced acute pain in the left leg, and fallen back into the chair. She has had osteoporosis for several years and is also a known diabetic. An X-ray revealed a fracture of the lower third of the shaft of the femur. A routine preoperative chest X-ray showed a few strands of atelectasis and a small cloudy area that may have represented mild pleural effusion. A cast was applied to the leg to immobilize the fracture. Her blood sugar was monitored throughout the stay. The physician documented spontaneous fracture secondary to osteoporosis.

34. A patient with a five-year history of emphysema was brought to the hospital's emergency department in acute respiratory failure. Endotracheal intubation was carried out in the emergency department, and the patient placed on mechanical ventilation. She was then admitted to unit 400, where she remained on the ventilator for three days and then was taken off the ventilator without a weaning period. She was discharged on the fifth hospital day.

35. A patient in acute respiratory failure was brought to the hospital by ambulance with ventilator in place. In the ambulance, an endotracheal tube was inserted into the patient. He had a long history of congestive heart failure, and studies confirmed that he was in congestive failure, with pleural effusion and acute pulmonary edema. The patient was treated with diuretics, and his cardiac condition was brought back into an acceptable range. He continued on ventilation for four days and was weaned on the fifth day. The physician was questioned regarding the reason for the admission, and she indicated that the patient was admitted for the respiratory failure.

36. A fourteen-year-old student was referred by the school health department for professional evaluation of a suspected mental disorder. According to the school counselor, he did not communicate well with other students and had demonstrated what the counselor felt was antisocial behavior generally. No evidence of mental disorder was found, and no other diagnosis to explain the student's apparent problems was identified.

37. A patient with hypertensive and diabetic chronic kidney disease who is on chronic dialysis is admitted because of dialysis disequilibrium (electrolyte imbalance).

38. A patient who has had arteriosclerotic disease of the right lower extremity with intermittent claudication for three years recently progressed to ulceration, and is now admitted with ulceration and gangrene of the toes of the right foot resulting from the arteriosclerosis. A transmetatarsal amputation of the right toes was performed, and the patient left the operating room in good condition.

39. A two-year-old child with a severe cough was admitted to the hospital with a history of having experienced malaise, loss of appetite, and cough for several days. In addition to the cough, he was experiencing some shortness of breath, and a chest X-ray showed an acute pneumonia. Sputum cultures showed B. pertussis. He was started on IV antibiotics and became afebrile on the fifth hospital day. A repeat chest X-ray was negative on the sixth hospital day, and the cough had partially cleared. He was discharged on the eighth day to be cared for at home and followed as an outpatient.

40. A ten-year-old boy was admitted because of severe cellulitis of the left leg. He had gone on a hiking trip in the nearby forest with his scout troop a week earlier and now has a painful reddened area on the left leg. He stated that there was a good deal of thorny brush and that he had several minor thorn punctures but had experienced no problem with them. The day before admission he had developed a painful swollen area that had become worse during the night. A diagnosis of cellulitis due to Streptococcus A was made and antibiotics were administered. The wound itself was evaluated but did not appear to need specific treatment. The area on the leg progressively healed. The patient was discharged to continue the antibiotic series at home and will be seen in the office in one week.

41. An unconscious patient was admitted with concussion and a skull fracture and subdural hematoma after falling from a high diving board and hitting the side of the pool. Drainage of the subdural space was carried out by incision and the fracture reduced. The patient left the operating room in fair condition but died the following day.

42. A patient was admitted because of increasing confusion and memory loss, which his family was unable to deal with. The patient was disoriented and unable to furnish any information. He was diagnosed as having senile dementia with Alzheimer's disease and was transferred to a nursing home.

43. Newborn twin girls, both living, were delivered in the hospital at 35 weeks, with extreme immaturity and weight of 850 grams for twin #1 and 900 grams for twin #2. Both were transferred to the neonatal intensive care nursery with a diagnosis of extreme immaturity.

44. A patient with a long history of angina pectoris came to the emergency department complaining of increasing anginal pain that he could not relieve with nitroglycerin and rest. The pain had occurred again about an hour ago and has been increasing in severity. Cardiac catheterization done recently showed some occlusion of the right coronary artery. It was decided to go ahead with a percutaneous transluminal coronary angioplasty, using a thrombolytic agent, in the hope of averting what appeared to be an impending myocardial infarction. The procedure was carried out without incident and the infarction was averted, but the patient did have an occlusion of the coronary artery.

45. A patient was admitted to the hospital with unstable angina that had been increasing in severity since the previous day. He was placed on bed rest and telemetry, and IV nitroglycerin was administered. An EKG showed some paroxysmal tachycardia as well, and so IV heparin was added to his medication program. His angina returned to its normal status, and the tachycardia was not shown on repeat studies at the end of one week. The patient was discharged to be seen by a visiting nurse over the next two weeks to supervise his medication regimen, and an appointment with his physician was made for two weeks later.

46. A patient who had been HIV positive for several years was seen in his physician's office with skin lesions over his back suggestive of HIV-related Kaposi's sarcoma. He was admitted for incisional biopsy, which confirmed the diagnosis.

47. A patient was admitted through the emergency department with acute right flank pain and was taken to surgery for removal of a ruptured appendix. At the time of the appendectomy, generalized peritonitis was observed along with some suspicious nodules on the head of the pancreas. A needle biopsy was performed while the abdomen was open; a diagnosis of carcinoma of the pancreas was made on the basis of the pathological examination.

48. A patient with a long history of type 1 diabetes mellitus was admitted in hyperosmolar coma with blood sugars out of control. Modification of the insulin regimen was instituted and the patient was monitored carefully throughout her stay. The coma cleared on the first hospital day, and the patient was brought into control over the next four days. In addition to this acute metabolic condition, she also had a diagnosis of diabetic nephropathy, with the complication identified as nephrotic syndrome. The patient was discharged on a modified insulin regimen and will be followed by a visiting nurse until the new program stabilizes.

49. A patient was admitted with severe decubitus ulcer on the left buttock, with extensive necrotic tissue and gangrene. She was taken to the operating room, where the surgeon carefully excised the necrotic tissue. The ulcer site was then treated with antibiotic ointment and gauze bandage, and the patient was returned to the nursing unit, where the wound was monitored carefully and additional antibiotic treatment was administered. By the fourth day, healing was beginning to close the area, but treatment was continued until discharge on the seventh day. The family was advised to use an egg crate mattress and to turn the patient regularly. The patient was scheduled for an outpatient visit in one week.

50. A patient with a diagnosis of end-stage renal disease due to type 1 diabetes mellitus was admitted for her first hemodialysis session. A central venous catheter was placed and hemodialysis carried out. Patient tolerated the procedure well and will continue receiving hemodialysis on a regular schedule.

ANSWERS TO FINAL REVIEW EXERCISE

1. 451.19   Thrombophlebitis of femoral vein

    E932.2   Therapeutic use of estrogen

    89.58   Plethysmogram

    Comment: Although the physician listed both thrombus and thrombophlebitis in the diagnosis, the code for thrombophlebitis includes the thrombosis; therefore, no additional code is assigned. Because this condition is an adverse effect of estrogen use, an E code for the medication is assigned.

2. 577.0   Acute pancreatitis

    303.02   Acute alcoholic intoxication in alcoholism

    94.62   Alcohol detoxification

    Comment: The condition responsible for the admission was the acute pancreatitis. No code is assigned for the abdominal pain because it is integral to the acute pancreatitis. The observation for withdrawal, standby orders, and administration of multiple vitamins are sufficient to code detoxification, but no withdrawal delirium occurred and so only the code for acute intoxication in alcoholism is assigned. Documentation indicates that the pattern of use was episodic.

3. 307.1   Anorexia nervosa

    261   Severe malnutrition

    Comment: Code 261, Nutritional marasmus, should be assigned as an additional diagnosis for the severe malnutrition. For some anorexic patients, the weight loss is so severe that it leads to malnutrition. Code 261 further describes the severity of the patient's condition.

4. 820.31   Open pertrochanteric fracture, intertrochanteric section

    920   Contusion of face and scalp

    E881.0   Fall from ladder

    E849.0   Home

    79.35   Open reduction with internal fixation

    79.65   Debridement

    Comment: When several injuries are present, the most severe is designated as the principal diagnosis.

5. 284.8   Aplastic anemia

    198.5   Secondary malignant neoplasm of bone

    E933.1   Adverse effect of antineoplastic and immunosuppressive drugs

    V10.3   History of malignant neoplasm of breast

    99.04   Transfusion of packed cells

    Comment: The complication of anemia is designated the principal diagnosis because it is the condition that occasioned admission to the hospital and the thrust of treatment. A code is assigned for the metastasis to the bone and a history code to indicate the previous breast malignancy. Code E933.1 includes the chemotherapy as the external cause (adverse effect) of the aplastic anemia.

6. 575.11   Chronic cholecystitis

    599.0   Urinary tract infection, due to

    041.4   E. coli

    V64.1   Surgery not carried out because of contraindication

    Comment: The principal diagnosis does not change because the planned treatment was not carried out; therefore, the cholecystitis is the principal diagnosis. Code V64.1 is assigned to indicate that the planned surgery was canceled because of a contraindication, which was the urinary tract infection.

7. <u>V58.11</u>   Encounter for antineoplastic chemotherapy
    183.0   Malignant neoplasm of ovary
    482.0   Klebsiella pneumonia
    99.25   Injection or infusion of cancer chemotherapeutic substance

Comment: When a patient is receiving therapy for neoplastic disease, a code for that condition is assigned rather than a history code, even though resection may have been performed previously. Because the patient was admitted solely for chemotherapy, V58.11 remains the principal diagnosis even though the patient remained in the hospital because of the pneumonia. Code 183.0 is assigned as an additional code rather than a history code because the patient is still under treatment.

8. <u>183.0</u>   Malignant neoplasm of ovary
    65.39   Unilateral oophorectomy
    99.25   Chemotherapy

Comment: When adjunct therapy such as radiotherapy or chemotherapy is given during an admission in which definitive surgery was performed, the code for the neoplasm is designated as the principal diagnosis and no code from category V58 is assigned. No code is assigned for the laparotomy because it is the operative approach for the oophorectomy.

9. <u>276.51</u>   Dehydration
    174.9   Malignant neoplasm of breast, unspecified
    E933.1   Adverse effect of antineoplastic and immunosuppressive drugs
    99.25   Chemotherapy

Comment: Because this admission was for the sole purpose of treating the dehydration, a complication of the chemotherapy, dehydration is designated the principal diagnosis, with an additional code for the malignant neoplasm. Even though she received chemotherapy during her hospital stay, the admission was not solely for that purpose and so V58.11 is not assigned.

10. <u>562.13</u>   Diverticulitis of colon with hemorrhage
    276.8   Hypopotassemia

Comment: The presence of melena indicates that bleeding is associated with the diverticulitis, and fifth-digit 3 is used to indicate that there is associated hemorrhage. Bleeding in a patient with diverticulitis is presumed to be due to the diverticulitis unless the physician specifies that it is due to a different cause. No code is assigned for the abdominal pain as it is implicit in the diagnosis. The low potassium was treated and therefore is a reportable diagnosis.

11. <u>714.0</u>   Rheumatoid arthritis
    359.6   Symptomatic inflammatory myopathy in disease classified elsewhere

Comment: No code for the joint pain is assigned because it is a characteristic component of rheumatoid arthritis. An instructional note at code 714.0 indicates that code 359.6 should be assigned when this type of myopathy is also present.

12. <u>635.92</u>   Legally induced abortion, complete
    655.33   Suspected damage to fetus from viral disease in mother
    69.01   D & C for termination of pregnancy

Comment: Because the fetal condition was responsible for modifying the treatment of the mother, the code for it is assigned to explain the rationale for the abortion. Fifth digit 3 is assigned because this is an antepartum condition.

13. <u>656.81</u>   Fetal distress
    74.0   Classical cesarean section
    V27.0   Single liveborn

Comment: In this case, the fetal distress affected the management of the mother, leading to the decision to deliver by cesarean.

14. <u>428.0</u>   Congestive heart failure

      411.1   Intermediate coronary syndrome

Comment: Because both conditions equally meet the criteria for principal diagnosis, either may be listed first.

15. <u>V71.4</u>   Observation following other accident

      922.31   Contusion of back

      913.0   Abrasion without mention of infection

      E812.0   Motor vehicle accident involving collision with another vehicle, driver

Comment: When the patient is admitted for observation for a possible serious injury such as an intracranial injury, the V71 code is assigned as the principal diagnosis even when minor injuries are present. In this case, the purpose of admission was to observe the patient; the minor injuries would not have required hospital admission. Additional codes are assigned for the minor injuries.

16. <u>942.34</u>   Third-degree burn of back

      943.21   Second-degree burn of forearm

      E891.3   Burning caused by conflagration

      E849.3   Industrial place and premises

Comment: When several burns are present, the burn of the highest degree takes precedence; therefore, the third-degree burn of the back is designated as the principal diagnosis. When more than one degree of burn occurs at the same site, only the code for the highest degree is assigned; therefore, only the second degree of the forearm is coded.

17. <u>153.3</u>   Malignant neoplasm of sigmoid colon

      197.7   Malignant neoplasm of liver, specified as secondary

      45.76   Sigmoidectomy

      50.11   Needle biopsy of liver

Comment: No code is assigned for the exploratory laparotomy because it is the operative approach for the sigmoidectomy. End-to-end anastomosis is included in the code for the colon resection. A needle biopsy performed during open surgery is coded as a closed biopsy.

18. <u>996.64</u>   Urinary sepsis due to indwelling urinary catheter

      038.11   Staphylococcal septicemia, staphylococcus aureus septicemia

      995.91   Sepsis

      599.0   Urinary tract infection, site not specified

      E879.6   Other procedures without mention of misadventure at the time of procedure as the cause of abnormal reaction of patient or of later complication, Urinary catheterization

      97.64   Removal of indwelling catheter

Comment: This infection was due to the presence of the indwelling catheter and is coded as an infection of that device. The physician also confirmed the diagnosis of sepsis. Code 038.11 is assigned for staphylococcus aureus sepsis instead of code 038.9. Code 995.91 is assigned along with code 038.11 to further describe sepsis.

19. <u>648.23</u>   Anemia complicating pregnancy

      280.9   Iron-deficiency anemia, unspecified

      99.04   Transfusion of packed cells

Comment: Code 648.23 from chapter 11 is assigned as the principal diagnosis because the anemia is complicating the pregnancy. Fifth digit 3 is assigned as this is an antepartum complication. Code 280.9 is also assigned to provide greater specificity as to the type of anemia.

20. <u>433.10</u>   Occlusion of carotid artery

    38.12   Endarterectomy of other vessel of head and neck (carotid artery)

    39.61   Cardiopulmonary bypass (extracorporeal circulation)

    Comment: Fifth digit 0 is assigned because there is no mention of infarction associated with the carotid occlusion. The carotid artery is included in the surgery code for "other vessels of head and neck." An instructional note with code 38.1x indicates that an additional code of 39.61 should be assigned when extracorporeal circulation is used during the endarterectomy.

21. <u>434.01</u>   Cerebral thrombosis with cerebral infarction

    780.01   Coma

    342.90   Hemiplegia

    Comment: A code for coma is assigned because it is not integral to a diagnosis of cerebral thrombosis. Codes for neurological deficits that clear by discharge are not coded and so no code for aphasia is assigned. A code for the hemiparesis is assigned because it was still present at discharge. Fifth digit 0 is assigned because there is no mention of whether the hemiparesis affected the dominant or nondominant side.

22. <u>531.30</u>   Acute gastric ulcer without mention of hemorrhage or perforation

    45.13   Esophagogastroduodenoscopy

    Comment: No code is assigned for the abdominal pain because it is integral to gastric ulcer.

23. <u>250.03</u>   Diabetes mellitus, type 1, out of control

    410.32   Inferolateral myocardial infarction, subsequent episode of care

    Comment: Fifth digit 3 is used to indicate that the diabetes mellitus was out of control. A patient admitted four weeks after an acute myocardial infarction will always require clinical evaluation; in this case, a specific diagnostic study was performed also. Fifth digit 2 indicates that this is a subsequent admission for the infarction.

24. <u>429.71</u>   Acquired cardiac septal defect

    410.02   Subsequent episode of care for anteroseptal myocardial infarction

    35.61   Repair of septal defect with tissue graft

    39.61   Cardiopulmonary bypass

    Comment: Although seven weeks have elapsed since the infarction, it is coded and reported (subsequent episode). A code for infarction is assigned through the eighth week following its occurrence. It required continuing evaluation and monitoring during the stay. Fifth digit 2 is assigned to indicate that this is a subsequent episode of care for this infarction. No code is assigned for the thoracotomy because it is the operative approach for the repair.

25. <u>389.2</u>   Mixed conductive and sensorineural hearing loss

    20.98   Implantation of multiple channel cochlear prosthetic device

    Comment: Because a combination code including both types of hearing loss is provided, only code 389.2 is assigned rather than individual codes for the hearing loss.

26. <u>996.81</u>   Complication of transplanted kidney

    55.23   Closed biopsy of kidney

    Comment: Transplant rejection is coded as a complication of the transplanted organ. A percutaneous biopsy is a closed biopsy.

27. <u>821.01</u>   Closed fracture of shaft of femur

    79.05   Closed reduction of fracture of femur without internal fixation

Comment: When the diagnostic statement does not indicate whether the fracture is open or closed, *ICD-9-CM* classifies it as closed. Application of skeletal traction is included in the code for closed reduction, and no additional code is assigned.

28. <u>414.01</u>   Arteriosclerosis of native coronary artery

    411.1   Unstable angina

    37.23   Combined right- and left-heart catheterization

Comment: When the purpose of admission for a patient with unstable angina is to determine the underlying cause, the code for the underlying condition is designated as the principal diagnosis.

29. <u>414.01</u>   Arteriosclerosis of native coronary artery

    36.12   Aortocoronary bypass of two coronary arteries

    36.15   Single internal mammary–coronary artery bypass

    36.17   Abdominal–coronary artery bypass

    39.61   Cardiopulmonary bypass

    39.64   Intraoperative cardiac pacemaker

Comment: Four coronary artery bypass grafts were placed, two of which were aortocoronary, one an internal mammary–coronary artery, and one an abdominal–coronary bypass. Codes are assigned for the cardiopulmonary bypass and the intraoperative pacemaker.

30. <u>803.62</u>   Open skull fracture with cerebral laceration and contusion, with brief loss of consciousness

    E881.1   Fall from scaffolding

    E849.3   Industrial place and premises (building under construction)

    02.02   Elevation of skull fracture fragments

Comment: *ICD-9-CM* provides a combination code that includes both the fracture and the cerebral lacerations and contusions. Debridement of compound (open) fracture of the skull is included in the code for fracture reduction.

31. <u>701.4</u>   Keloid scar

    906.6   Late effect of burn of hand

    E929.4   Late effect of accident caused by fire

    86.4   Radical excision of skin lesion

    86.61   Full-thickness skin graft to hand

Comment: The residual keloid is sequenced first, with code 906.6 indicating that it is a late effect of a burn of the wrist and hand. Because the condition is a late effect, the E code must also be a late effect code. No code is assigned for excision of skin for the graft because the exclusion note for 86.91 indicates that it is not to be used when skin for the graft is excised during the same episode of care in which the graft is applied.

32. <u>980.0</u>   Poisoning by ethyl alcohol

    969.4   Poisoning by Valium

    780.09   Other alteration of consciousness (stupor)

    E860.0   Accidental poisoning by alcoholic beverage

    E853.2   Accidental poisoning by benzodiazepine-based tranquilizer (Valium)

    E849.0   Home

Comment: Although the Valium was used correctly, the fact that alcohol was also taken during the same period of time makes this a poisoning. Because two substances were involved, two poisoning codes and two E codes are assigned. Either poisoning code can be designated as principal diagnosis.

33. <u>733.15</u>   Pathological fracture of other specified part of the femur

    733.00   Osteoporosis, unspecified

    250.00   Diabetes mellitus, unspecified type

    93.53   Application of cast

Comment: Spontaneous fractures such as this are always classified as pathological. Although the osteoporosis was not treated, it is the underlying cause of the fracture and a code is needed for complete coding. No codes are assigned for the atelectasis or possible pleural effusion because these represent X-ray findings only, without further evaluation or treatment. The diabetes was monitored and so a code is assigned.

34. <u>518.81</u>   Respiratory failure

    492.8   Emphysema

    96.71   Continuous mechanical ventilation for less than 96 consecutive hours

    96.04   Insertion of endotracheal tube

Comment: Respiratory failure associated with chronic pulmonary disease, such as emphysema, can be designated as the principal diagnosis. The patient was on mechanical ventilation only three days, a total of less than 96 hours. A code is assigned for the tube insertion because it was performed in the emergency department of the hospital with immediate admission.

35. 518.81   Acute respiratory failure

    <u>428.0</u>   Congestive heart failure

    96.72   Continuous mechanical ventilation for 96 hours or more

Comment: When a patient is admitted with respiratory failure and another acute condition (e.g., congestive heart failure), the principal diagnosis will not be the same in every situation. Selection of the principal diagnosis will depend on the circumstances of admission. In this instance, the physician had to be queried to determine whether the congestive heart failure or the respiratory failure was responsible for the admission. Pleural effusion and acute pulmonary edema are part of congestive heart failure, and no additional codes are assigned for these conditions. Time counting for mechanical ventilation begins at time of admission when the ventilator is already in use. No code is assigned for the endotracheal tube insertion because it was done in the ambulance and cannot be reported by the hospital.

36. V71.02   Observation for possible mental disorder, adolescent antisocial behavior

    94.08   Other psychologic evaluation and testing

Comment: It is appropriate to use category V71 when a patient is seen for evaluation and no diagnosis is made. If the suspected diagnosis or a related diagnosis had been established, including a significant symptom, the code for that condition would be assigned rather than the code from category V71.

37. <u>276.9</u>   Electrolyte and fluid disorders, not elsewhere classified

    403.91   Hypertensive chronic kidney disease with chronic kidney disease stage V or end-stage renal disease

    585.6   End-stage renal disease

    250.40   Diabetes mellitus with renal manifestations

    V45.1   Dialysis status

    E879.1   Other procedures without mention of misadventure at the time of procedure as the cause of abnormal reaction of patient or of later complication, Kidney dialysis

Comment: When chronic kidney disease is the result of both hypertension and diabetes mellitus, both 403.xx and 250.4x are assigned. Because the patient has hypertensive chronic kidney disease and is on chronic dialysis, codes 403.x1 and 585.6 are assigned. Code E879.1 is assigned to indicate that the dialysis is responsible for the condition. The fact that the patient is receiving regular dialysis is significant, so the code for dialysis status can be assigned.

38. <u>440.24</u>   Atherosclerosis of the extremities with gangrene

    707.15   Ulcer of other part of foot

    84.12   Amputation through foot

Comment: Code 440.24 includes gangrene. An additional code may be assigned for the ulceration. A transmetatarsal amputation is coded as amputation through the foot as indicated in the Alphabetic Index and in the inclusion note for code 84.12.

39. <u>033.0</u>   Whooping cough due to B. pertussis

    484.3   Pneumonia in whooping cough

Comment: Whooping cough is the condition resulting from infection by B. pertussis. When pneumonia is associated with whooping cough, both the Alphabetic Index and the instructional note indicate that dual codes must be assigned, with the code for whooping cough sequenced first.

40. <u>682.6</u>   Cellulitis of leg

    891.1   Open wound of leg, complicated

    041.01   Bacterial infection due to group A Streptococcus

    E920.8   Accident caused by other specified piercing instrument (thorn)

    E849.8   Other specified place (forest)

Comment: In this case, the minor puncture wounds did not require treatment at the time they occurred and would not have required hospital care; therefore, the cellulitis is designated as the principal diagnosis. The wounds were evaluated, however, and so a code for the injury is assigned. Because of this infection, the open wound is classified as complicated.

41. <u>803.25</u> Closed skull fracture with subdural hematoma

    E883.0   Accident from diving into water (swimming pool)

    E849.4   Place of recreation or sport

    02.02   Elevation of skull fracture fragments

    01.31   Incision and drainage of subdural space

Comment: The subdural hematoma is included in code 803.25. No code is assigned for concussion when there is skull fracture with intracranial injury. Fifth digit 5 is used because the patient was unconscious on admission, never regained consciousness, and expired the following day. Two procedure codes are needed, one for the fracture reduction and one for the incision and drainage of the hematoma.

42. <u>331.0</u>   Alzheimer's disease

    294.10   Dementia in disease classified elsewhere without behavioral disturbance

Comment: When dementia is associated with Alzheimer's disease, the code for Alzheimer's disease is sequenced first, followed by code 294.10.

43. Twin #1: <u>V31.00</u> Liveborn twin, mate liveborn, born in hospital without mention of cesarean delivery

           765.03 Extreme immaturity, weight 750–999 grams

           765.28 35–36 Completed weeks of gestation

   Twin #2: V31.00 Liveborn twin, mate liveborn, born in hospital without mention of cesarean delivery

           765.03 Extreme immaturity, weight 750–999 grams

           765.28 35–36 Completed weeks of gestation

Comment: A code from categories V30–V39 is always designated as the principal diagnosis for the episode in which birth occurs. A fifth digit is assigned to indicate whether the delivery was by cesarean; in this case, it was not. An additional code is assigned to indicate extreme immaturity, with a fifth digit indicating the weight.

44. <u>411.81</u> Coronary occlusion without myocardial infarction

    00.66   Percutaneous transluminal coronary angioplasty

    00.40   Procedure on single vessel

    99.10   Injection or infusion of thrombolytic agent

Comment: The code for intermediate artery syndrome (411.1) is not assigned when a code from 411.8x is also assigned. Code 00.66 is assigned for the PTCA, with code 00.40 indicating that the PTCA was done on a single vessel. The infusion of a thrombolytic agent is reported separately using code 99.10.

45. <u>411.1</u>   Intermediate coronary syndrome
    427.2   Paroxysmal tachycardia, unspecified
    89.52   Electrocardiogram

    Comment: In this case, no studies were done to identify the underlying pathology and no surgical intervention was undertaken. Therefore, the unstable angina is the principal diagnosis. Typically, tests such as EKGs, x-rays, and laboratory tests are not coded in the inpatient setting.

46. <u>042</u>   Human immunodeficiency virus (HIV) disease
    176.0   Kaposi's sarcoma of skin
    86.11   Biopsy of skin

    Comment: When the patient is admitted for treatment of a condition due to HIV infection, the code for the infection is designated as the principal diagnosis, with an additional code for the related condition.

47. <u>540.0</u>   Acute appendicitis with generalized peritonitis
    157.0   Malignant neoplasm of pancreas, Head of pancreas
    47.09   Appendectomy
    52.11   Percutaneous biopsy of pancreas

    Comment: The code for the appendicitis is designated the principal diagnosis because it was clearly the condition that occasioned the admission. The code for the malignant neoplasm is also assigned, but there is no guideline that suggests that a malignancy takes any precedence in a situation of this type. A needle biopsy done in the course of an open surgical procedure is coded as a closed biopsy.

48. <u>250.23</u>   Diabetes mellitus, type 1, with hyperosmolarity, out of control
    250.43   Diabetes mellitus, type 1 out of control, with nephropathy
    581.81   Nephrotic syndrome in disease classified elsewhere

    Comment: The code for diabetes mellitus with hyperosmolarity includes the associated coma. Although a diagnosis of diabetic nephropathy was also established during this episode of care, it was the coma that occasioned the admission; therefore, it is designated as the principal diagnosis. Both diabetes codes use fifth digit 3 to indicate that it is type 1 and that it was also out of control.

49. <u>707.05</u>   Decubitus ulcer, buttock
    785.4   Gangrene
    86.22   Excisional debridement

    Comment: The code for gangrene must be sequenced following the code for the ulcer because it is a chapter 16 code (symptom) and the responsible condition is identified. Cutting away of necrotic tissue is considered to be an excisional debridement.

50. <u>V56.0</u>   Admitted for extracorporeal dialysis
    250.41   Diabetes mellitus, type 1, with renal manifestation
    585.6   End-stage renal disease
    39.95   Hemodialysis
    38.95   Venous catheterization for renal dialysis

    Comment: Code V56.0 is the principal diagnosis because this admission was solely for the purpose of dialysis. The fact that the venous catheter was inserted does not affect principal diagnosis assignment when the catheterization is followed by dialysis. A code for the diabetes mellitus is assigned with fourth digit 4 to indicate the presence of a kidney complication and fifth digit 1 to indicate that it is type 1 and not described as being out of control. The end-stage renal disease is the manifestation of the diabetes and the condition for which the dialysis is performed. Procedure codes are assigned for both the catheter insertion and the hemodialysis.

AHA
Coding Clinic™
for ICD-9-CM

ICD-9-CM Official Guidelines
for Coding and Reporting

Effective December 1, 2005
Narrative changes appear in bold text.
Items underlined have been moved
within the guidelines since April 2005.
The guidelines include the updated V
Code Table.

The Centers for Medicare and Medicaid Services (CMS) and the National Center for Health Statistics (NCHS), two departments within the U.S. Federal Government's Department of Health and Human Services (DHHS) provide the following guidelines for coding and reporting using the International Classification of Diseases, 9th Revision, Clinical Modification (ICD-9-CM). These guidelines should be used as a companion document to the official version of the ICD-9-CM as published on CD-ROM by the U.S. Government Printing Office (GPO).

These guidelines have been approved by the four organizations that make up the Cooperating Parties for the ICD-9-CM: the American Hospital Association (AHA), the American Health Information Management Association (AHIMA), CMS, and NCHS. These guidelines are included on the official government version of the ICD-9-CM, and also appear in *"Coding Clinic for ICD-9-CM"* published by the AHA.

These guidelines are a set of rules that have been developed to accompany and complement the official conventions and instructions provided within the ICD-9-CM itself. These guidelines are based on the coding and sequencing instructions in Volumes I, II and III of ICD-9-CM, but provide additional instruction. Adherence to these guidelines when assigning ICD-9-CM diagnosis and procedure codes is required under the Health Insurance Portability and Accountability Act (HIPAA). The diagnosis codes (Volumes 1-2) have been adopted under HIPAA for all healthcare settings. Volume 3 procedure codes have been adopted for inpatient procedures reported by hospitals. A joint effort between the healthcare provider and the coder is essential to achieve complete and accurate documentation, code assignment, and reporting of diagnoses and procedures. These guidelines have been developed to assist both the healthcare provider and the coder in identifying those diagnoses and procedures that are to be reported. The importance of consistent, complete documentation in the medical record cannot be overemphasized. Without such documentation accurate coding cannot be achieved. The entire record should be reviewed to determine the specific reason for the encounter and the conditions treated.

The term encounter is used for all settings, including hospital admissions. In the context of these guidelines, the term provider is used throughout the guidelines to mean physician or any qualified health care practitioner who is legally accountable for establishing the patient's diagnosis. Only this set of guidelines, approved by the Cooperating Parties, is official.

The guidelines are organized into sections. Section I includes the structure and conventions of the classification and general guidelines that apply to the entire classification, and chapter-specific guidelines that correspond to the chapters as they are arranged in the classification. Section II includes guidelines for selection of principal diagnosis for nonoutpatient settings. Section III includes guidelines for reporting additional diagnoses in nonoutpatient settings. Section IV is for outpatient coding and reporting.

ICD-9-CM Official Guidelines for Coding and Reporting

Section I. Conventions, general coding guidelines and chapter specific guidelines

A. Conventions for the ICD-9-CM
  1. Format
  2. Abbreviations
     a. Index abbreviations
     b. Tabular abbreviations
  3. Punctuation
  4. Includes and Excludes Notes and Inclusion terms
  5. Other and Unspecified codes
     a. "Other" codes
     b. "Unspecified" codes
  6. Etiology/manifestation convention ("code first," "use additional code" and "in diseases classified elsewhere" notes)
  7. "And"
  8. "With"
  9. "See" and "See Also"
B. General Coding Guidelines
  1. Use of Both Alphabetic Index and Tabular List
  2. Locate each term in the Alphabetic Index
  3. Level of Detail in Coding
  4. Code or codes from 001.0 through V84.8
  5. Selection of codes 001.0 through 999.9
  6. Signs and symptoms
  7. Conditions that are an integral part of a disease process
  8. Conditions that are not an integral part of a disease process
  9. Multiple coding for a single condition
  10. Acute and Chronic Conditions
  11. Combination Code
  12. Late Effects
  13. Impending or Threatened Condition
C. Chapter-Specific Coding Guidelines
  1. Chapter 1: Infectious and Parasitic Diseases (001-139)
     a. Human Immunodeficiency Virus (HIV) Infections
     b. Septicemia, Systemic Inflammatory Response Syndrome (SIRS), Sepsis, Severe Sepsis, and Septic Shock

2. Chapter 2: Neoplasms (140-239)
   a. Treatment directed at the malignancy
   b. Treatment of secondary site
   c. Coding and sequencing of complications
   d. Primary malignancy previously excised
   e. Admissions/Encounters involving chemotherapy and radiation therapy
   f. Admission/encounter to determine extent of malignancy
   g. Symptoms, signs, and ill-defined conditions listed in Chapter 16
3. Chapter 3: Endocrine, Nutritional, and Metabolic Diseases and Immunity Disorders (240-279)
   a. Diabetes mellitus
4. **Chapter 4: Diseases of Blood and Blood Forming Organs (280-289)**
   a. **Anemia of chronic disease**
5. Chapter 5: Mental Disorders (290-319)
   Reserved for future guideline expansion
6. Chapter 6: Diseases of Nervous System and Sense Organs (320-389)
   Reserved for future guideline expansion
7. Chapter 7: Diseases of Circulatory System (390-459)
   a. Hypertension
   b. Cerebral infarction/stroke/cerebrovascular accident (CVA)
   c. Postoperative cerebrovascular accident
   d. Late Effects of Cerebrovascular Disease
   e. **Acute myocardial infarction (AMI)**
8. Chapter 8: Diseases of Respiratory System (460-519)
   a. Chronic Obstructive Pulmonary Disease [COPD] and Asthma
   b. Chronic Obstructive Pulmonary Disease [COPD] and Bronchitis
9. Chapter 9: Diseases of Digestive System (520-579)
   Reserved for future guideline expansion
10. Chapter 10: Diseases of Genitourinary System (580-629)
    a. **Chronic kidney disease**
11. Chapter 11: Complications of Pregnancy, Childbirth, and the Puerperium (630-677)
    a. General Rules for Obstetric Cases
    b. Selection of OB Principal or First-listed Diagnosis

   c. Fetal Conditions Affecting the Management
      of the Mother
   d. HIV Infection in Pregnancy, Childbirth and the
      Puerperium
   e. Current Conditions Complicating Pregnancy
   f. Diabetes mellitus in pregnancy
   g. Gestational diabetes
   h. Normal Delivery, Code 650
   i. The Postpartum and Peripartum Periods
   j. Code 677, Late effect of complication of
      pregnancy
   k. Abortions

12. Chapter 12: Diseases Skin and Subcutaneous
    Tissue (680-709)
    Reserved for future guideline expansion

13. Chapter 13: Diseases of Musculoskeletal and
    Connective Tissue (710-739)
    Reserved for future guideline expansion

14. Chapter 14: Congenital Anomalies (740-759)
   a. Codes in categories 740-759, Congenital
      Anomalies

15. Chapter 15: Newborn (Perinatal) Guidelines (760-779)
   a. General Perinatal Rules
   b. Use of codes V30-V39
   c. Newborn transfers
   d. Use of category V29
   e. Use of other V codes on perinatal records
   f. Maternal Causes of Perinatal Morbidity
   g. Congenital Anomalies in Newborns
   h. Coding Additional Perinatal Diagnoses
   i. Prematurity and Fetal Growth Retardation
   j. Newborn sepsis

16. Chapter 16: Signs, Symptoms and Ill-Defined
    Conditions (780-799)
    Reserved for future guideline expansion

17. Chapter 17: Injury and Poisoning (800-999)
   a. Coding of Injuries
   b. Coding of Fractures
   c. Coding of Burns
   d. Coding of Debridement of Wound, Infection,
      or Burn

  e. Adverse Effects, Poisoning and Toxic Effects
  f. Complications of care
 18. Classification of Factors Influencing Health Status
   and Contact with Health Service (Supplemental V01-V84)
  a. Introduction
  b. V codes use in any healthcare setting
  c. V Codes indicate a reason for an encounter
  d. Categories of V Codes
  e. V Code Table
 19. Supplemental Classification of External Causes of Injury
   and Poisoning (E-codes, E800-E999)
  a. General E Code Coding Guidelines
  b. Place of Occurrence Guideline
  c. Adverse Effects of Drugs, Medicinal and
   Biological Substances Guidelines
  d. Multiple Cause E Code Coding Guidelines
  e. Child and Adult Abuse Guideline
  f. Unknown or Suspected Intent Guideline
  g. Undetermined Cause
  h. Late Effects of External Cause Guidelines
  i. Misadventures and Complications of Care
   Guidelines
  j. Terrorism Guidelines

Section II. Selection of Principal Diagnosis
 A. Codes for symptoms, signs, and ill-defined conditions
 B. Two or more interrelated conditions, each potentially
   meeting the definition for principal diagnosis
 C. Two or more diagnoses that equally meet the definition
   for principal diagnosis
 D. Two or more comparative or contrasting conditions
 E. A symptom(s) followed by contrasting/comparative diagnoses
 F. Original treatment plan not carried out
 G Complications of surgery and other medical care
 H. Uncertain diagnosis
 I. Admission from Observation Unit
  1. Admission Following Medical Observation
  2. Admission Following Postoperative Observation
 J. Admission from Outpatient Surgery

Section III. Reporting Additional Diagnoses
A. Previous conditions
B. Abnormal findings
C. Uncertain diagnosis

Section IV. Diagnostic Coding and Reporting Guidelines for Outpatient Services
A. Selection of first-listed condition
    1. Outpatient Surgery
    2. Observation Stay
B. Codes from 001.0 through V84.8
C. Accurate reporting of ICD-9-CM diagnosis codes
D. Selection of codes 001.0 through 999.9
E. Codes that describe symptoms and signs
F. Encounters for circumstances other than a disease or injury
G. Level of Detail in Coding
    1. ICD-9-CM codes with 3, 4, or 5 digits
    2. Use of full number of digits required for a code
H. ICD-9-CM code for the diagnosis, condition, problem, or other reason for encounter/visit
I. "Probable," "suspected," "questionable," "rule out," or "working diagnosis"
J. Chronic diseases
K. Code all documented conditions that coexist
L. Patients receiving diagnostic services only
M. Patients receiving therapeutic services only
N. Patients receiving preoperative evaluations only
O. Ambulatory surgery
P. Routine outpatient prenatal visits

Section I. Conventions, general coding guidelines and chapter specific guidelines

The conventions, general guidelines and chapter-specific guidelines are applicable to all health care settings unless otherwise indicated.

A. Conventions for the ICD-9-CM

The conventions for the ICD-9-CM are the general rules for use of the classification independent of the guidelines. These conventions are incorporated within the index and tabular of the ICD-9-CM as instructional notes. The conventions are as follows:

1. Format:

The ICD-9-CM uses an indented format for ease in reference

2. Abbreviations

a. Index abbreviations

NEC   "Not elsewhere classifiable"
This abbreviation in the index represents "other specified" when a specific code is not available for a condition the index directs the coder to the "other specified" code in the tabular.

b. Tabular abbreviations

NEC   "Not elsewhere classifiable"
This abbreviation in the tabular represents "other specified". When a specific code is not available for a condition the tabular includes an NEC entry under a code to identify the code as the "other specified" code (See Section I.A.5.a. "Other" codes).

NOS   "Not otherwise specified"
This abbreviation is the equivalent of unspecified.
(See Section I.A.5.b. "Unspecified" codes)

3. Punctuation

[ ] Brackets are used in the tabular list to enclose synonyms, alternative wording or explanatory phrases. Brackets are used in the index to identify manifestation codes. (See Section I.A.6. "Etiology/manifestations")

( ) Parentheses are used in both the index and tabular to enclose supplementary words that may be present or absent in the statement of a disease or procedure without affecting the code number to which it is assigned. The terms within the parentheses are referred to as nonessential modifiers.

: Colons are used in the Tabular list after an incomplete term which needs one or more of the modifiers following the colon to make it assignable to a given category.

4. **Includes and Excludes Notes and Inclusion terms**

Includes: This note appears immediately under a three-digit code title to further define, or give examples of, the content of the category.

Excludes: An excludes note under a code indicates that the terms excluded from the code are to be coded elsewhere. In some cases the codes for the excluded terms should not be used in conjunction with the code from which it is excluded. An example of this is a congenital condition excluded from an acquired form of the same condition. The congenital and acquired codes should not be used together. In other cases, the excluded terms may be used together with an excluded code. An example of this is when fractures of different bones are coded to different codes. Both codes may be used together if both types of fractures are present.

Inclusion terms: List of terms are included under certain four and five digit codes. These terms are the conditions for which that code number is to be used. The terms may be synonyms of the code title, or, in the case of "other specified" codes, the terms are a list of the various conditions assigned to that code. The inclusion terms are not necessarily exhaustive. Additional terms found only in the index may also be assigned to a code.

5. **Other and Unspecified codes**
   a. **"Other" codes**
      Codes titled "other" or "other specified" (usually a code with a 4th digit 8 or fifth digit 9 for diagnosis codes) are for use when the information in the medical record provides detail for which a specific code does not exist. Index entries with NEC in the line designate "other" codes in the tabular. These index entries represent specific disease entities for which no specific code exists so the term is included within an "other" code.

   b. **"Unspecified" codes**
      Codes (usually a code with a 4th digit 9 or 5th digit 0 for diagnosis codes) titled "unspecified" are for use when the information in the medical record is insufficient to assign a more specific code.

6. **Etiology/manifestation convention ("code first," "use additional code" and "in diseases classified elsewhere" notes)**

   Certain conditions have both an underlying etiology and multiple body system manifestations due to the underlying etiology. For such conditions, the ICD-9-CM has a coding convention that requires the underlying condition be sequenced first followed by the manifestation. Wherever such a combination exists, there is a "use additional code" note at the etiology code, and a "code first" note at the manifestation code. These instructional notes indicate the proper sequencing order of the codes, etiology followed by manifestation.

   In most cases the manifestation codes will have in the code title, "in diseases classified elsewhere." Codes with this title are a component of the etiology/ manifestation convention. The code title indicates that it is a manifestation code. "In diseases classified elsewhere" codes are never permitted to be used as first listed or principal diagnosis codes. They must be used in conjunction with an underlying condition code and they must be listed following the underlying condition.

There are manifestation codes that do not have "in diseases classified elsewhere" in the title. For such codes a "use additional code" note will still be present and the rules for sequencing apply.

In addition to the notes in the tabular, these conditions also have a specific index entry structure. In the index both conditions are listed together with thc etiology code first followed by the manifestation codes in brackets. The code in brackets is always to be sequenced second.

The most commonly used etiology/manifestation combinations are the codes for Diabetes mellitus, category 250. For each code under category 250 there is a use additional code note for the manifestation that is specific for that particular diabetic manifestation. Should a patient have more than one manifestation of diabetes, more than one code from category 250 may be used with as many manifestation codes as are needed to fully describe the patient's complete diabetic condition. The **category** 250 diabetes codes should be sequenced first, followed by the manifestation codes.

"Code first" and "Use additional code" notes are also uscd as scquencing rules in the classification for certain codes that are not part of an etiology/ manifestation combination. See Section I.B.9. "Multiple coding for a single condition."

7. **"And"**
The word "and" should be interpreted to mean either "and" or "or" when it appears in a title.

8. **"With"**
The word "with" in the alphabetic index is sequenced immediately following the main term, not in alphabetical order.

9. **"See" and "See Also"**
The "see" instruction following a main term in the index indicates that another term should be referenced. It is necessary to go to the main term referenced with the "see" note to locate the correct code.

A "see also" instruction following a main term in the index instructs that there is another main term that may also be referenced that may provide additional index entries that may be useful. It is not necessary to follow the "see also" note when the original main term provides the necessary code.

B. General Coding Guidelines

1. Use of Both Alphabetic Index and Tabular List

Use both the Alphabetic Index and the Tabular List when locating and assigning a code. Reliance on only the Alphabetic Index or the Tabular List leads to errors in code assignments and less specificity in code selection.

2. Locate each term in the Alphabetic Index

Locate each term in the Alphabetic Index and verify the code selected in the Tabular List. Read and be guided by instructional notations that appear in both the Alphabetic Index and the Tabular List.

3. Level of Detail in Coding

Diagnosis and procedure codes are to be used at their highest number of digits available.

ICD-9-CM diagnosis codes are composed of codes with either 3, 4, or 5 digits. Codes with three digits are included in ICD-9-CM as the heading of a category of codes that may be further subdivided by the use of fourth and/or fifth digits, which provide greater detail.

A three-digit code is to be used only if it is not further subdivided. Where fourth-digit subcategories and/or fifth-digit subclassifications are provided, they must be assigned. A code is invalid if it has not been coded to the full number of digits required for that code. For example, Acute myocardial infarction, code 410, has fourth digits that describe the location of the infarction (e.g., 410.2, Of inferolateral wall), and fifth digits that identify the episode of care. It would be incorrect to report a code in category 410 without a fourth and fifth digit.

ICD-9-CM Volume 3 procedure codes are composed of codes with either 3 or 4 digits. Codes with two digits are included in ICD-9-CM as the heading of a category of codes that may be further subdivided by the use of third and/or fourth digits, which provide greater detail.

4. Code or codes from 001.0 through V84.8

The appropriate code or codes from 001.0 through V84.8 must be used to identify diagnoses, symptoms, conditions, problems, complaints or other reason(s) for the encounter/visit.

5. Selection of codes 001.0 through 999.9

The selection of codes 001.0 through 999.9 will frequently be used to describe the reason for the admission/encounter. These codes are from the section of ICD-9-CM for the classification of diseases and injuries (e.g., infectious and parasitic diseases; neoplasms; symptoms, signs, and ill-defined conditions, etc.).

6. Signs and symptoms

Codes that describe symptoms and signs, as opposed to diagnoses, are acceptable for reporting purposes when a related definitive diagnosis has not been established (confirmed) by the provider. Chapter 16 of ICD-9-CM, Symptoms, Signs, and Ill-defined conditions (codes 780.0 - 799.9) contain many, but not all codes for symptoms.

7. Conditions that are an integral part of a disease process

Signs and symptoms that are integral to the disease process should not be assigned as additional codes.

8. Conditions that are not an integral part of a disease process

Additional signs and symptoms that may not be associated routinely with a disease process should be coded when present.

9. Multiple coding for a single condition

In addition to the etiology/manifestation convention that requires two codes to fully describe a single condition that affects multiple body systems, there are other single conditions that also require more than one code. "Use additional code" notes are found in the tabular at codes that are not part of an etiology/manifestation pair where a secondary code is useful to fully describe a condition. The sequencing rule is the same as the etiology/manifestation pair, "use additional code" indicates that a secondary code should be added.

For example, for infections that are not included in chapter 1, a secondary code from category 041, Bacterial infection in conditions classified elsewhere and of unspecified site, may be required to identify the bacterial organism causing the infection. A "use additional code" note will normally be found at the infectious disease code, indicating a need for the organism code to be added as a secondary code.

"Code first" notes are also under certain codes that are not specifically manifestation codes but may be due to an underlying cause. When a "code first" note is present and an underlying condition is present the underlying condition should be sequenced first.

"Code, if applicable, any causal condition first", notes indicate that this code may be assigned as a principal diagnosis when the causal condition is unknown or not applicable. If a causal condition is known, then the code for that condition should be sequenced as the principal or first-listed diagnosis.

Multiple codes may be needed for late effects, complication codes and obstetric codes to more fully describe a condition. See the specific guidelines for these conditions for further instruction.

10. Acute and Chronic Conditions

If the same condition is described as both acute (subacute) and chronic, and separate subentries exist in the Alphabetic Index at the same indentation level, code both and sequence the acute (subacute) code first.

11. Combination Code

A combination code is a single code used to classify:
Two diagnoses, or
A diagnosis with an associated secondary process (manifestation)
A diagnosis with an associated complication

Combination codes are identified by referring to subterm entries in the Alphabetic Index and by reading the inclusion and exclusion notes in the Tabular List.

Assign only the combination code when that code fully identifies the diagnostic conditions involved or when the Alphabetic Index so directs. Multiple coding should not be used when the classification provides a combination code that clearly identifies all of the elements documented in the diagnosis. When the combination code lacks necessary specificity in describing the manifestation or complication, an additional code should be used as a secondary code.

12. Late Effects

A late effect is the residual effect (condition produced) after the acute phase of an illness or injury has terminated. There is no time limit on when a late effect code can be used. The residual may be apparent early, such as in cerebrovascular accident cases, or it may occur months or years later, such as that due to a previous injury. Coding of late effects generally requires two codes sequenced in the following order: The condition or nature of the late effect is sequenced first. The late effect code is sequenced second.

An exception to the above guidelines are those instances where the code for late effect is followed by a manifestation code identified in the Tabular List and title, or the late effect code has been expanded (at the fourth and fifth-digit levels) to include the manifestation(s). The code for the acute phase of an illness or injury that led to the late effect is never used with a code for the late effect.

13. Impending or Threatened Condition

Code any condition described at the time of discharge as "impending" or "threatened" as follows:
If it did occur, code as confirmed diagnosis.
If it did not occur, reference the Alphabetic Index to determine if the condition has a subentry term for "impending" or "threatened" and also reference main term entries for "Impending" and for "Threatened."
If the subterms are listed, assign the given code.

If the subterms are not listed, code the existing underlying condition(s) and not the condition described as impending or threatened.

C. Chapter-Specific Coding Guidelines

In addition to general coding guidelines, there are guidelines for specific diagnoses and/or conditions in the classification. Unless otherwise indicated, these guidelines apply to all health care settings. Please refer to Section II for guidelines on the selection of principal diagnosis.

1. Chapter 1: Infectious and Parasitic Diseases (001-139)

a. Human Immunodeficiency Virus (HIV) Infections

1) Code only confirmed cases

Code only confirmed cases of HIV infection/illness. This is an exception to the hospital inpatient guideline Section II, H.

In this context, "confirmation" does not require documentation of positive serology or culture for HIV; the provider's diagnostic statement that the patient is HIV positive, or has an HIV-related illness is sufficient.

2) Selection and sequencing of HIV codes

(a) Patient admitted for HIV-related condition

If a patient is admitted for an HIV-related condition, the principal diagnosis should be 042, followed by additional diagnosis codes for all reported HIV-related conditions.

(b) Patient with HIV disease admitted for unrelated condition

If a patient with HIV disease is admitted for an unrelated condition (such as a traumatic injury), the code for the unrelated condition (e.g., the nature of injury code) should be the principal diagnosis. Other diagnoses would be 042 followed by additional diagnosis codes for all reported HIV-related conditions.

(c) Whether the patient is newly diagnosed

Whether the patient is newly diagnosed or has had previous admissions/encounters for HIV conditions is irrelevant to the sequencing decision.

(d) Asymptomatic human immunodeficiency virus

V08 Asymptomatic human immunodeficiency virus [HIV] infection, is to be applied when the patient without any documentation of symptoms is listed as being "HIV positive," "known HIV," "HIV test positive," or similar terminology. Do not use this code if the term "AIDS" is used or if the patient is treated for any HIV-related illness or is described as having any condition(s) resulting from his/her HIV positive status; use 042 in these cases.

(e) Patients with inconclusive HIV serology

Patients with inconclusive HIV serology, but no definitive diagnosis or manifestations of the illness, may be assigned code 795.71, Inconclusive serologic test for Human Immunodeficiency Virus [HIV].

(f) Previously diagnosed HIV-related illness

Patients with any known prior diagnosis of an HIV-related illness should be coded to 042. Once a patient has developed an HIV-related illness, the patient should always be assigned code 042 on every subsequent admission/encounter. Patients previously diagnosed with any HIV illness (042) should never be assigned to 795.71 or V08.

(g) HIV Infection in Pregnancy, Childbirth and the Puerperium

During pregnancy, childbirth or the puerperium, a patient admitted (or presenting for a health care encounter) because of an HIV-related illness should receive a principal diagnosis code of 647.6X, Other specified infectious and parasitic diseases in the mother classifiable elsewhere, but complicating the pregnancy, childbirth or the puerperium, followed by 042 and the code(s) for the HIV-related illness(es). Codes from Chapter 15 always take sequencing priority.

Patients with asymptomatic HIV infection status admitted (or presenting for a health care encounter) during pregnancy, childbirth, or the puerperium should receive codes of 647.6X and V08.

(h) Encounters for testing for HIV

If a patient is being seen to determine his/her HIV status, use code V73.89, Screening for other specified viral disease. Use code V69.8, Other problems related to lifestyle, as a secondary code if an asymptomatic patient is in a known high risk group for HIV. Should a patient with signs or symptoms or illness, or a confirmed HIV related diagnosis be tested for HIV, code the signs and symptoms or the diagnosis. An additional counseling code V65.44 may be used if counseling is provided during the encounter for the test.

When a patient returns to be informed of his/her HIV test results use code V65.44, HIV counseling, if the results of the test are negative.

If the results are positive but the patient is asymptomatic use code V08, Asymptomatic HIV infection. If the results are positive and the patient is symptomatic use code 042, HIV infection, with codes for the HIV related symptoms or diagnosis. The HIV counseling code may also be used if counseling is provided for patients with positive test results.

b. Septicemia, Systemic Inflammatory Response Syndrome (SIRS), Sepsis, Severe Sepsis, and Septic Shock

1) Sepsis as principal diagnosis or secondary diagnosis

(a) Sepsis as principal diagnosis

If sepsis is present on admission, and meets the definition of principal diagnosis, the underlying systemic infection code (e.g., 038.xx, 112.5, etc) should be assigned as the principal diagnosis, followed by code 995.91, Systemic inflammatory response syndrome due to infectious process without organ dysfunction, as required by the sequencing rules in the Tabular List. Codes from subcategory 995.9 can never be assigned as a principal diagnosis.

(b) Sepsis as secondary diagnoses

When sepsis develops during the encounter (it was not present on admission), the sepsis codes may be assigned as secondary diagnoses, following the sequencing rules provided in the Tabular List.

(c) Documentation unclear as to whether sepsis present on admission

If the documentation is not clear whether the sepsis was present on admission, the provider should be queried. After provider query, if sepsis is determined at that point to have met the definition of principal diagnosis, the underlying systemic infection (038.xx, 112.5, etc.) may be used as principal diagnosis along with code 995.91, Systemic inflammatory response syndrome due to infectious process without organ dysfunction.

2) Septicemia/Sepsis

In most cases, it will be a code from category 038, Septicemia, that will be used in conjunction with a code from subcategory 995.9 such as the following:

(a) Streptococcal sepsis

If the documentation in the record states streptococcal sepsis, codes 038.0 and code 995.91 should be used, in that sequence.

(b) Streptococcal septicemia

If the documentation states streptococcal septicemia, only code 038.0 should be assigned; however, the provider should be queried whether the patient has sepsis, an infection with SIRS.

(c) Sepsis or SIRS must be documented
Either the term sepsis or SIRS must be documented, to assign a code from subcategory 995.9.

3) Terms sepsis, severe sepsis, or SIRS
If the terms sepsis, severe sepsis, or SIRS are used with an underlying infection other than septicemia, such as pneumonia, cellulitis or a nonspecified urinary tract infection, a code from category 038 should be assigned first, then code 995.91, followed by the code for the initial infection. The use of the terms sepsis or SIRS indicates that the patient's infection has advanced to the point of a systemic infection so the systemic infection should be sequenced before the localized infection. The instructional note under subcategory 995.9 instructs to assign the underlying systemic infection first.

Note: The term urosepsis is a nonspecific term. If that is the only term documented then only code 599.0 should be assigned based on the default for the term in the ICD-9-CM index, in addition to the code for the causal organism if known.

4) Severe sepsis
For patients with severe sepsis, the code for the systemic infection (e.g., 038.xx, 112.5, etc) or trauma should be sequenced first, followed by either code 995.92, Systemic inflammatory response syndrome due to infectious process with organ dysfunction, or code 995.94, Systemic inflammatory response syndrome due to noninfectious process with organ dysfunction. Codes for the specific organ dysfunctions should also be assigned.

5) Septic shock
(a) Sequencing of septic shock
Septic shock is a form of organ dysfunction associated with severe sepsis. A code for the initiating underlying systemic infection followed by a code for SIRS (code 995.92) must be assigned before the code for septic shock. As noted in the

sequencing instructions in the Tabular List, the code for septic shock cannot be assigned as a principal diagnosis.

(b) Septic Shock without documentation of severe sepsis
Septic shock cannot occur in the absence of severe sepsis. A code from subcategory 995.9 must be sequenced before the code for septic shock. The use additional code notes and the code first note provide sequencing instructions.

6) Sepsis and septic shock associated with abortion
Sepsis and septic shock associated with abortion, ectopic pregnancy, and molar pregnancy are classified to category codes in Chapter 11 (630-639).

7) Negative or inconclusive blood cultures
Negative or inconclusive blood cultures do not preclude a diagnosis of septicemia or sepsis in patients with clinical evidence of the condition, however, the provider should be queried.

8) Newborn sepsis
See Section I.C.15.j for information on the coding of newborn sepsis.

9) Sepsis due to a Postprocedural Infection
Sepsis resulting from a postprocedural infection is a complication of care. For such cases code 998.59, Other postoperative infections, should be coded first followed by the appropriate codes for the sepsis. The other guidelines for coding sepsis should then be followed for the assignment of additional codes.

10) External cause of injury codes with SIRS
An external cause code is not needed with codes 995.91, Systemic inflammatory response syndrome due to infectious process without organ dysfunction, or code 995.92, Systemic inflammatory response syndrome due to infectious process with organ dysfunction.

Refer to Section I.C.19.a.7 for instructions on the use of external cause of injury codes with codes for SIRS resulting from trauma.

2. **Chapter 2: Neoplasms (140-239)**
   <u>General guidelines</u>
   Chapter 2 of the ICD-9-CM contains the codes for most benign and all malignant neoplasms. Certain benign neoplasms, such as prostatic adenomas, may be found in the specific body system chapters. To properly code a neoplasm it is necessary to determine from the record if the neoplasm is benign, in-situ, malignant, or of uncertain histologic behavior. If malignant, any secondary (metastatic) sites should also be determined.

   The neoplasm table in the Alphabetic Index should be referenced first. However, if the histological term is documented, that term should be referenced first, rather than going immediately to the Neoplasm Table, in order to determine which column in the Neoplasm Table is appropriate. For example, if the documentation indicates "adenoma," refer to the term in the Alphabetic Index to review the entries under this term and the instructional note to "see also neoplasm, by site, benign." The table provides the proper code based on the type of neoplasm and the site. It is important to select the proper column in the table that corresponds to the type of neoplasm. The tabular should then be referenced to verify that the correct code has been selected from the table and that a more specific site code does not exist.

   See Section I. C. 18.d.4. for information regarding V codes for genetic susceptibility to cancer.

   a. **Treatment directed at the malignancy**
      If the treatment is directed at the malignancy, designate the malignancy as the principal diagnosis.

   b. **Treatment of secondary site**
      When a patient is admitted because of a primary neoplasm with metastasis and treatment is directed toward the secondary site only, the secondary neoplasm is designated as the principal diagnosis even though the primary malignancy is still present.

c. Coding and sequencing of complications

Coding and sequencing of complications associated with the malignancies or with the therapy thereof are subject to the following guidelines:

1) Anemia associated with malignancy

When admission/encounter is for management of an anemia associated with the malignancy, and the treatment is only for anemia, the **appropriate** anemia **code (such as code 285.22, Anemia in neoplastic disease)** is designated at the principal diagnosis and is followed by the appropriate code(s) for the malignancy.

Code 285.22 may also be used as a secondary code if the patient suffers from anemia and is being treated for the malignancy.

2) Anemia associated with chemotherapy, <u>immunotherapy and radiation therapy</u>

When the admission/encounter is for management of an anemia associated with chemotherapy, **immunotherapy** or radiotherapy and the only treatment is for the anemia, the anemia is sequenced first followed by **code E933.1. The appropriate neoplasm code should be assigned as an additional code.**

3) Management of dehydration due to the malignancy

When the admission/encounter is for management of dehydration due to the malignancy or the therapy, or a combination of both, and only the dehydration is being treated (intravenous rehydration), the dehydration is sequenced first, followed by the code(s) for the malignancy.

4) Treatment of a complication resulting from a surgical procedure

When the admission/encounter is for treatment of a complication resulting from a surgical procedure, designate the complication as the principal or first-listed diagnosis if treatment is directed at resolving the complication.

d. Primary malignancy previously excised

When a primary malignancy has been previously excised or eradicated from its site and there is no further treatment directed to that site and there is no evidence of any existing primary malignancy, a code from category V10, Personal history of malignant neoplasm, should be used to indicate the former site of the malignancy. Any mention of extension, invasion, or metastasis to another site is coded as a secondary malignant neoplasm to that site. The secondary site may be the principal or first-listed with the V10 code used as a secondary code.

e. Admissions/Encounters involving chemotherapy, <u>immunotherapy</u> and radiation therapy

1) Episode of care involves surgical removal of neoplasm

When an episode of care involves the surgical removal of a neoplasm, primary or secondary site, followed by adjunct chemotherapy or radiation treatment **during the same episode of care**, the neoplasm code should be assigned as principal or first-listed diagnosis, using codes in the 140-198 series or where appropriate in the 200-203 series.

2) Patient admission/encounter solely for administration of chemotherapy, <u>immunotherapy</u> <u>and radiation therapy</u>

If a patient admission/encounter is solely for the administration of chemotherapy, **immunotherapy** or radiation therapy **assign** code V58.0, Encounter for radiation therapy, or **V58.11,** Encounter for **antineoplastic** chemotherapy, **or V58.12, Encounter for antineoplastic immunotherapy as** the first-listed or principal diagnosis. If a patient receives **more than one of these therapies during the same admission, more than one of these codes may be assigned, in any sequence.**

3) **Patient admitted for radiotherapy/chemotherapy
   and immunotherapy and develops complications**
   When a patient is admitted for the purpose of
   radiotherapy, **immunotherapy** or chemotherapy and
   develops complications such as uncontrolled nausea and
   vomiting or dehydration, the principal or first-listed
   diagnosis is V58.0, Encounter for radiotherapy, or V58.1**1**,
   **Encounter for antineoplastic chemotherapy, or
   V58.12, Encounter for antineoplastic
   immunotherapy,** followed by any codes for the
   complications.

   See Section I.C.18.d.7. for additional information
   regarding aftercare V codes.

f. **Admission/encounter to determine extent of
   malignancy**
   When the reason for admission/encounter is to determine the
   extent of the malignancy, or for a procedure such as
   paracentesis or thoracentesis, the primary malignancy or
   appropriate metastatic site is designated as the principal or
   first-listed diagnosis, even though chemotherapy or
   radiotherapy is administered.

g. **Symptoms, signs, and ill-defined conditions listed in
   Chapter 16**
   Symptoms, signs, and ill-defined conditions listed in Chapter
   16 characteristic of, or associated with, an existing primary or
   secondary site malignancy cannot be used to replace the
   malignancy as principal or first-listed diagnosis, regardless of
   the number of admissions or encounters for treatment and
   care of the neoplasm.

   **See Section I.C.18.d.14, Encounter for prophylactic
   organ removal.**

3. **Chapter 3: Endocrine, Nutritional, and Metabolic
   Diseases and Immunity Disorders (240-279)**

a. **Diabetes mellitus**
   Codes under category 250, Diabetes mellitus, identify
   complications/manifestations associated with diabetes

mellitus. A fifth-digit is required for all category 250 codes to identify the type of diabetes mellitus and whether the diabetes is controlled or uncontrolled.

1) **Fifth-digits for category 250:**
   The following are the fifth-digits for the codes under category 250:

   0   type II or unspecified type, not stated as uncontrolled
   1   type I, [juvenile type], not stated as uncontrolled
   2   type II or unspecified type, uncontrolled
   3   type I, [juvenile type], uncontrolled

   The age of a patient is not the sole determining factor, though most type I diabetics develop the condition before reaching puberty. For this reason type I diabetes mellitus is also referred to as juvenile diabetes.

2) **Type of diabetes mellitus not documented**
   If the type of diabetes mellitus is not documented in the medical record the default is type II.

3) **Diabetes mellitus and the use of insulin**
   All type I diabetics must use insulin to replace what their bodies do not produce. However, the use of insulin does not mean that a patient is a type I diabetic. Some patients with type II diabetes mellitus are unable to control their blood sugar through diet and oral medication alone and do require insulin. If the documentation in a medical record does not indicate the type of diabetes but does indicate that the patient uses insulin, the appropriate fifth-digit for type II must be used. For type II patients who routinely use insulin, code V58.67, Long-term (current) use of insulin, should also be assigned to indicate that the patient uses insulin. Code V58.67 should not be assigned if insulin is given temporarily to bring a type II patient's blood sugar under control during an encounter.

4) **Assigning and sequencing diabetes codes and associated conditions**
When assigning codes for diabetes and its associated conditions, the code(s) from category 250 must be sequenced before the codes for the associated conditions. The diabetes codes and the secondary codes that correspond to them are paired codes that follow the etiology/manifestation convention of the classification (See Section I.A.6., Etiology/manifestation convention). Assign as many codes from category 250 as needed to identify all of the associated conditions that the patient has. The corresponding secondary codes are listed under each of the diabetes codes.

(a) **Diabetic retinopathy/diabetic macular edema**
Diabetic macular edema, code 362.07, is only present with diabetic retinopathy. Another code from subcategory 362.0, Diabetic retinopathy, must be used with code 362.07. Codes under subcategory 362.0 are diabetes manifestation codes, so they must be used following the appropriate diabetes code.

5) **Diabetes mellitus in pregnancy and gestational diabetes**
(a) For diabetes mellitus complicating pregnancy, see Section I.C.11.f., Diabetes mellitus in pregnancy.

(b) For gestational diabetes, see Section I.C.11, g., Gestational diabetes.

6) **Insulin pump malfunction**
(a) **Underdose of insulin due insulin pump failure**
An underdose of insulin due to an insulin pump failure should be assigned 996.57, Mechanical complication due to insulin pump, as the principal or first listed code, followed by the appropriate diabetes mellitus code based on documentation.

(b) **Overdose of insulin due to insulin pump failure**
The principal or first listed code for an encounter due to an insulin pump malfunction resulting in an

overdose of insulin, should also be 996.57, Mechanical complication due to insulin pump, followed by code 962.3, Poisoning by insulins and antidiabetic agents, and the appropriate diabetes mellitus code based on documentation.

4. **Chapter 4: Diseases of Blood and Blood Forming Organs (280-289)**
   a. **Anemia of chronic disease**
   Subcategory 285.2, Anemia in chronic illness, has codes for anemia in chronic kidney disease, code 285.21; anemia in neoplastic disease, code 285.22; and anemia in other chronic illness, code 285.29. These codes can be used as the principal/first listed code if the reason for the encounter is to treat the anemia. They may also be used as secondary codes if treatment of the anemia is a component of an encounter, but not the primary reason for the encounter. When using a code from subcategory 285 it is also necessary to use the code for the chronic condition causing the anemia.

   1) **Anemia in chronic kidney disease**
   When assigning code 285.21, Anemia in chronic kidney disease. It is also necessary to assign a code from category 585, Chronic kidney disease, to indicate the stage of chronic kidney disease. See I.C.10.a. Chronic kidney disease (CKD).

   2) **Anemia in neoplastic disease**
   When assigning code 285.22, Anemia in neoplastic disease, it is also necessary to assign the neoplasm code that is responsible for the anemia. Code 285.22 is for use for anemia that is due to the malignancy, not for anemia due to antineoplastic chemotherapy drugs, which is an adverse effect. See I.C.2.c.1. Anemia associated with malignancy. See I.C.2.c.2. Anemia associated with chemotherapy, immunotherapy and radiation therapy. See I.C.17.e.1. Adverse effects.

5. **Chapter 5: Mental Disorders (290-319)**
   Reserved for future guideline expansion

6. **Chapter 6: Diseases of Nervous System and Sense Organs (320-389)**
   Reserved for future guideline expansion

7. **Chapter 7: Diseases of Circulatory System (390-459)**
   a. **Hypertension**
   Hypertension Table
   The Hypertension Table, found under the main term, "Hypertension", in the Alphabetic Index, contains a complete listing of all conditions due to or associated with hypertension and classifies them according to malignant, benign, and unspecified.

   1) **Hypertension, Essential, or NOS**
      Assign hypertension (arterial) (essential) (primary) (systemic) (NOS) to category code 401 with the appropriate fourth digit to indicate malignant (.0), benign (.1), or unspecified (.9). Do not use either .0 malignant or .1 benign unless medical record documentation supports such a designation.

   2) **Hypertension with Heart Disease**
      Heart conditions (425.8, 429.0-429.3, 429.8, 429.9) are assigned to a code from category 402 when a causal relationship is stated (due to hypertension) or implied (hypertensive). Use an additional code from category 428 to identify the type of heart failure in those patients with heart failure. More than one code from category 428 may be assigned if the patient has systolic or diastolic failure and congestive heart failure.

      The same heart conditions (425.8, 429.0-429.3, 429.8, 429.9) with hypertension, but without a stated casual relationship, are coded separately. Sequence according to the circumstances of the admission/encounter.

   3) **Hypertensive Kidney Disease**
      Assign codes from category 403, Hypertensive **kidney** disease, when conditions classified to categories 585-587

are present. Unlike hypertension with heart disease, ICD-9-CM presumes a cause-and-effect relationship and classifies renal failure with hypertension as hypertensive **kidney** disease.

4) **Hypertensive Heart and <u>Kidney</u> Disease**
Assign codes from combination category 404, Hypertensive heart and **kidney** disease, when both hypertensive **kidney** disease and hypertensive heart disease are stated in the diagnosis. Assume a relationship between the hypertension and the **kidney** disease, whether or not the condition is so designated. Assign an additional code from category 428, to identify the type of heart failure. More than one code from category 428 may be assigned if the patient has systolic or diastolic failure and congestive heart failure.

5) **Hypertensive Cerebrovascular Disease**
First assign codes from 430-438, Cerebrovascular disease, then the appropriate hypertension code from categories 401-405.

6) **Hypertensive Retinopathy**
Two codes are necessary to identify the condition. First assign the code from subcategory 362.11, Hypertensive retinopathy, then the appropriate code from categories 401-405 to indicate the type of hypertension.

7) **Hypertension, Secondary**
Two codes are required: one to identify the underlying etiology and one from category 405 to identify the hypertension. Sequencing of codes is determined by the reason for admission/encounter.

8) **Hypertension, Transient**
Assign code 796.2, Elevated blood pressure reading without diagnosis of hypertension, unless patient has an established diagnosis of hypertension. Assign code 642.3x for transient hypertension of pregnancy.

9) Hypertension, Controlled

Assign appropriate code from categories 401-405. This diagnostic statement usually refers to an existing state of hypertension under control by therapy.

10) Hypertension, Uncontrolled

Uncontrolled hypertension may refer to untreated hypertension or hypertension not responding to current therapeutic regimen. In either case, assign the appropriate code from categories 401-405 to designate the stage and type of hypertension. Code to the type of hypertension.

11) Elevated Blood Pressure

For a statement of elevated blood pressure without further specificity, assign code 796.2, Elevated blood pressure reading without diagnosis of hypertension, rather than a code from category 401.

b. Cerebral infarction/stroke/cerebrovascular accident (CVA)

The terms stroke and CVA are often used interchangeably to refer to a cerebral infarction. The terms stroke, CVA, and cerebral infarction NOS are all indexed to the default code 434.91, Cerebral artery occlusion, unspecified, with infarction. Code 436, Acute, but ill-defined, cerebrovascular disease, should not be used when the documentation states stroke or CVA.

c. Postoperative cerebrovascular accident

A cerebrovascular hemorrhage or infarction that occurs as a result of medical intervention is coded to 997.02, Iatrogenic cerebrovascular infarction or hemorrhage. Medical record documentation should clearly specify the cause-and-effect relationship between the medical intervention and the cerebrovascular accident in order to assign this code. A secondary code from the code range 430-432 or from a code from subcategories 433 or 434 with a fifth digit of "1" should also be used to identify the type of hemorrhage or infarct.

This guideline conforms to the use additional code note instruction at category 997. Code 436, Acute, but ill-defined, cerebrovascular disease, should not be used as a secondary code with code 997.02.

d. Late Effects of Cerebrovascular Disease

1) Category 438, Late Effects of Cerebrovascular disease

Category 438 is used to indicate conditions classifiable to categories 430-437 as the causes of late effects (neurologic deficits), themselves classified elsewhere. These "late effects" include neurologic deficits that persist after initial onset of conditions classifiable to 430-437. The neurologic deficits caused by cerebrovascular disease may be present from the onset or may arise at any time after the onset of the condition classifiable to 430-437.

2) Codes from category 438 with codes from 430-437

Codes from category 438 may be assigned on a health care record with codes from 430-437, if the patient has a current cerebrovascular accident (CVA) and deficits from an old CVA.

3) Code V12.59

Assign code V12.59 (and not a code from category 438) as an additional code for history of cerebrovascular disease when no neurologic deficits are present.

e. Acute myocardial infarction (AMI)

1) ST elevation myocardial infarction (STEMI) and non ST elevation myocardial infarction (NSTEMI)
The ICD-9-CM codes for acute myocardial infarction (AMI) identify the site, such as anterolateral wall or true posterior wall. Subcategories 410.0-410.6 and 410.8 are used for ST elevation myocardial infarction (STEMI). Subcategory 410.7, Subendocardial infarction, is used for non ST elevation myocardial infarction (NSTEMI) and nontransmural MIs.

2) **Acute myocardial infarction, unspecified**
Subcategory 410.9 is the default for the unspecified term acute myocardial infarction. If only STEMI or transmural MI without the site is documented, query the provider as to the site, or assign a code from subcategory 410.9.

3) **AMI documented as nontransmural or subendocardial but site provided**
If an AMI is documented as nontransmural or subendocardial, but the site is provided, it is still coded as a subendocardial AMI. If NSTEMI evolves to STEMI, assign the STEMI code. If STEMI converts to NSTEMI due to thrombolytic therapy, it is still coded as STEMI.

8. **Chapter 8: Diseases of Respiratory System (460-519)**
   a. **Chronic Obstructive Pulmonary Disease [COPD] and Asthma**

1) **Conditions that comprise COPD and Asthma**
The conditions that comprise COPD are obstructive chronic bronchitis, subcategory 491.2, and emphysema, category 492. All asthma codes are under category 493, Asthma. Code 496, Chronic airway obstruction, not elsewhere classified, is a nonspecific code that should only be used when the documentation in a medical record does not specify the type of COPD being treated.

2) **Acute exacerbation of chronic obstructive bronchitis and asthma**
The codes for chronic obstructive bronchitis and asthma distinguish between uncomplicated cases and those in acute exacerbation. An acute exacerbation is a worsening or a decompensation of a chronic condition. An acute exacerbation is not equivalent to an infection superimposed on a chronic condition, though an exacerbation may be triggered by an infection.

3) **Overlapping nature of the conditions that comprise COPD and asthma**

   Due to the overlapping nature of the conditions that make up COPD and asthma, there are many variations in the way these conditions are documented. Code selection must be based on the terms as documented. When selecting the correct code for the documented type of COPD and asthma, it is essential to first review the index, and then verify the code in the tabular list. There are many instructional notes under the different COPD subcategories and codes. It is important that all such notes be reviewed to assure correct code assignment.

4) **Acute exacerbation of asthma and status asthmaticus**

   An acute exacerbation of asthma is an increased severity of the asthma symptoms, such as wheezing and shortness of breath. Status asthmaticus refers to a patient's failure to respond to therapy administered during an asthmatic episode and is a life threatening complication that requires emergency care. If status asthmaticus is documented by the provider with any type of COPD or with acute bronchitis, the status asthmaticus should be sequenced first. It supersedes any type of COPD including that with acute exacerbation or acute bronchitis. It is inappropriate to assign an asthma code with 5th digit 2, with acute exacerbation, together with an asthma code with 5th digit 1, with status asthmatics. Only the 5th digit 1 should be assigned.

b. **Chronic Obstructive Pulmonary Disease [COPD] and Bronchitis**

   1) **Acute bronchitis with COPD**

      Acute bronchitis, code 466.0, is due to an infectious organism. When acute bronchitis is documented with COPD, code 491.22, Obstructive chronic bronchitis with acute bronchitis, should be assigned. It is not necessary to also assign code 466.0. If a medical record documents acute bronchitis with COPD with acute exacerbation, only code 491.22 should be assigned. The acute bronchitis included in code 491.22 supersedes the acute exacerbation. If a medical record documents COPD with acute exacerbation without mention of acute bronchitis, only code 491.21 should be assigned.

9. **Chapter 9: Diseases of Digestive System (520-579)**
Reserved for future guideline expansion

10. **Chapter 10: Diseases of Genitourinary System (580-629)**
    a. **Chronic kidney disease**
       1) **Stages of chronic kidney disease (CKD)**
          The ICD-9-CM classifies CKD based on severity. The severity of CKD is designated by stages I-V. Stage II, code 585.2, equates to mild CKD; stage III, code 585.3, equates to moderate CKD; and stage IV, code 585.4, equates to severe CKD. Code 585.6, End stage renal disease (ESRD), is assigned when the provider has documented end-stage-renal disease (ESRD).

          If both a stage of CKD and ESRD are documented, assign code 585.6 only.

       2) **Chronic kidney disease and kidney transplant status**
          Patients who have undergone kidney transplant may still have some form of CKD because the kidney transplant may not fully restore kidney function. Code V42.0 may be assigned with the appropriate CKD code for patients who are status post kidney transplant, based on the patient's post-transplant stage. The use additional code note under category 585 provides this instruction.

          Use of a 585 code with V42.0 does not necessarily indicate transplant rejection or failure. Patients with mild or moderate CKD following a transplant should not be coded as having transplant failure, unless it is documented in the medical record. For patients with severe CKD or ESRD it is appropriate to assign code 996.81, Complications of transplanted organ, kidney transplant, when

kidney transplant failure is documented. If a post kidney transplant patient has CKD and it is unclear from the documentation whether there is transplant failure or rejection it is necessary to query the provider.

3) **Chronic kidney disease with other conditions**
Patients with CKD may also suffer from other serious conditions, most commonly diabetes mellitus and hypertension. The sequencing of the CKD code in relationship to codes for other contributing conditions is based on the conventions in the tabular list.
See I.C.3.a.4 for sequencing instructions for diabetes.
See I.C.4.a.1. for anemia in CKD.
See I.C.7.a.3 for hypertensive kidney disease.
See I.C.17.f.1.b. Transplant complications, for instructions on coding of documented rejection or failure.

11. **Chapter 11: Complications of Pregnancy, Childbirth, and the Puerperium (630-677)**

a. **General Rules for Obstetric Cases**

1) **Codes from chapter 11 and sequencing priority**
Obstetric cases require codes from chapter 11, codes in the range 630-677, Complications of Pregnancy, Childbirth, and the Puerperium. Chapter 11 codes have sequencing priority over codes from other chapters. Additional codes from other chapters may be used in conjunction with chapter 11 codes to further specify conditions. Should the provider document that the pregnancy is incidental to the encounter, then code V22.2 should be used in place of any chapter 11 codes. It is the provider's responsibility to state that the condition being treated is not affecting the pregnancy.

2) **Chapter 11 codes used only on the maternal record**
Chapter 11 codes are to be used only on the maternal record, never on the record of the newborn.

3) Chapter 11 fifth-digits
Categories 640-648, 651-676 have required fifth-digits, which indicate whether the encounter is antepartum, postpartum and whether a delivery has also occurred.

4) Fifth-digits, appropriate for each code
The fifth-digits, which are appropriate for each code number, are listed in brackets under each code. The fifth-digits on each code should all be consistent with each other. That is, should a delivery occur all of the fifth-digits should indicate the delivery.

b. Selection of OB Principal or First-listed Diagnosis

1) Routine outpatient prenatal visits
For routine outpatient prenatal visits when no complications are present codes V22.0, Supervision of normal first pregnancy, and V22.1, Supervision of other normal pregnancy, should be used as the first-listed diagnoses. These codes should not be used in conjunction with chapter 11 codes.

2) Prenatal outpatient visits for high-risk patients
For prenatal outpatient visits for patients with high-risk pregnancies, a code from category V23, Supervision of high-risk pregnancy, should be used as the principal or first-listed diagnosis. Secondary chapter 11 codes may be used in conjunction with these codes if appropriate.

3) Episodes when no delivery occurs
In episodes when no delivery occurs, the principal diagnosis should correspond to the principal complication of the pregnancy, which necessitated the encounter. Should more than one complication exist, all of which are treated or monitored, any of the complications codes may be sequenced first.

4) When a delivery occurs
When a delivery occurs, the principal diagnosis should correspond to the main circumstances or complication of the delivery. In cases of cesarean delivery, the selection of the principal diagnosis should correspond to the

reason the cesarean delivery was performed unless the reason for admission/encounter was unrelated to the condition resulting in the cesarean delivery.

5) Outcome of delivery

An outcome of delivery code, V27.0-V27.9, should be included on every maternal record when a delivery has occurred. These codes are not to be used on subsequent records or on the newborn record.

c. Fetal Conditions Affecting the Management of the Mother

1) Codes from category 655

Known or suspected fetal abnormality affecting management of the mother, and category 656, Other fetal and placental problems affecting the management of the mother, are assigned only when the fetal condition is actually responsible for modifying the management of the mother, i.e., by requiring diagnostic studies, additional observation, special care, or termination of pregnancy. The fact that the fetal condition exists does not justify assigning a code from this series to the mother's record.

2) In utero surgery

In cases when surgery is performed on the fetus, a diagnosis code from category 655, Known or suspected fetal abnormalities affecting management of the mother, should be assigned identifying the fetal condition. Procedure code 75.36, Correction of fetal defect, should be assigned on the hospital inpatient record.

No code from Chapter 15, the perinatal codes, should be used on the mother's record to identify fetal conditions. Surgery performed in utero on a fetus is still to be coded as an obstetric encounter.

d. HIV Infection in Pregnancy, Childbirth and the Puerperium

During pregnancy, childbirth or the puerperium, a patient admitted because of an HIV-related illness should receive a principal diagnosis of 647.6X, Other specified infectious and parasitic diseases in the mother classifiable elsewhere, but complicating the pregnancy, childbirth or the puerperium, followed by 042 and the code(s) for the HIV-related illness(es).

Patients with asymptomatic HIV infection status admitted during pregnancy, childbirth, or the puerperium should receive codes of 647.6X and V08.

e. Current Conditions Complicating Pregnancy
Assign a code from subcategory 648.x for patients that have current conditions when the condition affects the management of the pregnancy, childbirth, or the puerperium. Use additional secondary codes from other chapters to identify the conditions, as appropriate.

f. Diabetes mellitus in pregnancy
Diabetes mellitus is a significant complicating factor in pregnancy. Pregnant women who are diabetic should be assigned code 648.0x, Diabetes mellitus complicating pregnancy, and a secondary code from category 250, Diabetes mellitus, to identify the type of diabetes.

Code V58.67, Long-term (current) use of insulin, should also be assigned if the diabetes mellitus is being treated with insulin.

g. Gestational diabetes
Gestational diabetes can occur during the second and third trimester of pregnancy in women who were not diabetic prior to pregnancy. Gestational diabetes can cause complications in the pregnancy similar to those of pre-existing diabetes mellitus. It also puts the woman at greater risk of developing diabetes after the pregnancy. Gestational diabetes is coded to 648.8x, Abnormal glucose tolerance. Codes 648.0x and 648.8x should never be used together on the same record.

Code V58.67, Long-term (current) use of insulin, should also be assigned if the gestational diabetes is being treated with insulin.

h. Normal Delivery, Code 650

1) Normal delivery

Code 650 is for use in cases when a woman is admitted for a full-term normal delivery and delivers a single, healthy infant without any complications antepartum, during the delivery, or postpartum during the delivery episode. Code 650 is always a principal diagnosis. It is not to be used if any other code from chapter 11 is needed to describe a current complication of the antenatal, delivery, or perinatal period. Additional codes from other chapters may be used with code 650 if they are not related to or are in any way complicating the pregnancy.

2) Normal delivery with resolved antepartum complication

Code 650 may be used if the patient had a complication at some point during her pregnancy, but the complication is not present at the time of the admission for delivery.

3) V27.0, Single liveborn, outcome of delivery

V27.0, Single liveborn, is the only outcome of delivery code appropriate for use with 650.

i. The Postpartum and Peripartum Periods

1) Postpartum and peripartum periods

The postpartum period begins immediately after delivery and continues for six weeks following delivery. The peripartum period is defined as the last month of pregnancy to five months postpartum.

2) Postpartum complication

A postpartum complication is any complication occurring within the six-week period.

3) Pregnancy-related complications after six-week period

Chapter 11 codes may also be used to describe pregnancy-related complications after the six-week period should the provider document that a condition is pregnancy related.

4) **Postpartum complications occurring during the same admission as delivery**
Postpartum complications that occur during the same admission as the delivery are identified with a fifth digit of "2." Subsequent admissions/encounters for postpartum complications should be identified with a fifth digit of "4."

5) **Admission for routine postpartum care following delivery outside hospital**
When the mother delivers outside the hospital prior to admission and is admitted for routine postpartum care and no complications are noted, code V24.0, Postpartum care and examination immediately after delivery, should be assigned as the principal diagnosis.

6) **Admission following delivery outside hospital with postpartum conditions**
A delivery diagnosis code should not be used for a woman who has delivered prior to admission to the hospital. Any postpartum conditions and/or postpartum procedures should be coded.

j. **Code 677, Late effect of complication of pregnancy**
1) **Code 677**
Code 677, Late effect of complication of pregnancy, childbirth, and the puerperium is for use in those cases when an initial complication of a pregnancy develops a sequelae requiring care or treatment at a future date.

2) **After the initial postpartum period**
This code may be used at any time after the initial postpartum period.

3) **Sequencing of Code 677**
This code, like all late effect codes, is to be sequenced following the code describing the sequelae of the complication.

k. Abortions

1) Fifth-digits required for abortion categories

Fifth-digits are required for abortion categories 634-637. Fifth-digit 1, incomplete, indicates that all of the products of conception have not been expelled from the uterus. Fifth-digit 2, complete, indicates that all products of conception have been expelled from the uterus prior to the episode of care.

2) Code from categories 640-648 and 651-659

A code from categories 640-648 and 651-659 may be used as additional codes with an abortion code to indicate the complication leading to the abortion.

Fifth digit 3 is assigned with codes from these categories when used with an abortion code because the other fifth digits will not apply. Codes from the 660-669 series are not to be used for complications of abortion.

3) Code 639 for complications

Code 639 is to be used for all complications following abortion. Code 639 cannot be assigned with codes from categories 634-638.

4) Abortion with Liveborn Fetus

When an attempted termination of pregnancy results in a liveborn fetus assign code 644.21, Early onset of delivery, with an appropriate code from category V27, Outcome of Delivery. The procedure code for the attempted termination of pregnancy should also be assigned.

5) Retained Products of Conception following an abortion

Subsequent admissions for retained products of conception following a spontaneous or legally induced abortion are assigned the appropriate code from category 634, Spontaneous abortion, or 635 Legally induced abortion, with a fifth digit of "1" (incomplete). This advice is appropriate even when the patient was discharged previously with a discharge diagnosis of complete abortion.

12. **Chapter 12: Diseases Skin and Subcutaneous Tissue (680-709)**
   Reserved for future guideline expansion

13. **Chapter 13: Diseases of Musculoskeletal and Connective Tissue (710-739)**
   Reserved for future guideline expansion

14. **Chapter 14: Congenital Anomalies (740-759)**
   a. **Codes in categories 740-759, Congenital Anomalies**
      Assign an appropriate code(s) from categories 740-759, Congenital Anomalies, when an anomaly is documented. A congenital anomaly may be the principal/first listed diagnosis on a record or a secondary diagnosis.

      When a congenital anomaly does not have a unique code assignment, assign additional code(s) for any manifestations that may be present.

      When the code assignment specifically identifies the congenital anomaly, manifestations that are an inherent component of the anomaly should not be coded separately. Additional codes should be assigned for manifestations that are not an inherent component.

      Codes from Chapter 14 may be used throughout the life of the patient. If a congenital anomaly has been corrected, a personal history code should be used to identify the history of the anomaly. **Although present at birth, a congenital anomaly may not be identified until later in life. Whenever the condition is diagnosed by the physician, it is appropriate to assign a code from codes 740-759.**

      For the birth admission, the appropriate code from category V30, Liveborn infants, according to type of birth should be sequenced as the principal diagnosis, followed by any congenital anomaly codes, 740-759.

15. **Chapter 15: Newborn (Perinatal) Guidelines (760-779)**
   For coding and reporting purposes the perinatal period is defined as **before** birth through the 28th day following birth. The following guidelines are provided for reporting purposes. Hospitals may record other diagnoses as needed for internal data use.

---

a. **General Perinatal Rules**
   1) **Chapter 15 Codes**
      They are <u>never</u> for use on the maternal record. Codes from Chapter 11, the obstetric chapter, are never permitted on the newborn record. Chapter 15 code may be used throughout the life of the patient if the condition is still present.

   2) **Sequencing of perinatal codes**
      Generally, codes from Chapter 15 should be sequenced as the principal/first-listed diagnosis on the newborn record, with the exception of the appropriate V30 code for the birth episode, followed by codes from any other chapter that provide additional detail. The "use additional code" note at the beginning of the chapter supports this guideline. If the index does not provide a specific code for a perinatal condition, assign code 779.89, Other specified conditions originating in the perinatal period, followed by the code from another chapter that specifies the condition. Codes for signs and symptoms may be assigned when a definitive diagnosis has not been established.

   3) **Birth process or community acquired conditions**
      If a newborn has a condition that may be either due to the birth process or community acquired and the documentation does not indicate which it is, the default is due to the birth process and the code from Chapter 15 should be used. If the condition is community-acquired, a code from Chapter 15 should not be assigned.

   4) **Code all clinically significant conditions**
      All clinically significant conditions noted on routine newborn examination should be coded. A condition is clinically significant if it requires:
      - clinical evaluation; or
      - therapeutic treatment; or
      - diagnostic procedures; or
      - extended length of hospital stay; or
      - increased nursing care and/or monitoring; or
      - has implications for future health care needs

Note: The perinatal guidelines listed above are the same as the general coding guidelines for "additional diagnoses", except for the final point regarding implications for future health care needs. Codes should be assigned for conditions that have been specified by the provider as having implications for future health care needs. Codes from the perinatal chapter should not be assigned unless the provider has established a definitive diagnosis.

b. Use of codes V30-V39

When coding the birth of an infant, assign a code from categories V30-V39, according to the type of birth. A code from this series is assigned as a principal diagnosis, and assigned only once to a newborn at the time of birth.

c. Newborn transfers

If the newborn is transferred to another institution, the V30 series is not used at the receiving hospital.

d. Use of category V29

1) Assigning a code from category V29

Assign a code from category V29, Observation and evaluation of newborns and infants for suspected conditions not found, to identify those instances when a healthy newborn is evaluated for a suspected condition that is determined after study not to be present. Do not use a code from category V29 when the patient has identified signs or symptoms of a suspected problem; in such cases, code the sign or symptom.

A code from category V29 may also be assigned as a principal code for readmissions or encounters when the V30 code no longer applies. Codes from category V29 are for use only for healthy newborns and infants for which no condition after study is found to be present.

2) V29 code on a birth record

A V29 code is to be used as a secondary code after the V30, Outcome of delivery, code.

e. Use of other V codes on perinatal records
V codes other than V30 and V29 may be assigned on a perinatal or newborn record code. The codes may be used as a principal or first-listed diagnosis for specific types of encounters or for readmissions or encounters when the V30 code no longer applies.

See Section I.C.18 for information regarding the assignment of V codes.

f. Maternal Causes of Perinatal Morbidity
Codes from categories 760-763, Maternal causes of perinatal morbidity and mortality, are assigned only when the maternal condition has actually affected the fetus or newborn. The fact that the mother has an associated medical condition or experiences some complication of pregnancy, labor or delivery does not justify the routine assignment of codes from these categories to the newborn record.

g. Congenital Anomalies in Newborns
For the birth admission, the appropriate code from category V30, Liveborn infants according to type of birth, should be used, followed by any congenital anomaly codes, categories 740-759. Use additional secondary codes from other chapters to specify conditions associated with the anomaly, if applicable.

Also, see Section I.C.14 for information on the coding of congenital anomalies.

h. Coding Additional Perinatal Diagnoses
1) Assigning codes for conditions that require treatment
Assign codes for conditions that require treatment or further investigation, prolong the length of stay, or require resource utilization.

2) Codes for conditions specified as having implications for future health care needs
Assign codes for conditions that have been specified by the provider as having implications for future health care needs.

Note: This guideline should not be used for adult patients.

3) **Codes for newborn conditions originating in the perinatal period**
Assign a code for newborn conditions originating in the perinatal period (categories 760-779), as well as complications arising during the current episode of care classified in other chapters, only if the diagnoses have been documented by the responsible provider at the time of transfer or discharge as having affected the fetus or newborn.

i. **Prematurity and Fetal Growth Retardation**
Providers utilize different criteria in determining prematurity. A code for prematurity should not be assigned unless it is documented. The 5th-digit assignment for codes from category 764 and subcategories 765.0 and 765.1 should be based on the recorded birth weight and estimated gestational age.

A code from subcategory 765.2, Weeks of gestation, should be assigned as an additional code with category 764 and codes from 765.0 and 765.1 to specify weeks of gestation as documented by the provider in the record.

j. **Newborn sepsis**
Code 771.81, Septicemia [sepsis] of newborn, should be assigned with a secondary code from category 041, Bacterial infections in conditions classified elsewhere and of unspecified site, to identify the organism. It is not necessary to use a code from subcategory 995.9, Systemic inflammatory response syndrome (SIRS), on a newborn record. A code from category 038, Septicemia, should not be used on a newborn record. Code 771.81 describes the sepsis.

16. **Chapter 16: Signs, Symptoms and Ill-Defined Conditions (780-799)**
Reserved for future guideline expansion

17. Chapter 17: Injury and Poisoning (800-999)

a. Coding of Injuries

When coding injuries, assign separate codes for each injury unless a combination code is provided, in which case the combination code is assigned. Multiple injury codes are provided in ICD-9-CM, but should not be assigned unless information for a more specific code is not available. These codes are not to be used for normal, healing surgical wounds or to identify complications of surgical wounds.

The code for the most serious injury, as determined by the provider and the focus of treatment, is sequenced first.

1) Superficial injuries

Superficial injuries such as abrasions or contusions are not coded when associated with more severe injuries of the same site.

2) Primary injury with damage to nerves/blood vessels

When a primary injury results in minor damage to peripheral nerves or blood vessels, the primary injury is sequenced first with additional code(s) from categories 950-957, Injury to nerves and spinal cord, and/or 900-904, Injury to blood vessels. When the primary injury is to the blood vessels or nerves, that injury should be sequenced first.

b. Coding of Fractures

The principles of multiple coding of injuries should be followed in coding fractures. Fractures of specified sites are coded individually by site in accordance with both the provisions within categories 800-829 and the level of detail furnished by medical record content. Combination categories for multiple fractures are provided for use when there is insufficient detail in the medical record (such as trauma cases transferred to another hospital), when the reporting form limits the number of codes that can be used in reporting pertinent clinical data, or when there is insufficient specificity at the fourth-digit or fifth-digit level. More specific guidelines are as follows:

1) **Multiple fractures of same limb**
Multiple fractures of same limb classifiable to the same three-digit or four-digit category are coded to that category.

2) **Multiple unilateral or bilateral fractures of same bone**
Multiple unilateral or bilateral fractures of same bone(s) but classified to different fourth-digit subdivisions (bone part) within the same three-digit category are coded individually by site.

3) **Multiple fracture categories 819 and 828**
Multiple fracture categories 819 and 828 classify bilateral fractures of both upper limbs (819) and both lower limbs (828), but without any detail at the fourth-digit level other than open and closed type of fractures.

4) **Multiple fractures sequencing**
Multiple fractures are sequenced in accordance with the severity of the fracture. The provider should be asked to list the fracture diagnoses in the order of severity.

c. **Coding of Burns**
Current burns (940-948) are classified by depth, extent and by agent (E code). Burns are classified by depth as first degree (erythema), second degree (blistering), and third degree (full-thickness involvement).

1) **Sequencing of burn and related condition codes**
Sequence first the code that reflects the highest degree of burn when more than one burn is present.

(a) **When the reason for the admission or encounter is for treatment of external multiple burns, sequence first the code that reflects the burn of the highest degree.**

(b) **When a patient has both internal and external burns, the circumstances of admission govern the selection of the principal diagnosis or first-listed diagnosis.**

(c) **When a patient is admitted for burn injuries and other related conditions such as smoke inhalation and/or respiratory failure, the circumstances of admission govern the selection of the principal or first-listed diagnosis.**

2) **Burns of the same local site**
Classify burns of the same local site (three-digit category level, 940-947) but of different degrees to the subcategory identifying the highest degree recorded in the diagnosis.

3) **Nonhealing burns**
Nonhealing burns are coded as acute burns. Necrosis of burned skin should be coded as a nonhealed burn.

4) **Code 958.3, Posttraumatic wound infection**
Assign code 958.3, Posttraumatic wound infection, not elsewhere classified, as an additional code for any documented infected burn site.

5) **Assign separate codes for each burn site**
When coding burns, assign separate codes for each burn site. Category 946 Burns of Multiple specified sites, should only be used if the location of the burns are not documented. Category 949, Burn, unspecified, is extremely vague and should rarely be used.

6) **Assign codes from category 948, Burns**
Burns classified according to extent of body surface involved, when the site of the burn is not specified or when there is a need for additional data. It is advisable to use category 948 as additional coding when needed to provide data for evaluating burn mortality, such as that needed by burn units. It is also advisable to use category 948 as an additional code for reporting purposes when there is mention of a third-degree burn involving 20 percent or more of the body surface.

In assigning a code from category 948:

Fourth-digit codes are used to identify the percentage of total body surface involved in a burn (all degree).

Fifth-digits are assigned to identify the percentage of body surface involved in third-degree burn.

Fifth-digit zero (0) is assigned when less than 10 percent or when no body surface is involved in a third-degree burn.

Category 948 is based on the classic "rule of nines" in estimating body surface involved: head and neck are assigned nine percent, each arm nine percent, each leg 18 percent, the anterior trunk 18 percent, posterior trunk 18 percent, and genitalia one percent. Providers may change these percentage assignments where necessary to accommodate infants and children who have proportionately larger heads than adults and patients who have large buttocks, thighs, or abdomen that involve burns.

7) **Encounters for treatment of late effects of burns**
Encounters for the treatment of the late effects of burns (i.e., scars or joint contractures) should be coded to the residual condition (sequelae) followed by the appropriate late effect code (906.5-906.9). A late effect E code may also be used, if desired.

8) **Sequelae with a late effect code and current burn**
When appropriate, both a sequelae with a late effect code, and a current burn code may be assigned on the same record (when both a current burn and sequelae of an old burn exist).

d. **Coding of Debridement of Wound, Infection, or Burn**
Excisional debridement involves an excisional debridement (surgical removal or cutting away), as opposed to a mechanical (brushing, scrubbing, washing) debridement.

For coding purposes, excisional debridement is assigned to code 86.22.

Nonexcisional debridement is assigned to code 86.28.

e. **Adverse Effects, Poisoning and Toxic Effects**
The properties of certain drugs, medicinal and biological substances or combinations of such substances, may cause toxic reactions. The occurrence of drug toxicity is classified in ICD-9-CM as follows:

1) **Adverse Effect**
When the drug was correctly prescribed and properly administered, code the reaction plus the appropriate code from the E930-E949 series. Codes from the E930-E949 series must be used to identify the causative substance for an adverse effect of drug, medicinal and biological substances, correctly prescribed and properly administered. The effect, such as tachycardia, delirium, gastrointestinal hemorrhaging, vomiting, hypokalemia, hepatitis, renal failure, or respiratory failure, is coded and followed by the appropriate code from the E930-E949 series.

Adverse effects of therapeutic substances correctly prescribed and properly administered (toxicity, synergistic reaction, side effect, and idiosyncratic reaction) may be due to (1) differences among patients, such as age, sex, disease, and genetic factors, and (2) drug-related factors, such as type of drug, route of administration, duration of therapy, dosage, and bioavailability.

2) **Poisoning**
(a) **Error was made in drug prescription**
Errors made in drug prescription or in the administration of the drug by provider, nurse, patient, or other person, use the appropriate poisoning code from the 960-979 series.

(b) **Overdose of a drug intentionally taken**
If an overdose of a drug was intentionally taken or administered and resulted in drug toxicity, it would be coded as a poisoning (960-979 series).

(c) **Nonprescribed drug taken with correctly prescribed and properly administered drug**
If a nonprescribed drug or medicinal agent was taken in combination with a correctly prescribed and properly administered drug, any drug toxicity or other reaction resulting from the interaction of the two drugs would be classified as a poisoning.

(d) **Sequencing of poisoning**
When coding a poisoning or reaction to the improper use of a medication (e.g., wrong dose, wrong substance, wrong route of administration) the poisoning code is sequenced first, followed by a code for the manifestation. If there is also a diagnosis of drug abuse or dependence to the substance, the abuse or dependence is coded as an additional code.

See Section I.C.3.a.6.b. if poisoning is the result of insulin pump malfunctions and Section I.C.19 for general use of E-codes.

3) **Toxic Effects**
(a) **Toxic effect codes**
When a harmful substance is ingested or comes in contact with a person, this is classified as a toxic effect. The toxic effect codes are in categories 980-989.

(b) **Sequencing toxic effect codes**
A toxic effect code should be sequenced first, followed by the code(s) that identify the result of the toxic effect.

(c) **External cause codes for toxic effects**
An external cause code from categories E860-E869 for accidental exposure, codes E950.6 or E950.7 for intentional self-harm, category E962 for assault, or categories E980-E982, for undetermined, should also be assigned to indicate intent.

f. **Complications of care**
   1) **Transplant complications**

   (a) **Transplant complications other than kidney**
   Codes under subcategory 996.8, Complications of transplanted organ, are for use for both complications and rejection of transplanted organs. A transplant complication code is only assigned if the complication affects the function of the transplanted organ. Two codes are required to fully describe a transplant complication, the appropriate code from subcategory 996.8 and a secondary code that identifies the complication.

   Preexisting conditions or conditions that develop after the transplant are not coded as complications unless they affect the function of the transplanted organs.

   Post-transplants surgical complications that do not relate to the function of the transplanted organ are classified to the specific complication. For example, a surgical wound dehiscence would be coded to the wound dehiscence, not as a transplant complication. Post-transplant patients who are seen for treatment unrelated to the transplanted organ should be assigned a code from category V42, Organ or tissue replaced by transplant, to identify the transplant status of the patient. A code from category V42 should never be used with a code from subcategory 996.8.

   (b) **Kidney transplant and chronic kidney disease**
   Patients with chronic kidney disease (CKD) following a transplant should not be assumed to have transplant failure or rejection unless it is documented by the provider. If documentation supports the presence of failure or rejection, then it is appropriate to assign code 996.81, Complications of transplanted organs, kidney followed by the appropriate CKD code.

18. Classification of Factors Influencing Health Status and Contact with Health Service (Supplemental V01-V84) Note: The chapter-specific guidelines provide additional information about the use of V codes for specified encounters.

a. **Introduction**

ICD-9-CM provides codes to deal with encounters for circumstances other than a disease or injury. The Supplementary Classification of Factors Influencing Health Status and Contact with Health Services (V01.0 - V84.8) is provided to deal with occasions when circumstances other than a disease or injury (codes 001-999) are recorded as a diagnosis or problem.

There are four primary circumstances for the use of V codes:

1) A person who is not currently sick encounters the health services for some specific reason, such as to act as an organ donor, to receive prophylactic care, such as inoculations or health screenings, or to receive counseling on health related issues.

(2) A person with a resolving disease or injury, or a chronic, long-term condition requiring continuous care, encounters the health care system for specific aftercare of that disease or injury (e.g., dialysis for renal disease; chemotherapy for malignancy; cast change). A diagnosis/symptom code should be used whenever a current, acute, diagnosis is being treated or a sign or symptom is being studied.

3) Circumstances or problems influence a person's health status but are not in themselves a current illness or injury.

4) Newborns, to indicate birth status

b. **V codes use in any healthcare setting**

V codes are for use in any healthcare setting. V codes may be used as either a first listed (principal diagnosis code in the inpatient setting) or secondary code, depending on the circumstances of the encounter. Certain V codes may only be used as first listed, others only as secondary codes. See Section I.C.18.e, **V Code Table.**

c. **V Codes indicate a reason for an encounter**
They are not procedure codes. A corresponding procedure code must accompany a V code to describe the procedure performed.

d. **Categories of V Codes**

1) **Contact/Exposure**
Category V01 indicates contact with or exposure to communicable diseases. These codes are for patients who do not show any sign or symptom of a disease but have been exposed to it by close personal contact with an infected individual or are in an area where a disease is epidemic. These codes may be used as a first listed code to explain an encounter for testing, or, more commonly, as a secondary code to identify a potential risk.

2) **Inoculations and vaccinations**
Categories V03-V06 are for encounters for inoculations and vaccinations. They indicate that a patient is being seen to receive a prophylactic inoculation against a disease. The injection itself must be represented by the appropriate procedure code. A code from V03-V06 may be used as a secondary code if the inoculation is given as a routine part of preventive health care, such as a well-baby visit.

3) **Status**
Status codes indicate that a patient is either a carrier of a disease or has the sequelae or residual of a past disease or condition. This includes such things as the presence of prosthetic or mechanical devices resulting from past treatment. A status code is informative, because the status may affect the course of treatment and its outcome. A status code is distinct from a history code. The history code indicates that the patient no longer has the condition.

A status code should not be used with a diagnosis code from one of the body system chapters, if the diagnosis code includes the information provided by the status code. For example, code V42.1, Heart transplant status, should not be used with code 996.83, Complications of transplanted heart. The status code does not provide additional information. The complication code indicates that the patient is a heart transplant patient.

The status V codes/categories are:

V02   Carrier or suspected carrier of infectious diseases
         Carrier status indicates that a person harbors the specific organisms of a disease without manifest symptoms and is capable of transmitting the infection.

V08   Asymptomatic HIV infection status
         This code indicates that a patient has tested positive for HIV but has manifested no signs or symptoms of the disease.

V09   Infection with drug-resistant microorganisms
         This category indicates that a patient has an infection that is resistant to drug treatment. Sequence the infection code first.

V21   Constitutional states in development

V22.2   Pregnant state, incidental
         This code is a secondary code only for use when the pregnancy is in no way complicating the reason for visit. Otherwise, a code from the obstetric chapter is required.

V26.5x   Sterilization status

V42   Organ or tissue replaced by transplant

V43   Organ or tissue replaced by other means

V44   Artificial opening status

V45   Other postsurgical states

V46   Other dependence on machines

V49.6   Upper limb amputation status

V49.7   Lower limb amputation status

V49.81   Postmenopausal status

V49.82   Dental sealant status

V49.83   Awaiting organ transplant status

V58.6 Long-term (current) drug use
This subcategory indicates a patient's continuous use of a prescribed drug (including such things as aspirin therapy) for the long-term treatment of a condition or for prophylactic use. It is not for use for patients who have addictions to drugs.

Assign a code from subcategory V58.6, Long-term (current) drug use, if the patient is receiving a medication for an extended period as a prophylactic measure (such as for the prevention of deep vein thrombosis) or as treatment of a chronic condition (such as arthritis) or a disease requiring a lengthy course of treatment (such as cancer). Do not assign a code from subcategory V58.6 for medication being administered for a brief period of time to treat an acute illness or injury (such as a course of antibiotics to treat acute bronchitis).

V83 Genetic carrier status
Genetic carrier status indicates that a person carries a gene, associated with a particular disease, which may be passed to offspring who may develop that disease. The person does not have the disease and is not at risk of developing the disease.

V84 Genetic susceptibility status
Genetic susceptibility indicates that a person has a gene that increases the risk of that person developing the disease.

Codes from category V84, Genetic susceptibility to disease, should not be used as principal or first-listed codes. If the patient has the condition to which he/she is susceptible, and that condition is the reason for the encounter, the code for the current condition should be sequenced first. If the patient is being seen for follow-

up after completed treatment for this condition, and the condition no longer exists, a follow-up code should be sequenced first, followed by the appropriate personal history and genetic susceptibility codes. If the purpose of the encounter is genetic counseling associated with procreative management, a code from subcategory V26.3, Genetic counseling and testing, should be assigned as the first-listed code, followed by a code from category V84.

Additional codes should be assigned for any applicable family or personal history. See Section I.C. 18.d.14 for information on prophylactic organ removal due to a genetic susceptibility.

Note: Categories V42-V46, and subcategories V49.6, V49.7 are for use only if there are no complications or malfunctions of the organ or tissue replaced, the amputation site or the equipment on which the patient is dependent.

4) **History (of)**

There are two types of history V codes, personal and family. Personal history codes explain a patient's past medical condition that no longer exists and is not receiving any treatment, but that has the potential for recurrence, and therefore may require continued monitoring. The exceptions to this general rule are category V14, Personal history of allergy to medicinal agents, and subcategory V15.0, Allergy, other than to medicinal agents. A person who has had an allergic episode to a substance or food in the past should always be considered allergic to the substance.

Family history codes are for use when a patient has a family member(s) who has had a particular disease that causes the patient to be at higher risk of also contracting the disease.

Personal history codes may be used in conjunction with follow-up codes and family history codes may be used in conjunction with screening codes to explain the need for a test or procedure. History codes are also acceptable on any medical record regardless of the reason for visit. A history of an illness, even if no longer present, is important information that may alter the type of treatment ordered.

The history V code categories are:

V10	Personal history of malignant neoplasm
V12	Personal history of certain other diseases
V13	Personal history of other diseases
	Except: V13.4, Personal history of arthritis, and V13.6, Personal history of congenital malformations. These conditions are life-long so are not true history codes.
V14	Personal history of allergy to medicinal agents
V15	Other personal history presenting hazards to health
	Except: V15.7, Personal history of contraception.
V16	Family history of malignant neoplasm
V17	Family history of certain chronic disabling diseases
V18	Family history of certain other specific diseases
V19	Family history of other conditions

5) **Screening**

Screening is the testing for disease or disease precursors in seemingly well individuals so that early detection and treatment can be provided for those who test positive for the disease. Screenings that are recommended for many subgroups in a population include: routine mammograms for women over 40, a fecal occult blood test for everyone over 50, an amniocentesis to rule out a fetal anomaly for pregnant women over 35, because the incidence of breast cancer and colon cancer in these subgroups is higher than in the general population, as is the incidence of Down's syndrome in older mothers.

The testing of a person to rule out or confirm a suspected diagnosis because the patient has some sign or symptom is a diagnostic examination, not a screening. In these cases, the sign or symptom is used to explain the reason for the test.

A screening code may be a first listed code if the reason for the visit is specifically the screening exam. It may also be used as an additional code if the screening is done during an office visit for other health problems. A screening code is not necessary if the screening is inherent to a routine examination, such as a pap smear done during a routine pelvic examination.

Should a condition be discovered during the screening then the code for the condition may be assigned as an additional diagnosis.

The V code indicates that a screening exam is planned. A procedure code is required to confirm that the screening was performed.

The screening V code categories:
V28   Antenatal screening
V73-V82   Special screening examinations

6) **Observation**
There are two observation V code categories. They are for use in very limited circumstances when a person is being observed for a suspected condition that is ruled out. The observation codes are not for use if an injury or illness or any signs or symptoms related to the suspected condition are present. In such cases the diagnosis/symptom code is used with the corresponding E code to identify any external cause.

The observation codes are to be used as principal diagnosis only. The only exception to this is when the principal diagnosis is required to be a code from the V30, Live born infant, category. Then the V29 observation code is sequenced after the V30 code. Additional codes may be used in addition to the observation code but only if they are unrelated to the suspected condition being observed.

The observation V code categories:

V29   Observation and evaluation of newborns for suspected condition not found
For the birth encounter, a code from category V30 should be sequenced before the V29 code.

V71   Observation and evaluation for suspected condition not found

7) Aftercare

Aftercare visit codes cover situations when the initial treatment of a disease or injury has been performed and the patient requires continued care during the healing or recovery phase, or for the long-term consequences of the disease. The aftercare V code should not be used if treatment is directed at a current, acute disease or injury, the diagnosis code is to be used in these cases. Exceptions to this rule are codes V58.0, Radiotherapy, and **codes from subcategory** V58.1, **Encounter for** chemotherapy **and immunotherapy for neoplastic conditions**. These codes are to be first listed, followed by the diagnosis code when a patient's encounter is solely to receive radiation therapy or chemotherapy for the treatment of a neoplasm. Should a patient receive both chemotherapy and radiation therapy during the same encounter code V58.0 and V58.1 may be used together on a record with either one being sequenced first.

The aftercare codes are generally first listed to explain the specific reason for the encounter. An aftercare code may be used as an additional code when some type of aftercare is provided in addition to the reason for admission and no diagnosis code is applicable. An example of this would be the closure of a colostomy during an encounter for treatment of another condition.

Certain aftercare V code categories need a secondary diagnosis code to describe the resolving condition or sequelae, for others, the condition is inherent in the code title.

Additional V code aftercare category terms include, fitting and adjustment, and attention to artificial openings.

Status V codes may be used with aftercare V codes to indicate the nature of the aftercare. For example code V45.81, Aortocoronary bypass status, may be used with code V58.73, Aftercare following surgery of the circulatory system, NEC, to indicate the surgery for which the aftercare is being performed. Also, a transplant status code may be used following code V58.44, Aftercare following organ transplant, to identify the organ transplanted. A status code should not be used when the aftercare code indicates the type of status, such as using V55.0, Attention to tracheostomy with V44.0, Tracheostomy status.

The aftercare V category/codes:

V52   Fitting and adjustment of prosthetic device and implant
V53   Fitting and adjustment of other device
V54   Other orthopedic aftercare
V55   Attention to artificial openings
V56   Encounter for dialysis and dialysis catheter care
V57   Care involving the use of rehabilitation procedures
V58.0   Radiotherapy
V58.11 Encounter for antineoplastic chemotherapy
V58.12 Encounter for antineoplastic immunotherapy
V58.3   Attention to surgical dressings and sutures
V58.41 Encounter for planned postoperative wound closure
V58.42 Aftercare, surgery, neoplasm
V58.43 Aftercare, surgery, trauma
V58.44 Aftercare involving organ transplant
V58.49 Other specified aftercare following surgery
V58.7x Aftercare following surgery
V58.81 Fitting and adjustment of vascular catheter
V58.82 Fitting and adjustment of nonvascular catheter
V58.83 Monitoring therapeutic drug
V58.89 Other specified aftercare

8) **Follow-up**
The follow-up codes are used to explain continuing surveillance following completed treatment of a disease, condition, or injury. They imply that the condition has been fully treated and no longer exists. They should not

be confused with aftercare codes that explain current treatment for a healing condition or its sequelae. Follow-up codes may be used in conjunction with history codes to provide the full picture of the healed condition and its treatment. The follow-up code is sequenced first, followed by the history code.

A follow-up code may be used to explain repeated visits. Should a condition be found to have recurred on the follow-up visit, then the diagnosis code should be used in place of the follow-up code.

The follow-up V code categories:
V24   Postpartum care and evaluation
V67   Follow-up examination

9) Donor

Category V59 is the donor codes. They are used for living individuals who are donating blood or other body tissue. These codes are only for individuals donating for others, not for self donations. They are not for use to identify cadaveric donations.

10) Counseling

Counseling V codes are used when a patient or family member receives assistance in the aftermath of an illness or injury, or when support is required in coping with family or social problems. They are not necessary for use in conjunction with a diagnosis code when the counseling component of care is considered integral to standard treatment.

The counseling V categories/codes:
V25.0   General counseling and advice for contraceptive management
V26.3   Genetic counseling
V26.4   General counseling and advice for procreative management
V61   Other family circumstances
V65.1   Person consulted on behalf of another person
V65.3   Dietary surveillance and counseling
V65.4   Other counseling, not elsewhere classified

11) Obstetrics and related conditions

See Section I.C.11., the Obstetrics guidelines for further instruction on the use of these codes.

V codes for pregnancy are for use in those circumstances when none of the problems or complications included in the codes from the Obstetrics chapter exist (a routine prenatal visit or postpartum care). Codes V22.0, Supervision of normal first pregnancy, and V22.1, Supervision of other normal pregnancy, are always first listed and are not to be used with any other code from the OB chapter.

The outcome of delivery, category V27, should be included on all maternal delivery records. It is always a secondary code.

V codes for family planning (contraceptive) or procreative management and counseling should be included on an obstetric record either during the pregnancy or the postpartum stage, if applicable.

Obstetrics and related conditions V code categories:

V22	Normal pregnancy
V23	Supervision of high-risk pregnancy Except: V23.2, Pregnancy with history of abortion. Code 646.3, Habitual aborter, from the OB chapter is required to indicate a history of abortion during a pregnancy.
V24	Postpartum care and evaluation
V25	Encounter for contraceptive management Except V25.0x (See Section I.C.18.d.11, Counseling)
V26	Procreative management Except V26.5x, Sterilization status, V26.3 and V26.4 (See Section I.C.18.d.11., Counseling)
V27	Outcome of delivery
V28	Antenatal screening (See Section I.C.18.d.6., Screening)

12) Newborn, infant and child
See Section I.C.15, the Newborn guidelines for further instruction on the use of these codes.

Newborn V code categories:
V20   Health supervision of infant or child
V29   Observation and evaluation of newborns for suspected condition not found (See Section I.C.18.d.7, Observation).
V30-V39   Liveborn infant according to type of birth

13) Routine and administrative examinations
The V codes allow for the description of encounters for routine examinations, such as, a general check-up, or, examinations for administrative purposes, such as, a pre-employment physical. The codes are for use as first listed codes only, and are not to be used if the examination is for diagnosis of a suspected condition or for treatment purposes. In such cases the diagnosis code is used. During a routine exam, should a diagnosis or condition be discovered, it should be coded as an additional code. Pre-existing and chronic conditions and history codes may also be included as additional codes as long as the examination is for administrative purposes and not focused on any particular condition.

Pre-operative examination V codes are for use only in those situations when a patient is being cleared for surgery and no treatment is given.

The V codes categories/code for routine and administrative examinations:

V20.2   Routine infant or child health check
        Any injections given should have a corresponding procedure code.
V70   General medical examination
V72   Special investigations and examinations Except V72.5 and V72.6

14) Miscellaneous V codes

The miscellaneous V codes capture a number of other health care encounters that do not fall into one of the other categories. Certain of these codes identify the reason for the encounter, others are for use as additional codes that provide useful information on circumstances that may affect a patient's care and treatment.

Prophylactic Organ Removal

For encounters specifically for prophylactic removal of breasts, ovaries, or another organ due to a genetic susceptibility to cancer or a family history of cancer, the principal or first listed code should be a code from subcategory V50.4, Prophylactic organ removal, followed by the appropriate genetic susceptibility code and the appropriate family history code.

If the patient has a malignancy of one site and is having prophylactic removal at another site to prevent either a new primary malignancy or metastatic disease, a code for the malignancy should also be assigned in addition to a code from subcategory V50.4. A V50.4 code should not be assigned if the patient is having organ removal for treatment of a malignancy, such as the removal of the testes for the treatment of prostate cancer.

Miscellaneous V code categories/codes:

V07	Need for isolation and other prophylactic measures
V50	Elective surgery for purposes other than remedying health states
V58.5	Orthodontics
V60	Housing, household, and economic circumstances
V62	Other psychosocial circumstances
V63	Unavailability of other medical facilities for care
V64	Persons encountering health services for specific procedures, not carried out
V66	Convalescence and Palliative Care
V68	Encounters for administrative purposes
V69	Problems related to lifestyle

15) Nonspecific V codes

Certain V codes are so nonspecific, or potentially redundant with other codes in the classification, that there can be little justification for their use in the inpatient setting. Their use in the outpatient setting should be limited to those instances when there is no further documentation to permit more precise coding. Otherwise, any sign or symptom or any other reason for visit that is captured in another code should be used.

Nonspecific V code categories/codes:

V11   Personal history of mental disorder
       A code from the mental disorders chapter, with an in remission fifth-digit, should be used.
V13.4 Personal history of arthritis
V13.6 Personal history of congenital malformations
V15.7 Personal history of contraception
V23.2 Pregnancy with history of abortion
V40   Mental and behavioral problems
V41   Problems with special senses and other special functions
V47   Other problems with internal organs
V48   Problems with head, neck, and trunk
V49   Problems with limbs and other problems
       Exceptions:
           V49.6 Upper limb amputation status
           V49.7 Lower limb amputation status
           V49.81 Postmenopausal status
           V49.82 Dental sealant status
           V49.83 Awaiting organ transplant status
V51   Aftercare involving the use of plastic surgery
V58.2 Blood transfusion, without reported diagnosis
V58.9 Unspecified aftercare
V72.5 Radiological examination, NEC
V72.6 Laboratory examination
       Codes V72.5 and V72.6 are not to be used if any sign or symptoms, or reason for a test is documented. See Section IV.K. and Section IV.L. of the Outpatient guidelines.

V Code Table
Items in bold indicate a change from the April 2005 table.
Items underlined have been moved within the table since April 2005.

FIRST LISTED: V codes/categories/subcategories which are only acceptable as principal/first listed.

Codes:

V22.0	Supervision of normal first pregnancy
V22.1	Supervision of other normal pregnancy
V46.12	Encounter for respirator dependence during power failure
V46.13	**Encounter for weaning from respirator [ventilator]**
V56.0	Extracorporeal dialysis
V58.0	Radiotherapy

V58.0 and V58.11 may be used together on a record with either one being sequenced first, when a patient receives both chemotherapy and radiation therapy during the same encounter code.

V58.11	**Encounter for antineoplastic chemotherapy**

V58.0 and **V58.11** may be used together on a record with either one being sequenced first, when a patient receives both chemotherapy and radiation therapy during the same encounter code.

V58.12	**Encounter for antineoplastic immunotherapy**

Categories/Subcategories:

V20	Health supervision of infant or child
V24	Postpartum care and examination
V29	Observation and evaluation of newborns for suspected condition not found
	Exception: A code from the V30-V39 may be sequenced before the V29 if it is the newborn record.
V30-V39	Liveborn infants according to type of birth
<u>V57</u>	<u>Care involving use of rehabilitation procedures</u>
V59	Donors
V66	Convalescence and palliative care
	Exception: V66.7 Palliative care
V68	Encounters for administrative purposes
V70	General medical examination

	Exception: V70.7 Examination of participant in clinical trial
V71	Observation and evaluation for suspected conditions not found
V72	Special investigations and examinations
	Exceptions:

V72.4 Pregnancy examination or test
V72.5   Radiological examination, NEC
V72.6   Laboratory examination
V72.86 Encounter for blood typing

FIRST OR ADDITIONAL: V code categories/subcategories which may be either principal/first listed or additional codes

Codes:

V15.88	**History of fall**
V43.22	Fully implantable artificial heart status
V46.14	**Mechanical complication of respirator [ventilator]**
V49.81	Asymptomatic postmenopausal status (age-related) (natural)
V49.84	**Bed confiement status**
V49.89	Other specified conditions influencing health status
V70.7	Examination of participant in clinical trial
V72.5	Radiological examination, NEC
V72.6	Laboratory examination
V72.86	**Encounter for blood typing**

Categories/Subcategories:

V01	Contact with or exposure to communicable diseases
V02	Carrier or suspected carrier of infectious diseases
V03-06	Need for prophylactic vaccination and inoculations
V07	Need for isolation and other prophylactic measures
V08	Asymptomatic HIV infection status
V10	Personal history of malignant neoplasm
V12	Personal history of certain other diseases
V13	Personal history of other diseases
	Exception: V13.4 Personal history of arthritis
	V13.69 Personal history of other congenital malformations
V16-V19	Family history of disease
V23	Supervision of high-risk pregnancy
V25	Encounter for contraceptive management
V26	Procreative management
	Exception: V26.5 Sterilization status

V28	Antenatal screening
V45.7	Acquired absence of organ
<u>V49.6x</u>	<u>Upper limb amputation status</u>
<u>V49.7x</u>	<u>Lower limb amputation status</u>
V50	Elective surgery for purposes other than remedying health states
V52	Fitting and adjustment of prosthetic device and implant
V53	Fitting and adjustment of other device
V54	Other orthopedic aftercare
V55	Attention to artificial openings
V56	Encounter for dialysis and dialysis catheter care
	Exception: V56.0 Extracorporeal dialysis
~~V57~~	~~Care involving use of rehabilitation procedures~~
V58.3	Attention to surgical dressings and sutures
V58.4	Other aftercare following surgery
~~V58.6~~	~~Long-term (current) drug use~~
V58.7	Aftercare following surgery to specified body systems, not elsewhere classified
V58.8	Other specified procedures and aftercare
V61	Other family circumstances
V63	Unavailability of other medical facilities for care
V65	Other persons seeking consultation without complaint or sickness
V67	Follow-up examination
V69	Problems related to lifestyle
V72.4	**Pregnancy examination or test**
V73-V82	Special screening examinations
V83	Genetic carrier status

ADDITIONAL ONLY: V code categories/subcategories which may only be used as additional codes, not principal/first listed

Codes:

V13.61	Personal history of hypospadias
V22.2	Pregnancy state, incidental
V46.11	**Dependence on respirator, status**
V49.82	Dental sealant status
V49.83	Awaiting organ transplant status
V66.7	Palliative care

Categories/Subcategories:

V09	Infection with drug-resistant microorganisms
V14	Personal history of allergy to medicinal agents

V15	Other personal history presenting hazards to health
	Exception: V15.7 Personal history of contraception
	V15.88 History of fall
V21	Constitutional states in development
V26.5	Sterilization status
V27	Outcome of delivery
V42	Organ or tissue replaced by transplant
V43	Organ or tissue replaced by other means
	Exception: V43.22 Fully implantable artificial heart status
V44	Artificial opening status
V45	Other postsurgical states
	Exception: Subcategory V45.7 Acquired absence of organ
V46	Other dependence on machines
	Exception: V46.12 Encounter for respirator dependence during power failure
	V46.13 Encounter for weaning from respirator [ventilator]
~~V49.6x~~	~~Upper limb amputation status~~
~~V49.7x~~	~~Lower limb amputation status~~
<u>V58.6</u>	<u>Long-term current drug use</u>
V60	Housing, household, and economic circumstances
V62	Other psychosocial circumstances
V64	Persons encountering health services for specified procedure, not carried out
V84	Genetic susceptibility to disease
V85	**Body Mass Index**

NONSPECIFIC CODES AND CATEGORIES:

V11	Personal history of mental disorder
V13.4	Personal history of arthritis
V13.69	Personal history of congenital malformations
V15.7	Personal history of contraception
V40	Mental and behavioral problems
V41	Problems with special senses and other special functions
V47	Other problems with internal organs
V48	Problems with head, neck, and trunk
V49.0	**Deficiencies of limbs**
V49.1	**Mechanical problems with limbs**
V49.2	**Motor problems with limbs**
V49.3	**Sensory problems with limbs**
V49.4	**Disfigurements in limbs**
V49.5	**Other problems with limbs**

V49.9	**Unspecified condition influencing health status**
~~V49~~	~~Problems with limbs and other problems~~
	Exceptions:
	~~V49.6~~ ~~Upper limb amputation status~~
	~~V49.7~~ ~~Lower limb amputation status~~
	~~V49.81~~ ~~Postmenopausal status (age-related) (natural)~~
	~~V49.82~~ ~~Dental sealant status~~
	~~V49.83~~ ~~Awaiting organ transplant status~~
V51	Aftercare involving the use of plastic surgery
V58.2	Blood transfusion, without reported diagnosis
V58.5	Orthodontics
V58.9	Unspecified aftercare
V72.5	Radiological examination, NEC
V72.6	Laboratory examination

19. Supplemental Classification of External Causes of Injury and Poisoning (E-codes, E800-E999)

Introduction: These guidelines are provided for those who are currently collecting E codes in order that there will be standardization in the process. If your institution plans to begin collecting E codes, these guidelines are to be applied. The use of E codes is supplemental to the application of ICD-9-CM diagnosis codes. E codes are never to be recorded as principal diagnoses (first-listed in noninpatient setting) and are not required for reporting to CMS.

External causes of injury and poisoning codes (E codes) are intended to provide data for injury research and evaluation of injury prevention strategies. E codes capture how the injury or poisoning happened (cause), the intent (unintentional or accidental; or intentional, such as suicide or assault), and the place where the event occurred.

Some major categories of E codes include:
transport accidents
poisoning and adverse effects of drugs, medicinal substances
and biologicals
accidental falls
accidents caused by fire and flames
accidents due to natural and environmental factors
late effects of accidents, assaults or self injury

assaults or purposely inflicted injury
suicide or self-inflicted injury

These guidelines apply for the coding and collection of E codes from records in hospitals, outpatient clinics, emergency departments, other ambulatory care settings and provider offices, and nonacute care settings, except when other specific guidelines apply.

a. **General E Code Coding Guidelines**
    1) **Used with any code in the range of 001-V84.8**
        An E code may be used with any code in the range of 001-V84.8, which indicates an injury, poisoning, or adverse effect due to an external cause.

    2) **Assign the appropriate E code for all initial treatments**
        Assign the appropriate E code for the initial encounters of an injury, poisoning, or adverse effect of drugs, **not for subsequent treatment.**

    3) **Use the full range of E codes**
        Use the full range of E codes to completely describe the cause, the intent and the place of occurrence, if applicable, for all injuries, poisonings, and adverse effects of drugs.

    4) **Assign as many E codes as necessary**
        Assign as many E codes as necessary to fully explain each cause. If only one E code can be recorded, assign the E code most related to the principal diagnosis.

    5) **The selection of the appropriate E code**
        The selection of the appropriate E code is guided by the Index to External Causes, which is located after the alphabetical index to diseases and by Inclusion and Exclusion notes in the Tabular List.

    6) **E code can never be a principal diagnosis**
        An E code can never be a principal (first listed) diagnosis.

7) External cause code(s) with systemic inflammatory response syndrome (SIRS)
An external cause code(s) may be used with codes 995.93, Systemic inflammatory response syndrome due to noninfectious process without organ dysfunction, and 995.94, Systemic inflammatory response syndrome due to noninfectious process with organ dysfunction, if trauma was the initiating insult that precipitated the SIRS. The external cause(s) code should correspond to the most serious injury resulting from the trauma. The external cause code(s) should only be assigned if the trauma necessitated the admission in which the patient also developed SIRS. If a patient is admitted with SIRS but the trauma has been treated previously, the external cause codes should not be used.

b. Place of Occurrence Guideline
Use an additional code from category E849 to indicate the Place of Occurrence for injuries and poisonings. The Place of Occurrence describes the place where the event occurred and not the patient's activity at the time of the event.

Do not use E849.9 if the place of occurrence is not stated.

c. Adverse Effects of Drugs, Medicinal and Biological Substances Guidelines

1) Do not code directly from the Table of Drugs
Do not code directly from the Table of Drugs and Chemicals. Always refer back to the Tabular List.

2) Use as many codes as necessary to describe
Use as many codes as necessary to describe completely all drugs, medicinal or biological substances.

3) If the same E code would describe the causative agent
If the same E code would describe the causative agent for more than one adverse reaction, assign the code only once.

4) **If two or more drugs, medicinal or biological substances**
   If two or more drugs, medicinal or biological substances are reported, code each individually unless the combination code is listed in the Table of Drugs and Chemicals. In that case, assign the E code for the combination.

5) **When a reaction results from the interaction of a drug(s)**
   When a reaction results from the interaction of a drug(s) and alcohol, use poisoning codes and E codes for both.

6) **If the reporting format limits the number of E codes**
   If the reporting format limits the number of E codes that can be used in reporting clinical data, code the one most related to the principal diagnosis. Include at least one from each category (cause, intent, place) if possible.

   If there are different fourth digit codes in the same three digit category, use the code for "Other specified" of that category. If there is no "Other specified" code in that category, use the appropriate "Unspecified" code in that category.

   If the codes are in different three digit categories, assign the appropriate E code for other multiple drugs and medicinal substances.

7) **Codes from the E930-E949 series**
   Codes from the E930-E949 series must be used to identify the causative substance for an adverse effect of drug, medicinal and biological substances, correctly prescribed and properly administered. The effect, such as tachycardia, delirium, gastrointestinal hemorrhaging, vomiting, hypokalemia, hepatitis, renal failure, or respiratory failure, is coded and followed by the appropriate code from the E930-E949 series.

d. Multiple Cause E Code Coding Guidelines

If two or more events cause separate injuries, an E code should be assigned for each cause. The first listed E code will be selected in the following order:

E codes for child and adult abuse take priority over all other E codes. See Section I.C.19.e., Child and Adult abuse guidelines

E codes for terrorism events take priority over all other E codes except child and adult abuse

E codes for cataclysmic events take priority over all other E codes except child and adult abuse and terrorism.

E codes for transport accidents take priority over all other E codes except cataclysmic events and child and adult abuse and terrorism.

The first-listed E code should correspond to the cause of the most serious diagnosis due to an assault, accident, or self-harm, following the order of hierarchy listed above.

e. Child and Adult Abuse Guideline

1) Intentional injury

When the cause of an injury or neglect is intentional child or adult abuse, the first listed E code should be assigned from categories E960-E968, Homicide and injury purposely inflicted by other persons, (except category E967). An E code from category E967, Child and adult battering and other maltreatment, should be added as an additional code to identify the perpetrator, if known.

2) Accidental intent

In cases of neglect when the intent is determined to be accidental E code E904.0, Abandonment or neglect of infant and helpless person, should be the first listed E code.

f. Unknown or Suspected Intent Guideline

1) **If the intent (accident, self-harm, assault) of the cause of an injury or poisoning is unknown**
   If the intent (accident, self-harm, assault) of the cause of an injury or poisoning is unknown or unspecified, code the intent as undetermined E980-E989.

2) **If the intent (accident, self-harm, assault) of the cause of an injury or poisoning is questionable**
   If the intent (accident, self-harm, assault) of the cause of an injury or poisoning is questionable, probable or suspected, code the intent as undetermined E980-E989.

g. Undetermined Cause

When the intent of an injury or poisoning is known, but the cause is unknown, use codes: E928.9, Unspecified accident, E958.9, Suicide and self-inflicted injury by unspecified means, and E968.9, Assault by unspecified means.

These E codes should rarely be used, as the documentation in the medical record, in both the inpatient outpatient and other settings, should normally provide sufficient detail to determine the cause of the injury.

h. Late Effects of External Cause Guidelines

1) **Late effect E codes**
   Late effect E codes exist for injuries and poisonings but not for adverse effects of drugs, misadventures and surgical complications.

2) **Late effect E codes (E929, E959, E969, E977, E989, or E999.1)**
   A late effect E code (E929, E959, E969, E977, E989, or E999.1) should be used with any report of a late effect or sequela resulting from a previous injury or poisoning (905-909).

3) **Late effect E code with a related current injury**
   A late effect E code should never be used with a related current nature of injury code.

4) Use of late effect E codes for subsequent visits
Use a late effect E code for subsequent visits when a late effect of the initial injury or poisoning is being treated. There is no late effect E code for adverse effects of drugs.

Do not use a late effect E code for subsequent visits for follow-up care (e.g., to assess healing, to receive rehabilitative therapy) of the injury or poisoning when no late effect of the injury has been documented.

i. Misadventures and Complications of Care Guidelines

1) Code range E870-E876
Assign a code in the range of E870-E876 if misadventures are stated by the provider.

2) Code range E878-E879
Assign a code in the range of E878-E879 if the provider attributes an abnormal reaction or later complication to a surgical or medical procedure, but does not mention misadventure at the time of the procedure as the cause of the reaction.

j. Terrorism Guidelines
1) Cause of injury identified by the Federal Government (FBI) as terrorism
When the cause of an injury is identified by the Federal Government (FBI) as terrorism, the first-listed E-code should be a code from category E979, Terrorism. The definition of terrorism employed by the FBI is found at the inclusion note at E979. The terrorism E-code is the only E-code that should be assigned. Additional E codes from the assault categories should not be assigned.

2) Cause of an injury is suspected to be the result of terrorism
When the cause of an injury is suspected to be the result of terrorism a code from category E979 should not be assigned. Assign a code in the range of E codes based circumstances on the documentation of intent and mechanism.

3) **Code E979.9, Terrorism, secondary effects**
   Assign code E979.9, Terrorism, secondary effects, for conditions occurring subsequent to the terrorist event. This code should not be assigned for conditions that are due to the initial terrorist act.

4) **Statistical tabulation of terrorism codes**
   For statistical purposes these codes will be tabulated within the category for assault, expanding the current category from E960-E969 to include E979 and E999.1.

Section II. Selection of Principal Diagnosis

The circumstances of inpatient admission always govern the selection of principal diagnosis. The principal diagnosis is defined in the Uniform Hospital Discharge Data Set (UHDDS) as "that condition established after study to be chiefly responsible for occasioning the admission of the patient to the hospital for care."

The UHDDS definitions are used by hospitals to report inpatient data elements in a standardized manner. These data elements and their definitions can be found in the July 31, 1985, *Federal Register* (Vol. 50, No, 147), pp. 31038-40.

Since that time the application of the UHDDS definitions has been expanded to include all nonoutpatient settings (acute care, short term, long term care and psychiatric hospitals; home health agencies; rehab facilities; nursing homes, etc.).

In determining principal diagnosis the coding conventions in the ICD-9-CM, Volumes I and II take precedence over these official coding guidelines. (See Section I.A., Conventions for the ICD-9-CM).

The importance of consistent, complete documentation in the medical record cannot be overemphasized. Without such documentation the application of all coding guidelines is a difficult, if not impossible, task.

A. **Codes for symptoms, signs, and ill-defined conditions**
   Codes for symptoms, signs, and ill-defined conditions from Chapter 16 are not to be used as principal diagnosis when a related definitive diagnosis has been established.

B. **Two or more interrelated conditions, each potentially meeting the definition for principal diagnosis.**
   When there are two or more interrelated conditions (such as diseases in the same ICD-9-CM chapter or manifestations characteristically associated with a certain disease) potentially meeting the definition of principal diagnosis, either condition may be sequenced first, unless the circumstances of the admission, the therapy provided, the Tabular List, or the Alphabetic Index indicate otherwise.

C. Two or more diagnoses that equally meet the definition for principal diagnosis

In the unusual instance when two or more diagnoses equally meet the criteria for principal diagnosis as determined by the circumstances of admission, diagnostic workup and/or therapy provided, and the Alphabetic Index, Tabular List, or another coding guidelines does not provide sequencing direction, any one of the diagnoses may be sequenced first.

D. Two or more comparative or contrasting conditions.

In those rare instances when two or more contrasting or comparative diagnoses are documented as "either/or" (or similar terminology), they are coded as if the diagnoses were confirmed and the diagnoses are sequenced according to the circumstances of the admission. If no further determination can be made as to which diagnosis should be principal, either diagnosis may be sequenced first.

E. A symptom(s) followed by contrasting/comparative diagnoses

When a symptom(s) is followed by contrasting/comparative diagnoses, the symptom code is sequenced first. All the contrasting/comparative diagnoses should be coded as additional diagnoses.

F. Original treatment plan not carried out

Sequence as the principal diagnosis the condition, which after study occasioned the admission to the hospital, even though treatment may not have been carried out due to unforeseen circumstances.

G. Complications of surgery and other medical care

When the admission is for treatment of a complication resulting from surgery or other medical care, the complication code is sequenced as the principal diagnosis. If the complication is classified to the 996-999 series and the code lacks the necessary specificity in describing the complication, an additional code for the specific complication should be assigned.

H. Uncertain Diagnosis

If the diagnosis documented at the time of discharge is qualified as "probable", "suspected", "likely", "questionable", "possible", or "still to be ruled out", code the condition as if it existed or was established. The bases for these guidelines are the diagnostic workup, arrangements for further workup or observation, and initial therapeutic approach that correspond most closely with the established diagnosis.

Note: This guideline is applicable only to short-term, acute, long-term care and psychiatric hospitals.

I. Admission from Observation Unit

1. **Admission Following Medical Observation**
    When a patient is admitted to an observation unit for a medical condition, which either worsens or does not improve, and is subsequently admitted as an inpatient of the same hospital for this same medical condition, the principal diagnosis would be the medical condition which led to the hospital admission.

2. **Admission Following Post-Operative Observation**
    When a patient is admitted to an observation unit to monitor a condition (or complication) that develops following outpatient surgery, and then is subsequently admitted as an inpatient of the same hospital, hospitals should apply the Uniform Hospital Discharge Data Set (UHDDS) definition of principal diagnosis as "that condition established after study to be chiefly responsible for occasioning the admission of the patient to the hospital for care."

J. Admission from Outpatient Surgery
    When a patient receives surgery in the hospital's outpatient surgery department and is subsequently admitted for continuing inpatient care at the same hospital, the following guidelines should be followed in selecting the principal diagnosis for the inpatient admission:

    • If the reason for the inpatient admission is a complication, assign the complication as the principal diagnosis.
    • If no complication, or other condition, is documented as the reason for the inpatient admission, assign the reason for the outpatient surgery as the principal diagnosis.
    • If the reason for the inpatient admission is another condition unrelated to the surgery, assign the unrelated condition as the principal diagnosis.

Section III. Reporting Additional Diagnoses

GENERAL RULES FOR OTHER (ADDITIONAL) DIAGNOSES

For reporting purposes the definition for "other diagnoses" is interpreted as additional conditions that affect patient care in terms of requiring:

> clinical evaluation; or
> therapeutic treatment; or
> diagnostic procedures; or
> extended length of hospital stay; or
> increased nursing care and/or monitoring.

The UHDDS item #11-b defines Other Diagnoses as "all conditions that coexist at the time of admission, that develop subsequently, or that affect the treatment received and/or the length of stay. Diagnoses that relate to an earlier episode which have no bearing on the current hospital stay are to be excluded." UHDDS definitions apply to inpatients in acute care, short-term, long term care and psychiatric hospital setting. The UHDDS definitions are used by acute care short-term hospitals to report inpatient data elements in a standardized manner. These data elements and their definitions can be found in the July 31, 1985, Federal Register (Vol. 50, No, 147), pp. 31038-40.

Since that time the application of the UHDDS definitions has been expanded to include all nonoutpatient settings (acute care, short term, long term care and psychiatric hospitals; home health agencies; rehab facilities; nursing homes, etc).

The following guidelines are to be applied in designating "other diagnoses" when neither the Alphabetic Index nor the Tabular List in ICD-9-CM provide direction. The listing of the diagnoses in the patient record is the responsibility of the attending provider.

A. **Previous conditions**
   If the provider has included a diagnosis in the final diagnostic statement, such as the discharge summary or the face sheet, it should ordinarily be coded. Some providers include in the diagnostic statement resolved conditions or diagnoses and status-post procedures from previous admission that have no bearing on the current stay. Such conditions are not to be reported and are coded only if required by hospital policy.

However, history codes (V10-V19) may be used as secondary codes if the historical condition or family history has an impact on current care or influences treatment.

B. Abnormal findings

Abnormal findings (laboratory, x-ray, pathologic, and other diagnostic results) are not coded and reported unless the provider indicates their clinical significance. If the findings are outside the normal range and the attending provider has ordered other tests to evaluate the condition or prescribed treatment, it is appropriate to ask the provider whether the abnormal finding should be added.

Please note: This differs from the coding practices in the outpatient setting for coding encounters for diagnostic tests that have been interpreted by a provider.

C. Uncertain Diagnosis

If the diagnosis documented at the time of discharge is qualified as "probable", "suspected", "likely", "questionable", "possible", or "still to be ruled out", code the condition as if it existed or was established. The bases for these guidelines are the diagnostic workup, arrangements for further workup or observation, and initial therapeutic approach that correspond most closely with the established diagnosis.

Note: This guideline is applicable only to short-term, acute, long-term care and psychiatric hospitals.

Section IV. Diagnostic Coding and Reporting Guidelines for Outpatient Services

These coding guidelines for outpatient diagnoses have been approved for use by hospitals/ providers in coding and reporting hospital-based outpatient services and provider-based office visits.

Information about the use of certain abbreviations, punctuation, symbols, and other conventions used in the ICD-9-CM Tabular List (code numbers and titles), can be found in Section IA of these guidelines, under "Conventions Used in the Tabular List." Information about the correct sequence to use in finding a code is also described in Section I.

The terms encounter and visit are often used interchangeably in describing outpatient service contacts and, therefore, appear together in these guidelines without distinguishing one from the other.

Though the conventions and general guidelines apply to all settings, coding guidelines for outpatient and provider reporting of diagnoses will vary in a number of instances from those for inpatient diagnoses, recognizing that:

> The Uniform Hospital Discharge Data Set (UHDDS) definition of principal diagnosis applies only to inpatients in acute, short-term, long-term care and psychiatric hospitals.

> Coding guidelines for inconclusive diagnoses (probable, suspected, rule out, etc.) were developed for inpatient reporting and do not apply to outpatients.

A. Selection of first-listed condition

In the outpatient setting, the term first-listed diagnosis is used in lieu of principal diagnosis.

In determining the first-listed diagnosis the coding conventions of ICD-9-CM, as well as the general and disease specific guidelines take precedence over the outpatient guidelines.

Diagnoses often are not established at the time of the initial encounter/visit. It may take two or more visits before the diagnosis is confirmed.

The most critical rule involves beginning the search for the correct code assignment through the Alphabetic Index. Never begin searching initially in the Tabular List as this will lead to coding errors.

1. **Outpatient Surgery**
   When a patient presents for outpatient surgery, code the reason for the surgery as the first-listed diagnosis (reason for the encounter), even if the surgery is not performed due to a contraindication.

2. **Observation Stay**
   When a patient is admitted for observation for a medical condition, assign a code for the medical condition as the first-listed diagnosis.

   When a patient presents for outpatient surgery and develops complications requiring admission to observation, code the reason for the surgery as the first reported diagnosis (reason for the encounter), followed by codes for the complications as secondary diagnoses.

B. Codes from 001.0 through V84.8

The appropriate code or codes from 001.0 through V84.8 must be used to identify diagnoses, symptoms, conditions, problems, complaints, or other reason(s) for the encounter/visit.

C. Accurate reporting of ICD-9-CM diagnosis codes

For accurate reporting of ICD-9-CM diagnosis codes, the documentation should describe the patient's condition, using terminology which includes specific diagnoses as well as symptoms, problems, or reasons for the encounter. There are ICD-9-CM codes to describe all of these.

D. Selection of codes 001.0 through 999.9

The selection of codes 001.0 through 999.9 will frequently be used to describe the reason for the encounter. These codes are from the section of ICD-9-CM for the classification of diseases and injuries (e.g., infectious and parasitic diseases; neoplasms; symptoms, signs, and ill-defined conditions, etc.).

E. Codes that describe symptoms and signs

Codes that describe symptoms and signs, as opposed to diagnoses, are acceptable for reporting purposes when a diagnosis has not been established (confirmed) by the provider. Chapter 16 of ICD-9-CM, Symptoms, Signs, and Ill-defined conditions (codes 780.0 - 799.9) contain many, but not all codes for symptoms.

F. Encounters for circumstances other than a disease or injury

ICD-9-CM provides codes to deal with encounters for circumstances other than a disease or injury. The Supplementary Classification of factors Influencing Health Status and Contact with Health Services (V01.0- V84.8) is provided to deal with occasions when circumstances other than a disease or injury are recorded as diagnosis or problems.

G. Level of Detail in Coding

1. ICD-9-CM codes with 3, 4, or 5 digits

ICD-9-CM is composed of codes with either 3, 4, or 5 digits. Codes with three digits are included in ICD-9-CM as the heading of a category of codes that may be further subdivided by the use of fourth and/or fifth digits, which provide greater specificity.

2. Use of full number of digits required for a code

A three-digit code is to be used only if it is not further subdivided. Where fourth-digit subcategories and/or fifth-digit subclassifications are provided, they must be assigned. A code is invalid if it has not been coded to the full number of digits required for that code. See also discussion under Section I.b.3., General Coding Guidelines, Level of Detail in Coding.

H. ICD-9-CM code for the diagnosis, condition, problem, or other reason for encounter/visit

List first the ICD-9-CM code for the diagnosis, condition, problem, or other reason for encounter/visit shown in the medical record to be chiefly responsible for the services provided. List additional codes that describe any coexisting conditions. In some cases the first-listed diagnosis may be a symptom when a diagnosis has not been established (confirmed) by the physician.

I. "Probable", "suspected", "questionable", "rule out", or "working diagnosis"

Do not code diagnoses documented as "probable", "suspected," "questionable," "rule out," or "working diagnosis". Rather, code the condition(s) to the highest degree of certainty for that encounter/visit, such as symptoms, signs, abnormal test results, or other reason for the visit. **Please note:** This differs from the coding practices used by short-term, acute care, long-term care and psychiatric hospitals.

J. Chronic diseases

Chronic diseases treated on an ongoing basis may be coded and reported as many times as the patient receives treatment and care for the condition(s).

K. Code all documented conditions that coexist

Code all documented conditions that coexist at the time of the encounter/visit, and require or affect patient care treatment or management. Do not code conditions that were previously treated and no longer exist. However, history codes (V10-V19) may be used as secondary codes if the historical condition or family history has an impact on current care or influences treatment.

L. Patients receiving diagnostic services only

For patients receiving diagnostic services only during an encounter/ visit, sequence first the diagnosis, condition, problem, or other reason for encounter/visit shown in the medical record to be chiefly responsible for the outpatient services provided during the encounter/ visit. Codes for other diagnoses (e.g., chronic conditions) may be sequenced as additional diagnoses.

For outpatient encounters for diagnostic tests that have been interpreted by a physician, and the final report is available at the time of coding, code any confirmed or definitive diagnosis(es) documented in the interpretation. Do not code related signs and symptoms as additional diagnoses.

Please note: This differs from the coding practice in the hospital inpatient setting regarding abnormal findings on test results.

M. Patients receiving therapeutic services only

For patients receiving therapeutic services only during an encounter/visit, sequence first the diagnosis, condition, problem, or other reason for encounter/visit shown in the medical record to be chiefly responsible for the outpatient services provided during the encounter/visit. Codes for other diagnoses (e.g., chronic conditions) may be sequenced as additional diagnoses.

The only exception to this rule is that when the primary reason for the admission/encounter is chemotherapy, radiation therapy, or rehabilitation, the appropriate V code for the service is listed first, and the diagnosis or problem for which the service is being performed listed second.

N. Patients receiving preoperative evaluations only

For patients receiving preoperative evaluations only, sequence first a code from category V72.8, Other specified examinations, to describe the pre-op consultations. Assign a code for the condition to describe the reason for the surgery as an additional diagnosis. Code also any findings related to the pre-op evaluation.

O. Ambulatory surgery

For ambulatory surgery, code the diagnosis for which the surgery was performed. If the postoperative diagnosis is known to be different from the preoperative diagnosis at the time the diagnosis is confirmed, select the postoperative diagnosis for coding, since it is the most definitive.

P. Routine outpatient prenatal visits

For routine outpatient prenatal visits when no complications are present, codes V22.0, Supervision of normal first pregnancy, or V22.1, Supervision of other normal pregnancy, should be used as the principal diagnosis. These codes should not be used in conjunction with chapter 11 codes.

Index

Abbreviations, 13–14
Abdomen, internal injuries of, 323
Ablation of lung, 152
Abnormal findings, 24–25, 77
Abortion, 225–233
    complications associated with, 226–227
    fetal loss and retention of one or more fetuses, 229
    inadvertent, 228
    maternal condition as reason for, 228
    missed, 231
    multiple gestation following fetal reduction, 230
    procedures for, 230
    resulting in liveborn infant, 229
    types of, 225
Abuse, child and adult, 314–315
Accidents
    industrial, 6
    transport and vehicle, 311
Acquired diverticula, 160–161
Acute conditions, 41–42, 96, 120, 146, 151–152, 174, 255, 256
"Acute confusional state," 106
Acute metabolic complications, of diabetes mellitus, 96
Acute pulmonary edema, 151–152
Acute renal failure, 174
Acute renal insufficiency, 174
Addiction (drug dependence), 112, 342
Adhesions, intestinal and peritoneal, 163
Admission
    for complications associated with malignant neoplasm, 300
    for normal deliveries and other obstetric care, 210–212
    for prophylactic organ removal, 301–302
    for radiotherapy or chemotherapy, 300–301
    V codes and categories for, 64–67, 302
Admitting diagnosis, 19–21, 25
Adnexae. See Eye
Adult abuse, 314–315
Adult respiratory distress syndrome (ARDS), 150–151
Affective disorders, 107–108

Aftercare
    complications vs., 351
    management, coding, 64–65
    orthopedic, 320–321
"After study," 19–20
Age, relationship to codes, 236, 241–242
AIDS, 90–92. See also HIV infections
Alcohol abuse, 111–112, 342
Alcoholism (alcohol dependence), 111–112, 342
Alphabetic Index of Diseases and Injuries, 4, 6–7, 8–9, 31, 32, 35, 36, 37, 38, 42–43, 63, 235, 241, 345, 346
    references to Tabular List, 4–6
Alphabetic Index of Procedures, 4, 9–10, 31, 32, 35, 36, 37, 38, 48, 49–50
Alphabetization rules, 8–9
Altered mental state, 106
Alzheimer's disease, 106
Ambulatory care. See Outpatient services
American Health Information Management Association, 3
American Hospital Association, 3
Amnesia, transient global, 106–107
Amputations, 324
Anaphylactic shock, 325–326
"And," 17
Anemia, 119–122
    aplastic, 121
    of chronic disease, 121
    due to acute blood loss, 120
    iron-deficiency, 119
    sickle-cell, 122
Aneurysm, 262
Angina pectoris, 259
Angiocardiography, 273
Angioplasty
    of non-coronary vessels, 277
    percutaneous transluminal coronary, 276
Anorexia nervosa, 110
Aplastic anemia, 121
Appendicitis, 166
Appendix A, Morphology of Neoplasms, of Tabular List, 4
Appendix B, Glossary of Mental Disorders, of Tabular List, 4, 6

Appendix C, Classification of Drugs by American Hospital Formulary Service List Number and Their ICD-9-CM Equivalents, 6

Appendix D, Classification of Industrial Accidents According to Agency, 6

Aqueous misdirection, 136

Arteriosclerotic heart disease (ASHD). *See* Ischemic heart disease

Arthritis, 195, 196

Aspergillosis, 143

Asphyxia, 243–244

Aspiration biopsy, 52

Aspiration pneumonia, 143

Asthma, 146

Atelectasis, 148

Atheroembolism, 270

Atherosclerosis of extremities, 270

Automatic cardioverter/defibrillator, implant of, 274

Autonomic dysreflexia, 130

Back disorders, 195–196

Bacteremia, 85

Bak cage, 200

Barrett's esophagus, 158

Bilateral procedures, 50

Biliary stones (calculi), removal of, 161–162

Biliary system, diseases of, 161–162

Biopsies
  of breast, 180
  of bronchus and lung, 152
  coding, 52–53

Birth injury, fractures due to, 319

Births. *See also* Childbirth; Delivery; Perinatal conditions; Pregnancy
  classification of, 242

Blindness. *See* Eye

Blood and blood-forming organs, diseases of, 119–124

Blood pressure, elevated, 269

Blood vessel injuries, 323

Breast
  diseases of, 180–181
  reconstruction of, 181–182

Bronchitis
  acute exacerbation of chronic obstructive, 145
  with chronic obstructive bronchitis, 145

Bronchospasm, 146

Bronchus, biopsy of, 152

Brush biopsy, 52

Bulimia, 110

Bundle of His study, 273

Burns, 331–334
  anatomical site of, 331
  associated injuries and illnesses, 334
  depth of, 331–332
  extent of, 332–333
  external causes of, 333
  sequencing of codes for, 332
  sunburn, 333

Bypass, coronary. *See* Coronary artery bypass graft (CABG)

Canceled procedures, coding, 54–55

Carcinoma in situ, 288–289

Cardiac arrest, 262

Cardiac pacemaker therapy, 274–275

Cardiac resynchronization, 276

Cardiac resynchronization defibrillator, 276

Cardiogenic acute pulmonary edema, 151

Cardiomyopathy, 261

Cardiomyostimulation system, implantation of, 282

Cardioverter defibrillator implant, 274

Cataracts, 135

Category code, 4

CD-ROM format, of *ICD-9-CM*, 4

Cellulitis
  other, 189
  of the skin, 188–189

Centers for Medicare & Medicaid Services (CMS), 3

Central nervous system
  conditions affecting, 128, 130–131
  infectious diseases of, 127

Cerclage of cervix, 215

Cerebrovascular disorders, 262–264
  late effects of, 44, 263–264

Cervix
  cerclage of, 215
  dysplasia of, 179

Cesarean delivery, 211–212, 218–219

Chemotherapy, 300–301

Chest, internal injuries of, 323

Child. *See also* Infants; Newborns
  health supervision of, 246

Child abuse, 314–315

Childbirth, 207–221. *See also* Delivery
  conditions complicating, 214–215, 269
  late effect of, 216

Cholecystectomy, 161

Cholesterolosis, 161
Chronic conditions, 23, 41–42, 96–98, 145–146, 259–260
    anemia in, 121
Chronic ischemic heart disease, 259–260
Chronic kidney disease, 97, 173–176
    with diabetes mellitus, 97, 174–175
    end-stage renal disease and, 173–174
    with hypertension, 174–175, 267
    stages of, 173
Chronic obstructive pulmonary disease (COPD), 145–146
Circulatory system
    diseases of, 253–283
    miscellaneous conditions of, 271
    procedures involving, 273–280
    status V codes, 272
Classification of Drugs by American Hospital Formulary Service List Number and Their ICD-9-CM Equivalents, Appendix C, 6
Classification of Industrial Accidents According to Agency, Appendix D, 6
Classification system, 3
Clinical diagnoses, 3
Closed biopsy, 52
Closed classification system, 3
Coagulation defects, 123–124
"Code also," 48–49
"Code first underlying condition," 12–13, 37–38
"Code, If Applicable, Any Causal Condition First," 13, 39
Coding
    basic steps in, 31–33
    demonstrations, 32–33
    ethical, 26
    guidelines for, 35–44, 47–57, 407–488
    locating code entry in Alphabetic Index, 6–9, 31
    verifying code number in Tabular List, 32
Coding Clinic for ICD-9-CM, 3
Colon, 16
Colostomy, complications of, 160
Combination codes, 36–37, 42
Comparable conditions, 21
Comparative diagnoses, 21
Compensated heart failure, 261
Complex statement (diagnostic or procedural), 37
Complications, 345–352
    affecting specified body systems, not classified elsewhere, 350

vs. aftercare, 351
    due to internal device/implant/graft, 348–349
    locating codes in Alphabetic Index, 346
    postoperative conditions not classified as, 346–347
    surgical or medical care as external cause of, 352
Congenital anomalies, 235–237
    location of terms in Alphabetic Index, 235
    newborn with, 236
    patient age and, 236
Congenital deformities, vs. perinatal deformities, 236
Congenital diverticula, 160
Conjunctivitis, 133
Connecting words, 8–9, 36, 37, 49
Connective tissue, diseases of, 195–202
Constipation, 167
Consultation notes, 27
Contiguous sites, of malignant neoplasms, 292
Contraceptive management services, 219
    sterilization, 220
Contrasting conditions, 21
Contrasting diagnoses, 21
Corneal injury, 133
Coronary arteriosclerosis (atherosclerosis). *See* Ischemic heart disease
Coronary artery bypass graft (CABG), 277–280
Counseling, HIV, 91
Critical illness myopathy, 132
Critical illness polyneuropathy, 131
Cross-references, 14–15, 49
Current illness, late effect coding and, 44
Current Procedural Terminology (CPT) coding system, 47
Cyclosporiasis, 84
Cystic fibrosis, 101
Cystic kidney disease, 236–237
Cystoscopy, as operative approach, 177

Data items, 19–25
Data tabulation, 3
    basis for, 3
Deafness, 136–137
Debridement, 190
Decimal point, 4
Decompensated heart failure, 261
Defibrillator/cardioverter implant, 274

Deficiency anemias, 119

Delivery. *See also* Births; Childbirth
 cesarean, 211–212, 218–219
 normal, 210–211
 outcome of, 208–209
 procedures assisting, 218–219
 selection of principal diagnosis for, 210–212

Dementia, in conditions classified elsewhere, 105–106

Derangement, 197

Dermal regenerative graft, 190

Dermatitis, due to drugs, 187

Detail, coding to the highest level of, 35–36

Detoxification, 113, 114

Diabetes
 mellitus
  chronic kidney disease with, 174–175
  complications of, 96–98
  gestational, 98
  manifestations of, 96–99
  neonatal conditions associated with maternal, 98–99
  pregnancy complications, 98–99
  types of, 95–96
 secondary, 100

Diagnoses
 admitting, 19, 25
 with less-than-complete information, 28
 other than principal, 22–25
 principal, 19–21
 unconfirmed, 40–41

Diagnosis-related procedures, coding, 54

Diagnostic and Statistical Manual of Mental Disorders, 4, 6, 105

Diagnostic cardiac catheterization, 273

Diagnostic statement, 27

Dialysis, renal, 175–176

Diarrhea, 166–167

Dieulafoy lesions, 159

Digestive system, diseases of, 157–167

Discharge summary, 27–28

Discretionary multiple coding, 39

Dislocations, 322

Disseminated superficial actinic porokeratosis (DSAP), 189

Diverticulitis, 160

Diverticulosis, 160

Drug abuse, 112, 342. *See also* Substance abuse disorders

Drug dependence (addiction), 112, 342

Drug-resistant infections, 88

Drugs
 adverse effects of, 337–343
  decision tree for coding, 338
  E codes for, 338–340
  guidelines for code assignment, 339–340
  late effects of, 343
  unspecified, of therapeutic use, 342
 dermatitis due to, 187

Dual classification (dual coding), 13, 37–38

"Due to," 17

Dysplasia, of cervix and vulva, 180

Ear. *See* Hearing loss

Eating disorders, 110

E codes, 4, 63
 for adverse effects of drugs, 338–340
 external cause of injury and, 310–312

Ectopic pregnancy, 230–231

Ehrlichiosis, 84

Electrophysiologic stimulation and recording studies (EP studies), 274

Endocrine diseases, 95–100

Endometrial ablation, 180

Endometriosis, 179

Endoscopic approaches, 50

Endoscopic biopsy, 52

End-stage renal disease, 173–174, 175

Enterostomy, complications of, 160

Epiglottitis. *See* Supraglottitis

Epilepsy, 128

Episiotomy, 218

Eponyms, for surgical procedures, 49

Esophagitis, 158

Esophagostomy, complications of, 160

Essential modifiers, 15

Ethical coding and reporting, 26

Evolving myocardial infarction, 256

Excision
 of lesion, 189
 of organ or lesion, 49

Exclusion notes, 11, 12

External fixation, of fractures, 320

Extraocular muscles, operations on, 134

Eye
 diabetes and disease of, 97
 disorders of, 133–136

Failed procedure, 56
Fasciitis, 202
Fertility treatments. *See* Procreative
 management
Fetal and newborn aspiration, 244
Fetal distress, 243–244
Fetal pulse oximetry, 218
Fetus. *See also* Childbirth; Pregnancy
 conditions of, affecting pregnancy,
  213–214
 endocrine and metabolic disturbances
  specific to, 247
 hematological disorders of, 119
 in utero surgery performed on, 214
 maternal conditions affecting, 247
 monitoring, 218
Fifth-digit subclassification, 3, 4
 for abortion, 226
 decision process for assigning, 209
 for injuries, 309
 for musculoskeletal system/connective
  tissue diseases, 195
 in obstetrical experience, 208
First-degree burns, 331
Follow-up examinations, 65–66, 302
Forceps delivery, 218
Fourth-digit subcategories, 3, 4
Fractures, 315–322
 compression, 319
 dislocations and, 322
 due to birth injury, 319
 of extremities, 317
 orthopedic aftercare for, 320–321
 pathological, 198–199, 318
 procedures related to, 319–320
 skull, 316
 vertebral, 316

Gastrointestinal (GI) hemorrhage, 157–158
Gastrostomy, complications of, 160
General notes, 11
Genetic susceptibility to disease, 69–70
Genital prolapse, 179–180
Genitourinary system, diseases of, 171–181
Genitourinary tract, infections of, 171
Gestational diabetes, 98
Glands, neoplasms of, 297
Glaucoma, 136
Glossary of Mental Disorders,
 Appendix B, 4–6
Grafts
 complications due to, 348

coronary artery bypass grafts, 277–279
 dermal regenerative graft, 190
Gram-negative bacterial infection, 87
Gram-negative pneumonia, 142–143
Gram-positive bacteria, 87

Health Care Financing Administration
 (HCFA), 3
Health status codes, 69
Hearing devices, 137
Hearing loss, 136–137
Heart assist devices, 282
Heart disease. *See* Ischemic heart disease;
 Rheumatic heart disease
Heart failure, 151, 260–261
Heart transplantation, 283
Hematopoietic system, malignancies of, 297
Hematuria, 172
Hemiplegia/hemiparesis, 130
Hemolytic disease of newborn, 244–245
Hernias, of the abdominal cavity, 164
History section, 27
HIV infections, 90–92, 246
Hodgkin's disease, 297
Hospitals, coding by, 26
Hypercoagulable state, 123
Hypertension
 benign and malignant, 265–266
 chronic kidney disease with, 174, 267
 complicating pregnancy/childbirth/
  puerperium, 214–215, 269
 vs. elevated blood pressure, 269–270
 location of codes for, 266
 with other conditions, 268
Hypertensive heart and kidney disease, 267
Hypertensive heart disease, 266–267
Hypoglycemic reactions, 100
Hypothermia, 326

ICD-9-CM
 conventions, 11–17, 48–49
 differences between *ICD-10-CM* and,
  362
 differences between *ICD-10-PCS* and,
  370
 *Official Guidelines for Coding and
  Reporting*, 407–488
ICD-10-CM, 357–359, 361–368, 377,
  379–382
 data conversion issues with, 381–382
 (continued)

ICD-10-CM *(continued)*
   development of, 361
   differences between *ICD-9-CM* and, 362
   field testing of, 362–363
   modifications to information systems
      required by, 379–381
   personnel training in, 379
   preparing for implementation of, 377
   structure, format, and conventions,
      364–366
ICD-10-PCS, 357–359, 369–375, 377,
    379–382
   data conversion issues with, 381–382
   development of, 369–370
   differences between *ICD-9-CM* and, 370
   field testing of, 370–371
   mapping between *ICD-9-CM* and, 375
   modifications to information systems
      required by, 379–381
   personnel training in, 379
   preparing for implementation of, 377
   structure, format, and conventions,
      371–375
Ill-defined conditions, 75, 77
Immune-system disorders, 101
Immunoproliferative neoplasms, 297
Impending condition, 42–43
Implants
   automatic cardioverter/defibrillator, 274
   breast, 180–181
   of cardiomyostimulation system, 283
   complications due to, 348
   hemodynamic monitor, 283
   infusion pump and vascular access
      devices, 282
Inadvertent abortion, 228
Inclusion notes, 11–12
Incomplete procedures, coding, 55–56
Indention pattern, in Alphabetic Index, 6, 41
Index tables, 9
Indiscriminate coding, 40
Infants. *See also* Newborns; Perinatal
    conditions
   health supervision of, 247
   observation and evaluation of, 245–246
Infectious diseases, 83–92, 127
Infusion pump, implantable, 282–283
Injuries, 309–327
   abuse as cause of, 314–315
   amputations, 324
   blood vessel and nerve, 323
   burns and, 334
   corneal, 133

   dislocations, 322
   external cause of, 310–312, 325–326
   fifth-digit subclassifications for, 309
   foreign body and, 323
   fractures, 315–320
   internal, 323
   intracranial, 316
   late effects of, 43–44, 312, 326–327
   multiple coding of, 310
   open wounds, 323
   orthopedic aftercare, 320–321
   sequencing of codes for, 310
   superficial, 324
   trauma complications and, 324–325
Instructional notes, 11–13
Insulin-dependent diabetes mellitus
    (IDDM), 95–96
Insulin reactions, 100
Intent, external cause of injury and,
    311–312
Interbody fusion, 200
Internal device, complications due to, 348
Internal fixation, of fractures, 319–320
Internal injuries, 323
Interstitial pneumonia, 142
Intracranial injuries, 316
Intravascular imaging procedures, 273
Intussusception, reduction of, 167
Ischemic heart disease, 254–260
   acute and subacute, 257–258
   chronic, 259
   myocardial infarction and, 255–256

Joint replacement, 199–200

Kidney disease. *See* Chronic kidney disease
Kyphoplasty, 201

Labor. *See* Childbirth
Laparoscopic approaches, 50
Late effects, 43, 44, 84–85, 216, 263–264,
    312, 326–327, 343
   coding requirements for, 44
   vs. current illness or injury, 44
   locating codes, 43–44
Legionnaires disease, 142
Lesion, excision of, 49, 189–190
Leukemias, 297
Lobar pneumonia, 141
Low birth weight, 243

Lung, biopsy of, 152
Lymphatic system, malignancies of, 297
Lymph nodes, neoplasms of, 297

Malignant neoplasm of esophagus, 292
Mandatory multiple coding, 37–38
Manifestation code, 37–38
Maternal condition, as reason for
    abortion, 228
Mechanical ventilation, 153–154
Meconium aspiration syndrome,
    244
Medicaid reporting, UHDDS and, 19
Medical care. *See also* Complications
    complications of, not classified
        elsewhere, 350–351
    as external cause of complications, 352
Medical record as source document, 27–29
Medicare reimbursement, 26
Medicare reporting
    of procedures, 47
    UHDDS and, 19, 26
Medication record, 28
Mental disorders, 105–114
    psychiatric therapy for, 114
Metabolic encephalopathy, 106
Metastatic (metastasis), neoplasms
    described as, 293–294
Missed abortion, 231
Modifiers, essential and nonessential, 15
Molar pregnancy, 230–231
Morphology of Neoplasms, Appendix A, 4
"Multi-drug resistant," 88
Multiple axes classification system, 4
Multiple coding, 37–40
    discretionary, 39
    indiscriminate, 40
    mandatory, 37–38
Multiple diagnoses, 20–21
Multiple myeloma, 297
Musculoskeletal system, diseases of,
    195–202
Myocardial infarction, 255–258
    postmyocardial infarction syndrome
        and, 258

Narcolepsy, 130–131
National Center for Health Statistics, 3
NEC (not elsewhere classified), 13–14,
    36, 150
Needle biopsy, 52, 53

Neoplasms, 287–302
    behavior classifications for, 287–288
    benign, 287
    carcinoma in situ, 288
    locating codes for neoplastic disease,
        289–290
    malignant, 287
        basic types of, 291
        coding of solid, 292–294
        complications associated with, 300
        contiguous sites, 292
        of esophagus, 292
        follow-up examinations and, 302
        immunoproliferative, 297
        in lymphatic and hematopoietic
            systems, 297
        metastatic (metastasis), 293–294
        morphology classification of, 288–289
        sequencing of codes for neoplastic
            diseases, 299–301
        of uncertain behavior, 288
        of unspecified nature, 288
Neoplasm table, in Index of Diseases and
    Injuries, 290
Neoplastic diseases, 119, 289–290,
    299–301
Nerve injuries, 323
Nervous system. *See* Central nervous
    system; Peripheral nervous system,
    disorders of
Neuropathy, diabetic, 97
Newborns. *See also* Perinatal conditions
    birth classifications for, 242
    clinically significant conditions for, 242
    with congenital conditions, 236
    with diabetic mothers, 98
    endocrine and metabolic disturbances
        specific to, 247
    hematological disorders of, 119
    hemolytic disease of, 245
    with HIV-positive mother, 91, 246
    low birth weight, 243
    maternal conditions affecting, 246–247
    observation and evaluation of, 245–246
    postmaturity and, 243
    prematurity of, 243
    vaccination of, 247
New codes, 3
Noncardiogenic acute pulmonary edema,
    151–152
Nonessential modifiers, 15
Non-insulin-dependent diabetes mellitus
    (NIDDM), 95–96

Nonorganic mental disorders, 110
Nonpsychotic mental disorders, 109–110
Nonspecific V codes, 72
NOS (not otherwise specified), 14, 36
Not elsewhere classified. *See* NEC (not elsewhere classified)
Not otherwise specified. *See* NOS (not otherwise specified)
Numerical code, 3
Numerical entries, 8
Nutritional disorders, 101

Observation and evaluation admission, coding, 66–67
Observation and evaluation of newborns and infants, 245–246
Obstetric care. *See also* Abortion; Delivery; Pregnancy
    admission for, other than delivery, 212
Obstetric patient, with HIV infection, 92, 246
Ocular torticollis, 133
Official Guidelines for Coding and Reporting, 407–488
Open biopsy, 52–53
Open wounds, 323
Operations. *See also* Surgery and surgical care
    classification of, 3
    coding guidelines for, 47–57
    on extraocular muscles, 134
Operative approaches and closures, coding, 50
Organ, excision of, 49
Organic anxiety syndrome, 105
Organic brain syndrome, 105
Organic impotence, diabetes and, 98
Organism, subterms and, 83
Original treatment plan, 21
Orthopedic aftercare, 320–321
Other diagnoses
    with no supporting documentation, 22–23
    reporting guidelines for, 22–25
"Other specified," 14
Outpatient services. *See also* Aftercare; Follow-up examinations
    UHDDS criteria for, 26
    V codes for, 68–69
Over-coding, 26
Over-reporting, 26

Pacemaker therapy, 274–275
Palliative care admission, 67
Parasitic diseases, 83–92
Parentheses, 15
Parkinson's disease, 130
Pathological fractures, 198–199
Patient history codes, 69
Payment for health care, ethical coding/ reporting and, 26
Pelvis, internal injuries of, 323
Percutaneous balloon pulmonary valvuloplasty (PBPV), 276
Percutaneous transluminal coronary angioplasty (PTCA), 276
Performed procedure, 55–56
Perinatal conditions, 241–247
    fractures due to birth injury, 319
    guidelines for, 241
    hematological disorders, 119
    infections and, 246
    locating codes in Alphabetic Index, 241
    patient age and, 241–242
Perinatal deformities, vs. congenital deformities, 236
Perineal lacerations, 218
Peripheral nervous system, disorders of, 131
Peripheral vascular disease, diabetic, 97
Periventricular leukomalacia (PVL), 245
Pleural effusion, 148
Plica syndrome, 202
Pneumonia, 141–143
Poisoning, 337–343
    decision tree for coding, 338
    due to substance abuse or dependence, 342
    external cause codes assignment, 339–340
    late effects of, 343
    locations of codes and E codes for, 338–339
Postcholecystectomy syndrome, 161
Postmaturity of newborn, 243
Postmyocardial infarction syndrome, 258
Postoperative conditions not classified as complications, 346–347
Postpartum (puerperium), 207–221
    complications, 215–216
    conditions complicating, 214–215, 269
    late effect of complication of, 216
Pregnancy, 207–221, 225–231. *See also* Abortion; Childbirth; Contraceptive management services; Obstetric care
    conditions complicating, 98, 119, 214–215, 269

ectopic, 230–231
fetal conditions affecting, 213–214
late effect of complication of, 216
molar, 230–231
procedures for termination of, 230
Prematurity of newborn, 243
Preoperative evaluations, V codes for, 68
Previous conditions, 22
Principal diagnosis, 19–21
diagnosis other than, 22–25
selection guidelines, 20–21
selection of, 19–21, 113, 149–150, 210–212
signs and symptoms as, 75–76
V codes as, 64–72
Principal procedure, 48
Printed versions, of *ICD-9-CM*, 4
Problem codes, 69
Procedures
classification of, 3
coding guidelines for, 47–57
complications of, not classified elsewhere, 350
fracture-related, 319–320
involving circulatory system, 273–279
locating entry in Alphabetic Index, 29–30
locating terms in Alphabetic Index, 49–50
UHDDS for reporting requirements, 26
verifying code number in Tabular List, 31, 32
Procreative management, 221
Prolapse, genital, 178–179
Prostate disease and therapy, 178–180
Pseudarthrosis. *See* Refusion of spine
Psychiatric therapy, for mental disorders, 114
Psychophysiologic disorders, 110
Psychosis, alcohol- and drug-related, 112–113
Puerperium. *See* Postpartum (puerperium)
Pulmonary insufficiency, NEC, 151
Punctuation marks, 15–16

Radiotherapy, 300–301
Reduction of fractures, 319
References, from Alphabetical Index to Tabular List, 4
Refusion of spine, 201
Rehabilitation, 111, 112, 113, 114
coding, 64

Relational terms, 17
Renal complications, of diabetes, 97
Renal dialysis, 175–176
Renal disease, 173–175. *See also* Chronic kidney disease
Resection, 49
Residual codes, 3. *See also* NEC (not elsewhere classified); NOS (not otherwise specified)
Residual condition. *See* Late effects
Resistance, 88
Respiratory failure, 148–150
Respiratory system, diseases of, 141–153
Revised codes, 3
Rheumatic heart disease, 253
"Ruled out," 41
"Rule out," 40, 41

Schizophrenic disorders, 107
Screening examinations, 68–69
Secondary codes, 22, 38, 76–77
Secondary diabetes, 100
Second-degree burns, 331
Sections, 4
"See" (cross-reference), 14
"See also" (cross-reference), 14–15
"See category" (cross-reference), 15
"See condition" (cross-reference), 15
Sense organs, disorders of, 133–137
Sepsis, 85–87
severe, 85–87
Septicemia, 85–86
Septic shock, 86
Serologic testing, for HIV infection, 91
Severe acute respiratory syndrome (SARS), 84
Shunt procedures, coding, 56
Sickle-cell anemia, 122
Signs and symptoms, 75–77
Skin and subcutaneous tissue, diseases of, 187–190
Source document, medical record as, 27–29
Special investigative examinations, 68
Special symptoms or syndromes, of nonpsychotic mental disorders, 110
"(specified drug) resistant condition," 88
Spinal disc prostheses, 201–202
Spinal fusion, 200–201
Square brackets, 16
Status post, 69, 352
Status V codes, 69, 272
Stent insertions, coding, 56

Stereotactic radiosurgery, coding, 57

Sterilization, 220

Stress, reactions to, 109

Subacute condition, 41

Subacute ischemic heart disease, 258

Subcategories, 4

Substance abuse, poisoning due to, 342

Substance abuse disorders, 111–114
  principal diagnosis selection for, 113
  therapy for, 114

Subterms, 17, 49

Sunburn, 333

Supplementary classifications. *See* E codes;
  V codes

Supraglottitis, 145

Surgery and surgical care. *See also* Alphabetic Index of Procedures; Complications; Operations; Procedures; Tabular List of Procedures
  computer assisted surgery, 57
  as external cause of complications, 352
  inadvertent abortion and, 228
  reconstructive breast surgery, 180–181

Suspected conditions, 40

Symptom, followed by contrasting/comparative diagnoses, 21

Symptom codes, 75–77

Systemic inflammatory response syndrome (SIRS), 85–87

Table of Contents from *ICD-9-CM*, 5

Table of Drugs and Chemicals, 63

Tabular List and Alphabetic Index of Procedures, 3. *See also* Alphabetic Index of Procedures; Tabular List of Procedures

Tabular List of Diseases and Injuries, 4, 6, 31, 32, 35, 37, 63

Tabular List of Procedures, 9–10, 32, 35, 37, 48

Takotsubo syndrome, 261

Terrorism, 312

Third-degree burns, 332

Third-party payers, coding of, 26, 47

Thoracoscopic approaches, 50

Threatened condition, 42–43

Three-digit categories, 3, 4

Thrombosis and thrombophlebitis of veins of extremities, 270

Tick-bourne rickettsiosis, 84

Toxic shock syndrome, 87

Tracheostomy, complications of, 153

Transient global amnesia, 106–107

Transport accident, 311

Transurethral approach (TUR), 176

Trauma, 324–325. *See also* Injuries
  early complications of, 324
  inadvertent abortion and, 228

Treatment
  directed at primary site of neoplastic diseases, 299–300
  directed at secondary site of neoplastic diseases, 300

Tuberculosis, 85

Two-digit categories, 3

Two or more diagnoses meeting principal diagnosis definition, 20

Ulcers
  diabetes and, 98
  of the skin, 187–188
  of stomach and small intestine, 158

Unconfirmed diagnoses, coding, 40–41, 91

Uniform Hospital Discharge Data Set (UHDDS), 19–26, 27, 40
  for reporting procedures, 47–48

Unilateral procedures, 50

Unspecified codes, 14, 40

Urinary calculus (stone), removal of, 176

Urinary incontinence, 172–173

Urinary tract infection (UTI). *See* Genitourinary tract, infections of

"Use additional code," 13, 37, 39

Vaccination of newborns, 247

Vacuum extraction, 218

Vascular access devices, implantable, 282

V codes, 4, 31, 63–72
  nonspecific, 72
  status, 69, 272
  table (effective December 1, 2005), 70–72

Vehicle accident, 311

Vertebroplasty, 201

Visual impairment. *See* Eye

Volume 1. *See* Tabular List of Diseases and Injuries

Volume 2. *See* Alphabetic Index of Diseases and Injuries

Volume 3. *See* Alphabetic Index of Procedures; Tabular List of Procedures

Vulva, dysplasia of, 179